Exercise and Its Mediating Effects on Cognition

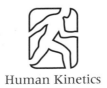

Human Kinetics

Aging, Exercise, and Cognition Series

VOLUME 2

Leonard W. Poon, PhD

Waneen W. Spirduso, EdD

Wojtek Chodzko-Zajko, PhD

SERIES EDITORS

Exercise and Its Mediating Effects on Cognition

WITHDRAWN

Waneen W. Spirduso, EdD
University of Texas at Austin

Leonard W. Poon, PhD
University of Georgia

Wojtek Chodzko-Zajko, PhD
University of Illinois at Urbana-Champaign

EDITORS

Human Kinetics

Library of Congress Cataloging-in-Publication Data

Exercise and its mediating effects on cognition / Waneen W. Spirduso, Leonard W. Poon, Wojtek Chodzko-Zajko, editors.
    p. cm. -- (Aging, exercise, and cognition series ; v. 2)
  Includes bibliographical references and index.
  ISBN-13: 978-0-7360-5786-8 (hard cover)
  ISBN-10: 0-7360-5786-2 (hard cover)
  1. Cognition--Effect of exercise on. 2. Exercise--Psychological aspects. I. Spirduso, Waneen Wyrick. II. Poon, Leonard W., 1942- III. Chodzko-Zajko, Wojtek J.
  BF311.E878 2007
  153--dc22

2007021385

ISBN-10: 0-7360-5786-2
ISBN-13: 978-0-7360-5786-8

Acquisitions Editor: Judy Patterson Wright, PhD; **Managing Editor:** Maureen Eckstein; **Assistant Editors:** Christine Horger and Christine Bryant Cohen; **Copyeditor:** Julie Anderson; **Proofreader:** Erin Cler; **Indexer:** Betty Frizzéll; **Permission Manager:** Carly Breeding; **Graphic Designer:** Nancy Rasmus; **Graphic Artist:** Dawn Sills; **Cover Designer:** Robert Reuther; **Photo Asset Manager:** Laura Fitch; **Photo Office Assistant:** Jason Allen; **Art Manager:** Kelly H. Hendren; **Illustrator:** Al Wilborn; **Printer:** Sheridan Books

Printed in the United States of America   10 9 8 7 6 5 4 3 2 1

Human Kinetics
Web site: www.HumanKinetics.com

United States: Human Kinetics
P.O. Box 5076
Champaign, IL 61825-5076
800-747-4457
e-mail: humank@hkusa.com

Canada: Human Kinetics
475 Devonshire Road Unit 100
Windsor, ON N8Y 2L5
800-465-7301 (in Canada only)
e-mail: orders@hkcanada.com

Europe: Human Kinetics
107 Bradford Road
Stanningley
Leeds LS28 6AT, United Kingdom
+44 (0) 113 255 5665
e-mail: hk@hkeurope.com

Australia: Human Kinetics
57A Price Avenue
Lower Mitcham, South Australia 5062
08 8372 0999
e-mail: info@hkaustralia.com

New Zealand: Human Kinetics
Division of Sports Distributors NZ Ltd.
P.O. Box 300 226 Albany
North Shore City
Auckland
0064 9 448 1207
e-mail: info@humankinetics.co.nz

CONTENTS

Contents

PREFACE

Historically, scientists believed that the brain functioned independently of the rest of the body, that what we were born with was what we had to work with, and that little could be done to deflect the inexorable damage done to the brain by the passage of time. Today we are beginning to understand that the brain is much more malleable than was ever thought, that neuronal networks are continually modified, that new neurons can be developed (neurogenesis), and that we can have substantial influence over our brain function.

This edited book is the second of a three-part series designed to assess our knowledge and define research directions regarding active living, cognitive functioning, and aging. Volume 1 of this series reviewed exercise and cognition, measurement issues, and physiological mechanisms that are relevant to this process among older adults. Volume 2 continues to expand our understanding by examining whether and how physical activity could indirectly affect cognitive function by influencing mediators that provide physical and mental resources for cognition: for example, by (a) enhancing physical energy levels by increasing sleep quality and enabling the intake of adequate amounts of food to maintain energy, (b) preventing or postponing disease states such as diabetes and chronic obstructive pulmonary disease, and (c) providing mechanisms that control anxiety and depression. This volume seeks to identify and study key sources of individual variations in exercise and cognition processes. Finally, volume 3 addresses neuropsychological mechanisms associated with exercise and cognition. This series is designed to create synergy across volumes and chapters.

Eighteen contributors met and produced this second volume. As in volume 1, volume 2 includes contributors who are experts in exercise, activity, cognition, neurobiological processes, and aging. Few contributors are experts in all areas, and the volume was produced to encourage synergy in addressing the complex issues involved in exercise, activity, and cognition in old age. Each of the experts prepared a draft review of the state of knowledge for his or her topic. Before coming together in a workshop to present and discuss the contents, all participants read the drafts. A working model was provided, and the experts were asked to relate their work to the model.

Two innovations were included by the editors in volume 2. At the beginning of each chapter, an introduction of the authors is provided followed by editors' notes on how the chapter fits into the general model introduced to organize the volume contents. Following each chapter, highlights of the chapter discussion are summarized to provide the reader a flavor of consensus or controversies associated with the topic. Consistent with volume 1, volume 2 is intended to serve as an up-to-date research reference as well as a classroom textbook on exercise, cognition, and aging.

The workshop was sponsored by the Institute of Gerontology at The University of Texas, the College of Education, the RGK Foundation, the Cain Foundation, the St. David's Foundation, and the Oscar and Anne Mauzy Regents Professorship, all of Austin, Texas. It was held at Austin Lakeway Inn and Resort, Austin, June 20 to 22, 2003. We acknowledge the valuable assistance and participation of Sandy Graham, Mina Rathbun, and Patty Coffman. Anne Marie Jennings was an important collaborator in organizing and editing the Editor's Discussion Summaries.

PART I

Models and Mediators of Exercise Effects on Cognition

CHAPTER 1

Using Resources and Reserves in an Exercise–Cognition Model

Waneen W. Spirduso, EdD; Leonard W. Poon, PhD;
and Wojtek Chodzko-Zajko, PhD

From previous research literature and many discussions, we know that aging affects cognitive functions, especially those associated with executive processing and functions of the frontal lobe. Not all cognitive processes decline, and those that do may not follow the same pattern of deterioration. In fact, different functions may express a wide variety of age-related states: no change (stability), as may be represented by cultural knowledge; disease-related change, which can be gradual or precipitous as expressed by Alzheimer's disease or other dementias; a steady decline in function, as occurs with most people's short-term memory; and even transient changes, such as occur following small transient ischemic strokes where function slowly recovers over time. Even what seem to be similar cognitive decrements in individuals may have different causes. Given these widely varying patterns of change, researchers have agreed that one thing is very clear: Both between- and within-individual variabilities increase throughout the adult age span.

Individual variability in cognitive functions such as memory and learning comes from many sources, some of which were summarized by Jenkins (1979). Jenkins' "tetrahedron" describes cognitive performances as summations of interactions among four domains: (1) the characteristics of the individual, such as age, skills, knowledge, health, and other resources; (2) cognitive strategies; (3) the nature of the material; and (4) criterion tasks such as recognition, recall, problem solving, and others (figure 1.1). Variations in the interactions of these factors produce inter- and intra-individual variabilities in cognitive performances.

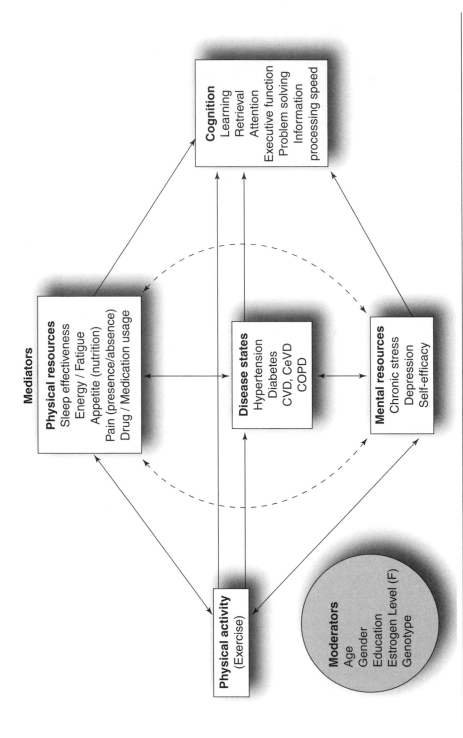

Figure 1.1 Working model of the role of mediators in exercise effects on cognition. F = female; CVD = cardiovascular disease; CeVD = cerebrovascular disease; COPD = chronic obstructive pulmonary disease.

We also know that exercise and physical activity are contextual factors that under specific conditions can improve cognitive functions. Direct influences, such as enhanced cerebrovascular function, are most frequently cited. However, it is highly probable that exercise also enhances cognition through its effects on mediator variables such as depression, sleep, appetite (diet), and energy levels and by postponing or preventing age-related diseases (e.g., diabetes, hypertension) known to affect cognition. It is thought that exercise affects both physical and mental resources or reserves, which in turn may create optimal conditions for cognitive function.

Hence, if we study how exercise could affect physical and mental resources that could in turn affect cognition, then we will begin to understand the facilitative mechanisms of exercise on cognition as individuals age. Indeed, cumulative indirect benefits via mediators may be more cognitively facilitating than direct effects.

The general strategy used to organize this volume was to (1) identify, using current knowledge, the paths—direct or indirect—through which exercise may influence cognition; (2) explore which mediators may most potently interact with aging, exercise, and cognition; (3) recommend directions that future research might take; and (4) determine whether a consensus statement regarding this topic can be generated from this review of the research literature. We propose that a way to study these paths is to identify key sources of individual variation or differences in exercise and cognition processes.

Model of the Effects of Exercise on Mediators of Cognition

To guide the reviews of the literature and the discussions that followed on individual variations in exercise and aging, we developed the model shown in figure 1.1. Some components of cognition that are most frequently studied in aging adults are shown in the right box labeled *Cognition*: attention, retrieval, information-processing speed, executive function, problem solving, and learning. Much of the research on this topic has been on potential direct influences of physical activity, such as increased brain oxygen availability and utilization attributable to improved cardiovascular function, increased glucose regulation, increased neural efficiency, neurotrophic enhancement, neurohormonal adaptations, and beneficial neural morphological changes. These mechanisms are shown in the model as a horizontal arrow directly from *Physical Activity* to *Cognition*.

However, the emphasis of this book is not on the direct and positive effects of exercise on cognition but rather on the indirect paths that exercise might take in positively affecting cognition: that is, how exercise may positively influence mediators of cognition, such as sleep, chronic disease, and depression and thereby indirectly improve cognition.

Mediators and Moderators— What Is the Difference?

Because mediators and moderators play such an important role in the model used by the authors of this book to address their topics, it was important to consider the definition, meaning, and use of mediators and moderators in the research literature of this field. These two terms have typically been used to describe a third variable that might affect the nature of the relationship between an independent variable and a dependent variable. In this model, mediating variables represent broader hypothetical constructs (depression, sleep, disease status) that influence the dependent variable of interest (cognition). Moderators are variables that partition independent variables into subgroups that establish its domains of maximal effectiveness in regard to a given dependent variable (age, gender, education).

The concept of mediators and moderators in models, however, is complex, and Jennifer Etnier (chapter 2) accepted the challenge to address this issue within the context of our model. She discusses various types of mediators, multiple mediator models, and micromediational chains and emphasizes the multiple interactions that most certainly occur among the mediators and the dependent variable of cognition. The interactions of exercise, mediators, and cognition are also influenced by powerful individual moderators such as gender, age, education level, estrogen level (in females), and genotype, shown in the circle in the lower left of figure 1.1.

The fact that most researchers routinely control for many of these mediators and moderators in their studies attests to their belief that these variables do indeed influence cognition and interact with exercise. It is also clear that many of these mediator variables are interrelated and may be based on similar mechanisms. For example, exercise benefits cognition by affecting serotonin and dopamine, and these transmitters also form the basis of a hypothesis to explain positive exercise effects on depression.

Effects of Exercise on Mediators of Cognition

Our hypothesized mediators of cognition are shown as the middle three boxes in figure 1.1: *Physical resources, Disease states*, and *Mental resources*. Physical resources are represented by *Sleep effectiveness, Energy and fatigue, Appetite (nutrition), Pain (presence or absence), and Drug/Medication usage*. The disease states included are several chronic diseases that have been shown to have substantial negative effects on cognition in older adults and have also been shown to be modifiable by exercise: *Hypertension, Diabetes, Cardiovascular disease (CVD), Cerebrovascular disease (CeVD), and Chronic obstructive pulmonary disease (COPD)*. *Mental resources*, the lowest box of the model, includes *Chronic stress, Depression*, and *Self-efficacy*. All of these can have negative effects on cognition, but self-efficacy can also be a positive force. Here it is shown as a mental resource, although Edward McAuley and Steriani Elavsky (chapter 5) argue that it should precede exercise, because exercise has a powerful influence on self-efficacy.

Exercise, Physical Resources, and Cognition

It has been claimed that exercise positively affects energy levels, sleep patterns, appetite, and other positive health behaviors (*Physical resources*, top box of figure 1.1). These resources include both the functional capacity of the system to perform cognitive tasks and the performance state, which is reflected in the ability of individuals to use their functional capacity. Individual differences and variability are dramatic in terms of both functional capacity and performance. Individuals vary widely in their innate levels of energy, their fatigability, the restorative efficiency of their sleep patterns, and their nutritional needs. Similarly, performance states vary widely both within individuals temporally and between individuals. We all have experienced physical states in which we believed that we did not have the energy to carry out a task, even though the task was mental and not physical. Extreme physical fatigue or sickness, for example, takes a toll on mental tasks. Who can study or do his income tax after a day of hard, physical work or when sick with the flu?

Phil Tomporowski (chapter 6) has suggested that energetics theory focuses on constructs that are used to describe the state of an organism (e.g., activation, arousal, fatigue) and that this theory may be applicable to the question of physical activity and cognition. Energetics theorists (e.g., Hockey, Coles, & Gaillard, 1986) suggest that mental performance is determined by (a) cognition—knowledge and skills (functional capacity), (b) conation—a willingness to expend physical or mental effort (performance state), and (c) affect—feelings and emotions (performance state). These constructs depend heavily on the role of physiologically based processes to explain individual differences in the availability of resources that are required for intensive and sustained goal-directed behavior. Regulation of behavior is explained in terms of brain structures and neurotransmitter systems and in terms of regulation of the autonomic nervous system. Optimal behavioral regulation and performance are assumed to be degraded when these physiological systems are impaired. The impairment of these physiological systems can come from two sources: (1) the workload engendered by the preparation and actual performance of a given task and (2) stressors that are not directly related to the task to be performed.

Sleep effectiveness is a more recognized physical resource that has been linked to health, physical activity, and cognitive function. Sleep is at the same time absolutely necessary for cognitive function and a serious problem in older adults. In chapter 9, Martita Lopez addresses the potential indirect effect that physical activity may have on cognition as it affects the quality of life, and in chapter 10, Michael Vitiello discusses mechanisms by which sleep enhances cognition and potential ways that physical activity might, by enhancing sleep, also influence cognition.

A sound nutritional status is thought to support optimum cognitive function, providing the nutrients necessary for optimum metabolic activities and high energy levels. In fact, Jim Joseph (chapter 8) builds a good case that certain combinations of antioxidant and anti-inflammatory polyphenolics that are found in fruits and vegetables may ameliorate age-related behavioral and neuronal deficits. Specifically, enhancing the diet with adequate amounts of berries such as blueberries and strawberries might have some benefit for certain types of cognition in old age. Many older adults, for various reasons that include immobility, poverty, poor appetite, ignorance, lack of interest, loss of olfactory sensitivity, gastrointestinal problems, and other illnesses, maintain an inadequate diet. It is highly likely that low levels of this physical resource contribute to poor cognition. Some suggestion has been made that physical activity may enhance appetite, thus enabling older adults to consume enough calories to increase their chance of obtaining recommended daily dietary requirements. However, this particular physical resource and its relationships to physical activity and cognition were not addressed in our workshop.

In the model (figure 1.1), these physical resources are shown to influence cognition, but at the same time they are affected by physical activity. Physical resources also affect mental resources and disease states, which influence cognition. Therefore, exercise can change physical resources, which enhance or degrade disease states, and mental resources, both of which affect cognition.

Prevention or Postponement of Disease States

It is frequently suggested that in addition to directly affecting brain function, exercise also enhances both physical and mental resources or reserves, which in turn may create optimal conditions for cognitive function. Thus, exercise plays an important role in preventing or postponing disease states (middle box of figure 1.1) such as hypertension (Hiro Tanaka and Miriam Cortez-Cooper, chapter 11), diabetes (Don Royall, chapter 12), and chronic obstructive pulmonary disease (Charles Emery, chapter 13) that are known to degrade cognition. Thus, exercise may mediate the negative effects of these and other diseases on cognitive function.

Exercise, Mental Resources, and Cognition

Mental resources are theoretical constructs that describe the notion of finite mental energy in the processing of information. Kahneman (1973) was one of the first to suggest that cognition requires mental effort and that arousal and attention play a large role in optimum cognitive performance. Attention is viewed as a limited capacity resource that is tapped to perform specific tasks, some more so than others. In chapter 6, Phil Tomporowski introduces energetics theory, which "assumes that human behavior can be conceptualized in terms of physiological and psychological states that can be self-regulated, human behavior is directed toward particular goal states, and the regulatory processes drawn upon to direct behavior involve costs to other regulatory processes" (Tomporowski, this volume).

Although mental resources are viewed as a limited capacity system, it is clear that they can be expanded in capacity. It has been shown that improvements in memory processes such as those reflected by the digit span test occur through extended practice. It also appears that limited resources can be replenished, as has been well documented in research on the importance of sleep and relaxation to cognitive performance. We know that cognition can be improved in older adults by the use of mnemonics and by pharmacological means. But the question that is most relevant to the model described in this book is whether physical activity, acute or chronic, can expand or replenish physical and mental resources.

Stress, Anxiety, and Depression

Other mental resource constructs that are important in cognitive function are stress, anxiety, and depression. Short-term stress can have some energizing, positive effects, but long-term stress that chronically and excessively mobilizes the stress response decreases physical and mental function, sometimes even to the extent of pathological development. In chapter 4, Nicole Berchtold describes the physiological response to stress, how stress affects mental function, and the effects of exercise on the stress system. She particularly focuses on the recent attention that brain-derived neurotrophic factor (BDNF) has attracted, because it promotes neuronal health and is a key mediator of synaptic efficacy, neuronal connectivity, and use-dependent plasticity. She reviews literature showing that stress may suppress hippocampal BDNF, which may account for many of the negative effects of stress on brain health and function. Conversely, exercise is a well-established intervention that rapidly increases hippocampal BDNF, protecting against stress-induced decreases in BDNF.

Psychological depression, which occurs with greater and greater frequency in the later decades of a person's life, has negative effects on cognition. As people age, they experience many emotionally negative events: the deaths of spouses, children, and relatives; losses of jobs; changes in their social roles; dramatic life changes such as retirement, downsizing their homes, and dealing with chronic disease; and losses of their ability to drive and be independent. Thus, late-onset depression is a serious problem for many people as they age. Depression can degrade both cognitive performance and cognitive functional capacity. In chapter 3, John Bartholomew and Joseph T. Ciccolo describe the importance of distinguishing between the transitory effects of depression on cognitive performance and the more lasting effects of depression on the cognition-related structures of the brain. Depression-related cognitive impairment has been demonstrated in both measures of functional capacity and cognitive performance. Deficits in cognitive performance could be caused by limitations in functional capacity that are brought about by structural change or neurological damage, or they could be attributable to the negative impact of episodes of depression on transient performance states.

Of great interest is whether physical activity or a systematic exercise program would, by increasing physical energy and endurance, also counteract the fatigue, loss of energy, and inability to concentrate that are all part of the clinical diagnosis of major depression. Each of these symptoms negatively affects performance on a very wide array of cognitive tasks. Bartholomew and Ciccolo detail many exercise-invoked changes in physical resources that might also decrease depression symptoms: changes in cerebral blood flow that might blunt the metabolic challenges to the brain during depression, enhanced neurotransmitters (particularly monoamines), enhanced neurogenesis to counteract structural damage, and improved function of the hypothalamic–pituitary–adrenal (HPA) axis.

Self-Efficacy

Edward McAuley and Steriani Elavsky (chapter 5) make the case that self-efficacy plays a potential mediating role in physical activity effects on anxiety, stress responses, and depression. They base their hypothesis on social cognitive theory, which takes the perspective that behavior, cognition, physiology, and environment all operate as interacting determinants of each other. Thus, the model guiding these discussions, which is biased toward being unidirectional, should also have arrows returning to exercise and physical activity not only from cognition but from most of the mediators as well. Because self-efficacy influences the initiation and the continuance of physical activity, it is a mental resource that should be viewed as preceding physical activity in this model. Conversely, self-efficacy is an outcome of physical activity and as an outcome enhances adherence to exercise and thus indirectly influences cognitive function via the beneficial effects of exercise on the various mediators such as physical resources, disease states, and mental resources.

Role of the Model in This Book and Visions for the Future

The model represents the strategy used by the organizers and participants of our Advanced Research Workshop to determine what we know about exercise, physical activity, and cognition; what the major technological and logistical barriers are to enhancing our understanding; and where we should go from here. For this reason, each of the following chapters was designed to provide background on how the variable of interest might be viewed as a mediator or moderator that could be influenced by exercise. Each review is followed by a list of discussions that we believe anyone interested in the chapter topic would also find intriguing and thought provoking. Next, we provide a list of important research technique or design problems that are impeding our understanding and that must be resolved before significant progress can be made. Third, suggestions are made for research directions that are most promising.

We proposed our hypothetical model as a means to provide points of reference and guide the thinking and discussion among colleagues working in the area of exercise and cognition among older adults. Indeed, several participants wanted to reverse the direction of the model, suggesting that cognition has a huge impact on exercise, physical activity, and physical function. Overall, our goal is the improvement of cognitive function and quality of life in older adults. As shown in figure 1.2, this is a long-term effort. This book is a contributor to step 1, the synthesis of research knowledge, from which we hope to improve research practice and formulate research questions that will lead to evidence-based approaches to working with older adults who are experiencing cognitive challenges. Ultimately, the goal is to influence public policy so that standards and guidelines that affect older adults will lead to the highest possible quality of life for all.

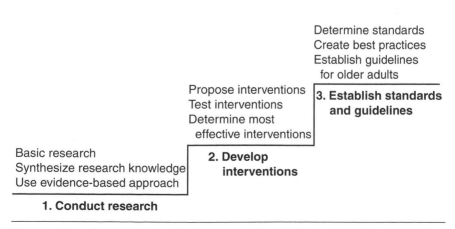

Figure 1.2 Three conceptualized actions (depicted as steps) that are used to improve the function and quality of life of older adults.

CHAPTER 2

Interrelationships of Exercise, Mediator Variables, and Cognition

Jennifer Etnier, PhD
Arizona State University

EDITORS' OVERVIEW

Dr. Etnier proposes that as our technical abilities continue to improve with regard to statistical techniques and innovations like structural and functional imaging techniques that allow us to noninvasively examine the mediators related to cerebral function and structure, it is likely that our knowledge in this area of research will increase rapidly. The identification of the mediators by which physical activity imparts its beneficial effects on cognition is of utmost importance. Until we have a better understanding of the precise mechanisms through which physical activity influences cognition, we cannot appropriately design exercise interventions to target these mechanisms. For example, if the effects are primarily mediated by changes in self-efficacy, then our programs should be designed first and foremost to increase self-efficacy. If, however, the effects are primarily mediated by changes in lipid profiles, then perhaps physical activity

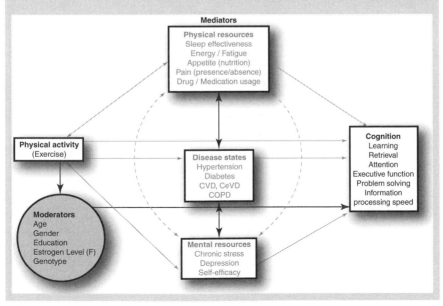

interventions provided in conjunction with dietary interventions may be most effective in attenuating age-related declines in cognition. Because the effects of physical activity on cognition appear to be fairly reliable and consistent, the next logical step for researchers is to clearly identify why this relationship exists so that those most at risk for cognitive decline can be identified and efficient, effective interventions can be implemented. The purpose of the workshop leading to this model was to review the literature on many of the potential lower-order mediators of the relationship between physical activity and cognition, with a goal of directing subsequent research using appropriate designs and techniques to confirm the mediational role of these variables.

The relationship between normal aging and cognitive performance is well established (e.g., Botwinick, 1977; Schaie, 1994) and suggests that as healthy, cognitively normal people age beyond 60 years, most show an age-related pattern of decline in cognitive performance. This age-related decline is of concern because of the increasing population of elderly adults and because of the implications of poor cognitive functioning.

The population of older adults is increasing at a disproportionately high rate that will result in the percentage of the U.S. population over the age of 65 reaching approximately 20% by the year 2025 (Science Directorate, 1993). Coupled with this increase in the population of older adults is the fact that older individuals have a likelihood of experiencing cognitive declines. These cognitive declines have implications for an aging workforce, for quality of life, and for the experience of clinical cognitive impairments. In particular, the rapid advances in technology that are occurring mandate that older adults maintain cognitive vitality and adaptability if they are to continue to participate in the workplace and in society as a whole (Crook et al., 1986). In addition, cognitive capabilities are an essential contributor to the overall quality of life of older adults (Fillit et al., 2002), and quality of life is recognized to be an important health outcome. Finally, the cognitive performance of healthy older adults predicts their future cognitive decline (Flicker, Ferris, & Reisberg, 1991; Swainson et al., 2001) and the likelihood of experiencing clinical declines (Ritchie, Artero, & Touchon, 2001). Given the increase in the population of older adults and the personal and social consequences of age-related cognitive declines, research related to the maintenance of cognitive functioning is of increasing relevance.

Although age-related declines in cognitive performance are undeniable, there are two important caveats to this statement. First, the cognitive deficits that are seen in nondemented older adults are typically limited to certain types of tasks. In particular, deficits are usually seen on tasks that require problem solving (e.g., Denney & Palmer, 1981; Denney, Pearce, & Palmer, 1982), have a large speeded component (e.g., Jacewicz & Hartley, 1987), rely on executive processing (e.g., Kramer et al., 1999), assess a variety of types of memory (e.g., Salthouse, 2003), or assess the acquisition and retention of novel skills (e.g., Etnier & Landers, 1997, 1998; Etnier, Romero, & Traustadottir, 2001). In contrast, nondemented older adults are typically able to maintain their long-term memory and the ability to perform tasks that are considered to be less effortful in terms of attentional demands (Hasher & Zacks, 1979). The unique pattern of cognitive declines that occur with age has provided insight into the areas of the brain that are implicated in aging, and this has helped us identify potential mediators of the relationship.

The second caveat regarding age-related declines in cognition is that there is substantial variability in the rate of these age-related declines, and, in fact, some older adults may never experience these declines. That is, some older adults may experience successful aging, which has been described as the evasion of disease and disability, continued engagement in social and productive activities, and sustained cognitive and physical functioning (Rowe & Kahn, 2000). Identifying genetic and lifestyle factors that predict successful aging is an important direction for researchers as we try to delineate risk factors for cognitive decline and as we develop behavioral interventions designed to attenuate cognitive decline.

Physical Activity, Exercise, and Aerobic Fitness

One behavioral variable that has been identified as being related to successful aging and more specifically to the maintenance of cognitive functioning is participation in physical activity. A substantial body of research literature has addressed the relationship between physical activity and cognition in older adults. Before reviewing this literature and discussing this relationship, we need to define the related terms of *physical activity, exercise,* and *physical fitness.*

Physical activity is defined as "bodily movement that is produced by the contraction of skeletal muscle and that substantially increases energy expenditure" (American College of Sports Medicine [ACSM], 2000, p. 4). Exercise is considered to be a subset of physical activity and describes those physically active behaviors that are conducted in a planned, structured fashion with a goal of maintaining or improving physical fitness. In contrast to these behaviors, physical fitness is defined as "a set of attributes that people have or achieve that relates to the ability to perform physical activity" (ACSM, 2000, p. 4). Physical fitness consists of aerobic fitness, muscular strength, muscular endurance, and flexibility (ACSM, 2000) and is determined by both genetic and behavioral factors. Thus, physical activity and exercise are terms used to describe behaviors that, depending on the type, frequency, and intensity, may or may not contribute to one or more components of physical fitness (Boutcher, 1993). In reviews of the scientific literature on physical activity and cognition, the distinction between physical activity and exercise has not always been made clear; therefore, to be as inclusive as possible, the broad term *physical activity* is used to represent physical activity and exercise for the remainder of this discussion.

Physical Activity and Cognition in Older Adults

The relationship between physical activity and cognitive functioning in older adults has been examined using a variety of experimental designs. Results from studies using cross-sectional designs have generally shown that older adults who are more physically active exhibit better cognitive performance than do older adults who are less physically active (Baylor & Spirduso, 1988; Christensen & Mackinnon, 1993; Clarkson-Smith & Hartley, 1989; Rikli & Busch, 1986; Spirduso, 1975; Spirduso, MacRae, MacRae, Prewitt, & Osborne, 1988). Thus, correlational evidence suggests that there is an association between physical activity and cognition in older adults.

In addition to these cross-sectional studies, six large-scale ($n > 1,000$) prospective studies have also been conducted with a goal of establishing a temporal relationship between current levels of physical activity and subsequent cognitive functioning. In these studies, physical activity and cognitive performance were assessed at baseline, and then cognitive performance was assessed again after a period of 2 to 8 years (Abbott et al., 2004; Albert et al., 1995; Laurin, Verreault, Lindsay, MacPherson, & Rockwood, 2001; Lytle, Vander Bilt, Pandav, Dodge, & Ganguli, 2004; Weuve et al., 2004; Yaffe, Barnes, Nevitt, Lui, & Covinsky, 2001). Results of these studies consistently indicated that higher levels of baseline physical activity predicted better maintenance of cognitive ability over the time period of observation. Thus, this evidence begins to suggest a causal relationship between physical activity and cognitive performance.

However, when the relationship between physical activity and cognitive performance has been examined in studies using chronic interventions, the effects have not been as consistent. Some studies have shown that increases in the physical activity levels of older adults result in concomitant improvements in cognitive performance (Dustman et al., 1984; Elsayed, Ismail, & Young, 1980; Emery, Schein, Hauck, & MacIntyre, 1998; Etnier & Berry, 2001; Hassmen, Ceci, & Backman, 1992; Hawkins, Kramer, & Capaldi, 1992; Khatri et al., 2001; Kramer et al., 1999; Moul, Goldman, & Warren, 1995; Palleschi et al., 1996; Rikli & Edwards, 1991; Stevenson & Topp, 1990; Williams & Lord, 1997). However, other researchers have found that physical activity interventions do not improve cognitive functioning (Barry, Steinmetz, Page, & Rodahl, 1966; Blumenthal et al., 1991; Blumenthal & Madden, 1988; Caplan, Ward, & Lord, 1993; Emery & Gatz, 1990; Hill, Storandt, & Malley, 1993; Madden, Blumenthal, Allen, & Emery, 1989; Normand, Kerr, & Metivier, 1987; Okumiya et al., 1996; Panton, Graves, Pollock, Hagberg, & Chen, 1990; Perri & Templer, 1985). Thus, when summarized using a traditional count analysis in which the conclusion of each study is scored as either supporting or failing to support the hypothesis, the results suggest equivocal findings for studies using chronic intervention designs (13 support the relationship, 11 fail to support the relationship). Fortunately, the interpretation of inconsistent findings from empirical research is facilitated by the use of meta-analytic techniques. These techniques, by allowing for the statistical compilation of results from many studies, result in a statistically powerful test of the hypothesis.

Colcombe and Kramer (2003) used meta-analytic techniques to review the studies that they considered to have used the strongest experimental designs in examining the effects of physical activity participation on cognition in older adults. They located 18 studies that used random assignment to either a chronic exercise intervention or an appropriate control condition. The results of their review indicated that older adults who participated in an intervention designed to increase physical activity levels showed improvements in cognitive performance of nearly one half of a standard deviation (effect size = 0.48). Of particular interest, their results also indicated that larger effects were apparent for cognitive tasks that required executive processes (effect size = 0.68). Thus, the meta-analytic findings indicate that when physical activity is manipulated in studies using true experimental designs, physical activity has a positive effect on cognitive performance, and larger effects are evident for particular types of cognitive tasks.

In summary, across empirical studies using cross-sectional and prospective designs, the results have been fairly consistent and suggest that there is a positive relationship between physical activity and cognition in older adults. Across studies using chronic interventions, the results have been mixed. However, when the most well-designed chronic interventions are reviewed using meta-analytic techniques, the results support a causative relationship between physical activity and cognition in older adults. Therefore, if we consider the existing evidence, it seems safe to say that there is a positive association between physical activity and cognition and that this relationship may be causative in nature. However, the next critical step for researchers is to identify the mechanisms that underlie this relationship so that we completely understand the precise nature of the relationship. That is, until we understand the mechanisms that explain the relationship between physical activity and cognition, we cannot with 100% certainty identify the aspect or aspects of physical activity that result in better cognitive performance and we cannot knowledgeably design interventions specifically to attenuate cognitive decline in older adults.

Of Moderators and Mediators

Before we engage in further discussion of the potentially complex model of the relationship between the independent variable of physical activity and the dependent variable of cognition, it is valuable to define the terms that are used to describe the various components of such a model. The terms *moderator* and *mediator* have typically been used to describe a third variable that might affect the nature of the relationship between the independent variable and the dependent variable (Baron & Kenny, 1986).

A moderator is defined as a third variable "which partitions a focal independent variable into subgroups that establish its domains of maximal effectiveness in regard to a given dependent variable" (Baron & Kenny, 1986, p. 1173). A moderator can be categorical or continuous in nature and affects either the direction or the strength of the relationship between the independent and dependent variables. In statistical terms (see figure 2.1), a variable is a moderator if the interaction of that variable and the independent variable has a significant effect on the dependent variable (i.e., if * is significant).

Many moderating variables are relevant to this discussion. First and foremost, age is thought to moderate the relationship between physical activity and cognition such that physical activity may be particularly beneficial for older adults and for children but may be less beneficial for young

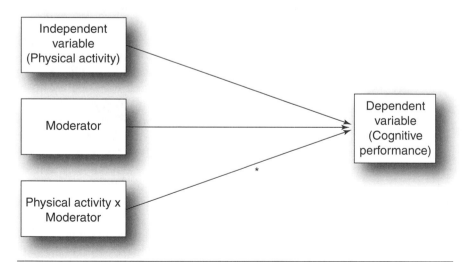

Figure 2.1 Single moderator model.

Adapted from R.M. Baron and D.A. Kenny, 1986, "The moderator-mediator variable distinction in social psychological research: Conceptual, strategic, and statistical considerations," *Journal of Personality and Social Psychology* 51(6):1173-1182.

to middle-aged adults (Etnier et al., 1997). Once we limit our focus to older adults, there are additional variables that may moderate the relationship between age and cognition and between physical activity and cognition. These possible moderators include gender, the estrogen status of women, ApoE-4 genotype (which is the genetic marker for Alzheimer's disease), and depression. The nature of these moderator effects is such that physical activity may be especially beneficial for the cognitive performance of women (particularly those who are postmenopausal and particularly those postmenopausal women who are on hormone replacement therapy), of ApoE-4 carriers, and of depressed individuals. The rationale for these effects is that these groups may be at most risk for cognitive decline and so may benefit the most from physical activity interventions.

In contrast, a mediator is defined as a third variable "which represents the generative mechanisms through which the focal independent variable is able to influence the dependent variable of interest" (Baron & Kenny, 1986, p. 1173). Mediators have also been referred to as indirect effects in the field of sociology and as surrogate effects or intermediate end point effects in the field of epidemiology (MacKinnon, Lockwood, Hoffman, West, & Sheets, 2002). Mediating variables are sometimes also referred to as mechanisms. However, some prefer to reserve the term *mechanism* for mediators that are directly quantifiable and that are biological in nature (e.g., serotonin, dopamine, number of synapses) and to use the term *mediators* for variables that represent broader hypothetical constructs (e.g., depression, self-efficacy, disease status). MacCorquodale and Meehl (1948) provided an eloquent discussion of variables that are considered to represent hypothetical constructs as opposed to variables that are quantifiable and that they referred to as intervening variables. For the purposes of this discussion, the term *mediator* is used to describe any third variable that could potentially explain the causal relationship between physical activity and cognition.

In statistical terms (see figure 2.2), Baron and Kenny (1986) define a variable as a mediator if the following hold true: (1) the independent variable is a significant predictor of the mediator (i.e., α is significant), (2) the independent variable is a significant predictor of the dependent variable (i.e., τ is significant), and (3) the mediator predicts a significant portion of the variance in the dependent variable after controlling for the independent variable (i.e., if β is significant after controlling for τ). However, some statisticians, including MacKinnon and colleagues (2002), suggest that the second requirement ignores the possibility that the mediated effect and the direct effect cancel each other out (resulting in a nonsignificant relationship between the independent variable and the dependent variable when the mediator is ignored) and suggest that only the first and third requirements are needed to establish mediation.

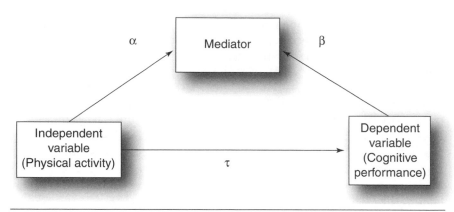

Figure 2.2   Single mediator model. Greek symbols represent regression coefficients for the paths between the identified variables.

Because the model of the relationship between physical activity and cognition is likely to be complex, identification of the mediators of the relationship is certain to be challenging. There are several sources of complexity in examining the relationship between physical activity and cognition. First, many possible mediators may explain the relationship between physical activity and cognition. These mediators can be categorized as being physiological, psychological, or behavioral or as being actual disease states of the individual. Second, the nature of the relationship is not likely to be represented by any single mediator acting directly on cognition. In fact, a multimediator model is likely in which physical activity affects cognition through several unique mediators (see figure 2.3).

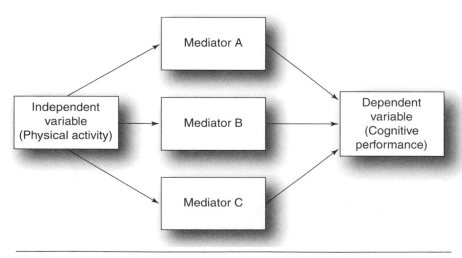

Figure 2.3   Model that includes multiple mediators (A, B, and C).

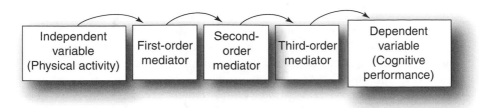

Figure 2.4 Model that includes a single micromediational chain.

Equally likely is a model that includes a single or multiple microme-diational chains that explain the effect of physical activity on cognition through cascading sequences of mediating processes (see figure 2.4). In a model that includes micromediational chains, the location of the media-tor in the causal chain can be described as first order, second order, third order, and so on.

Perhaps even more likely is a model of the relationship that is more complicated. For example, the model (see figure 2.5) may include both multiple mediators (mediators A and C) and mediators that function through micromediational chains (mediators B1 and B2).

A third complication in the elucidation of the model of physical activity and cognition is the fact that the role of the constructs in the model may not be unidimensional. Depression is an example of a variable that can play multiple roles in the model of the relationship between physical activity

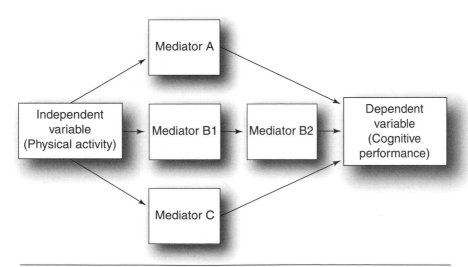

Figure 2.5 Model that includes multiple mediators (A and C) and micromedia-tional chains (B1 and B2).

and cognition. Depression can serve as a mediator of the relationship, can be a step in a micromediational chain, or can moderate the relationship. In addition, identification of the nature of these relationships is complicated by the chicken-and-egg nature of the question. Again, depression provides a perfect example of this issue. Low levels of physical activity may result in depression, which may (directly or through other mediators) affect cognitive performance. But equally possible is a model by which depression results in decreased levels of physical activity, which may (directly or through other mediators) influence cognitive performance.

Potential Mediators of the Physical Activity and Cognition Relationship

The potential mediators of the relationship between physical activity and cognition can be categorized using a variety of schemes. Here they are categorized as physiological, psychological, behavioral, or related to disease states of the individual.

Physiological mediators. The physiological mediators that have been proposed to explain the relationship include aerobic fitness, hormones (cortisol, estrogen, testosterone), lipid profiles, arterial stiffness, cerebral blood flow, blood pressure, cerebral structure, insulin-like growth factor I, catecholamines (epinephrine, norepinephrine), neurotransmitters (dopamine, serotonin), and neutrophins (brain-derived neurotrophin). These mediators may operate as single mediators or as relatively high-order mediators in a micromediational chain.

Psychological mediators. The potential psychological mediators include mediators that are likely to act as various steps in micromediational chains. The psychological mediators that may be early steps in these chains include depression, quality of life, pain, stress reactivity, and self-efficacy. The psychological mediators that are likely to act as either low- or high-order steps in micromediational chains include attentional control, inhibition control, speed–accuracy trade-offs, motivation, persistence, effort, and fatigue.

Behavioral mediators. The proposed behavioral mediators of the relationship include drug and medication use, sleep patterns, and eating habits. These mediators are likely to affect cognitive performance indirectly through their impact on subsequent mediators (from any category). It is also possible that these behaviors do not actually mediate the relationship between physical activity and cognition but rather are performed concurrently by physically active adults and exert their effects on cognition independently of physical activity.

Disease and health state mediators. It is possible that physical activity affects cognition through its influence on underlying disease states. These disease states may include Alzheimer's disease, diabetes, chronic obstructive pulmonary disease, cardiovascular disease, and hypertension. These mediators are likely to be lower-order steps in a micromediational chain.

State of the Literature Examining Mediators

Identifying potential mediators of the relationship between physical activity and cognition requires the use of appropriate experimental designs and suitable statistical analyses. Although the techniques for assessing mediation are not new and have been used regularly in the fields of sociology and psychology (MacKinnon, Lockwood, et al., 2002), the use of these techniques in exercise psychology has been rare. Most of the studies that have tested mediators have focused on exercise adherence and have tested models of the relationship between physical activity interventions and physical activity participation (see reviews by Baranowski, Anderson, & Carmack, 1998; Lewis, Marcus, Pate, & Dunn, 2002). To my knowledge, there is no study in the literature in which mediators of the relationship between physical activity and cognition have been statistically tested. In fact, an on-line search of the PubMed system conducted in April 2003 using combinations of the terms *mediation, mediator, cognition, cognitive, mental, fitness, exercise,* and *physical activity* supports this assertion because no studies could be found using these terms. Although experimental designs have been used that would allow for the testing of mediators, researchers have not used statistical techniques to actually test mediational processes.

Despite the lack of empirical study in which the necessary statistical techniques have been used to examine mediation, the literature does provide indirect evidence about the role of potential mediators of the relationship. Three major types of studies provide this indirect evidence. In general, these groups of studies provide examples of cases in which individual or pairs of relationships that are a part of the mediational model are tested, but the viability of the full mediational model is not assessed.

In one type of study, researchers have tested for differences between treatment groups and comparison groups on measures of cognition and on measures of the potential mediators. In other words, researchers have tested path α and path τ (see figure 2.2). When differences exist on both, authors have tended to conclude that this provides support for the mediator as a mechanism of the relationship. However, this interpretation is not precisely accurate because findings of this nature only provide an indication that mediation is possible and that authors have not used the appropriate statistical tests to determine whether these potential mediators actually statistically mediate the relationship between physical activity and cognition. Emery and Gatz (1990) came closer to testing mediation effects by manipulating physical activity levels and then examining correlations between physiological changes and cognitive changes as a result of the intervention. However, they again did not conduct the appropriate statistical tests to truly test for mediation.

A second type of indirect evidence for mediators of the physical activity–cognition relationship comes from studies in which physical activity levels have been manipulated and changes in potentially relevant mediator variables have been observed (i.e., α has been tested). Most of the mediators that are thought to possibly explain the positive relationship between physical activity and cognition have been tested using this method. These studies have been conducted with humans and with animals, and mediators from all categories have been examined. In general, there is support for the hypothesis that physical activity affects the proposed mediators that have been identified here. However, this evidence is clearly indirect because cognition has not been measured in studies of this type and so all of the pathways necessary to establish mediation have not been tested.

A third type of indirect evidence for mediation comes from studies in which potential mediators are correlated with cognition (i.e., β is tested), for example, studies in which levels of depression are correlated with cognitive performance. Again, although these studies provide a test of one of the necessary paths in the mediational model, they have not typically used physical activity as a means of manipulating depression while also studying cognition, and if they have included both of these variables, they have not statistically tested the mediational effect.

Thus, although there is indirect evidence suggesting that changes in physical activity alter some of the potential mediators, that changes in physical activity alter cognitive function, and that some of the potential mediators are correlated with cognitive performance, no studies could be located that have statistically tested the actual role of the potential mediator in the relationship between physical activity and cognition. Despite the dearth of direct evidence for mediators, aerobic fitness is one potential mediator that has been systematically tested with humans and is worthy of separate mention.

Evidence Relevant to the Potential Mediator of Aerobic Fitness

The relative wealth of research testing the role of aerobic fitness is likely attributable to the popularity of the cardiovascular fitness hypothesis as an explanation of many of the mental health benefits of physical activity. As applied to the area of cognition, the cardiovascular fitness hypothesis suggests that the increases in cardiovascular fitness that occur as a result of physical activity mediate the changes in cognitive performance. This hypothesis has been revised in other popular hypotheses to more clearly delineate the expected nature of the effects on cognition. Colcombe and Kramer (2003) described these as the speed hypothesis, the visuospatial hypothesis, the controlled-processing hypothesis, and the executive-control hypothesis. Regardless of which particular hypothesis one adopts, the common mediating variable in all of these hypotheses has been proposed to be fitness (and, more specifically, aerobic fitness). For this reason and for the purposes of this chapter, all of these hypotheses are considered to fall under the more general cardiovascular fitness hypothesis.

Indirect support for the cardiovascular fitness hypothesis is provided by findings from cross-sectional studies indicating that more aerobically fit adults perform better on cognitive tests than do less fit adults (e.g., Chodzko-Zajko, Schuler, Solomon, Heinl, & Ellis, 1992; Dustman et al., 1990; Offenbach, Chodzko-Zajko, & Ringel, 1990; van Boxtel et al., 1997) and from correlational studies in which measures of aerobic fitness have been found to be significantly related to measures of cognitive performance (e.g., Aleman et al., 2000; Era, Jokela, & Heikkinen, 1986; Izquierdo-Porrera & Waldstein, 2002). However, results from chronic interventions designed to increase aerobic fitness have been more equivocal. For example, some studies in which significant increases in aerobic fitness were obtained as a function of an exercise intervention found concomitant improvements in cognitive performance for their treatment groups (e.g., Dustman et al., 1984; Dustman, Emmerson, & Shearer, 1994; Emery et al., 1998). However, other researchers have also found significant gains in aerobic fitness as a result of an exercise intervention but have not found significant improvements in cognitive performance as a result of the intervention (e.g., Blumenthal et al., 1991; Madden et al., 1989).

Results from two meta-analytic reviews of the literature cited previously suggest that aerobic fitness does not mediate the relationship between physical activity and cognition. Colcombe and Kramer (2003) were able to test the influence of aerobic fitness on the effect sizes in their meta-analysis. Somewhat surprisingly, the size of the effect was not affected by the relative gain in aerobic fitness (coded as unreported, 5-11% gain in $\dot{V}O_2$max, and 12-25% gain in $\dot{V}O_2$max). This finding indicates that the cognitive performance gains realized as a function of increased physical activity did not differ as a function of the percentage of improvement in aerobic fitness. This conclusion is in agreement with that of another meta-analytic review of the literature that included studies with all age groups and found that there was no relationship between differences (or gains) in aerobic fitness and differences (or gains) in cognitive performance (Etnier, Nowell, Landers, & Sibley, 2006). Thus, when we think of a model with aerobic fitness as the sole mediator of the relationship (see figure 2.6) and evaluate the evidence relative to the criteria necessary to establish mediation, the existing evidence at this point does not seem to support the role of aerobic fitness as a mediator of the physical activity–cognition relationship. That is, there is strong evidence to support path α and there is evidence to support path τ. However, the support for path β is much more equivocal, and the actual mediational role of aerobic fitness has not been tested.

The fact that the studies using causative designs have been mixed and that two meta-analytic reviews failed to support a dose–response relation-

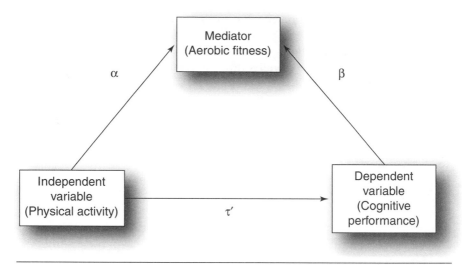

Figure 2.6 Aerobic fitness as the sole mediator of the physical activity–cognition relationship. Greek symbols represent regression coefficients for the paths between the identified variables.

ship between aerobic fitness and cognitive performance in older adults is an important finding that must be considered as we move toward identifying mechanisms that might underlie the relationship. It is, of course, possible that aerobic fitness does in fact mediate the relationship, but that the experimental designs and statistical techniques used have not been powerful enough to identify these effects (i.e., manipulation was not strong enough, measures of fitness were not precise enough, cognitive tests were not sensitive enough). It is equally possible that aerobic fitness only partially mediates the relationship between physical activity and cognition. This would suggest that other mediators or other steps in a micromediational chain between aerobic fitness and cognition must be identified to explain a significant percentage of the variance in cognitive performance. Whatever the case, the fact that the evidence for aerobic fitness is equivocal and that aerobic fitness may not best explain the relationship is especially important considering that much of the public health policy regarding recommended levels of physical activity (Corbin & Pangrazi, 1996; Institute of Medicine, 2002) has been formulated based on amounts of exercise necessary to produce fitness changes. If aerobic fitness does not, in fact, mediate the relationship with cognition, then it is possible that we are designing physical activity programs that are targeted toward the wrong mediating variable in terms of maintaining cognitive performance in older adults.

Direction for Future Study

The development of a model to explain how and why physical activity seems to benefit cognitive functioning is incredibly challenging, and there may not be a simple solution. In fact, Bäckman, Small, and Wahlin (2001) made a comment regarding the relationship between age and cognition that is equally relevant to the relationship between physical activity and cognition. They stated that the identification of a *single* biological parameter to explain the variance in cognitive functioning relative to age may be "doomed to fail, because of the inherent complexity at both the biological and behavioral level" (p. 364). These authors encouraged researchers to consider multiple factors at varying levels of analysis. This advice is equally relevant for researchers who investigate physical activity and cognition.

The clear implication of this discussion is that the first step in our quest to identify mediators of the relationship is, very simply, to conduct the appropriate statistical tests of these mediators. As mentioned, the positive relationship between physical activity and cognition has been reasonably well established through cross-sectional, prospective, and experimental studies. However, the designs and statistical techniques that have been used have not been predicated on a desire to test for mediation. In addition, many of the potential mediators of the relationship have often been treated merely as potential confounds of the relationship and have been controlled for rather than tested as mediators (e.g., depression by Etnier & Berry, 2001; Khatri et al., 2001). The clear direction for subsequent research is to use techniques that will allow for decisions to be made regarding the viability of particular variables as mediators of the relationship.

In particular, mediation analysis techniques need to be used to further our understanding of these relationships. Mediation analysis is a statistical tool that can be used with studies of any design. In fact, MacKinnon (2001) suggested that mediation techniques should be used in a program of research in which information is garnered from correlational studies and then is manipulated in randomized trials so that the key components of a program designed to affect the dependent variable can be identified. In a statement demonstrating the inherent complexity of this process, MacKinnon (2001) further suggested that we should "view the identification of mediating variables as a sustained research effort requiring a variety of experimental and nonexperimental approaches to identify mediating variables" (p. 9506). The use of statistical techniques to test mediation is straightforward and simply involves the use of repeated regression analyses. A variety of methods have been proposed to test mediational models, and MacKinnon, Lockwood, and colleagues (2002) provided a review of these models that includes information regarding their conceptual bases and their respective statistical power. Additional information regarding the

27

use of these statistical methods is readily available in the printed literature (see Baron & Kenny, 1986; Cheong, MacKinnon, & Khoo, 2003; Mac-Kinnon, 2001; MacKinnon, Lockwood, et al., 2002; MacKinnon, Taborga, & Morgan-Lopez, 2002) and through on-line resources (see http://www.public.asu.edu/~davidpm/ripl/mediate.htm; http://www.psych.ku.edu/preacher/sobel/sobel.htm; or use search key words mediation and David A. Kenny).

In addition to using the appropriate statistical techniques, study in this area would benefit from the use of longitudinal designs in which individuals are followed through their older years. These studies would allow for the examination of intraindividual change and would be especially valuable for distinguishing between normal differences that occur with aging and those that are not normal and that may be linked to important mediator variables. The identification of these potentially important mediator variables would then provide direction for subsequent research that has a causative design.

Ultimately, the implementation of true experimental studies that allow for conclusions regarding causation will be crucial to advance our understanding of the effects of physical activity on cognitive functioning. Willis (2001) recently provided a review of the factors that should be considered in designing such research and particularly emphasized that studies must be designed to elucidate the mechanisms that mediate the intervention. In designing these studies, we must consider one key issue if we are to truly advance our understanding of mediational processes. This issue is related to the choice of an appropriate control condition that differs from the treatment condition only by the independent variable. This may sound trivial, but given the host of physiological, psychological, behavioral, and disease state mechanisms that could potentially explain the relationship between physical activity and cognition, the selection and design of an appropriate control condition are actually very challenging. One of the goals of this workshop is to present the evidence with regard to the potential mediators of the relationship so that researchers will have the knowledge necessary to address this important issue when they design behavioral interventions.

Summary

As our technical abilities continue to improve with regard to statistical techniques and innovations like the structural and functional imaging techniques that allow for a noninvasive examination of the mediators related to cerebral function and structure, it is likely that our knowledge in this area of research will increase rapidly. Identification of the mediators by which physical activity imparts its beneficial effects on cognition is of utmost importance. Until we better understand the precise mechanisms through which physical activity influences cognition, we cannot appropriately design exercise interventions to target these mechanisms. That is, for example, if the effects are primarily mediated by changes in self-efficacy, then our programs should be designed first and foremost to increase self-efficacy. If, however, the effects are primarily mediated by changes in lipid profiles, then perhaps physical activity interventions provided in conjunction with dietary interventions may be most effective to attenuate age-related declines in cognition. Because the effects of physical activity on cognition for older adults appear to be reliable, consistent, and causal, the next logical step for researchers in this area is to clearly identify why this relationship exists so that those most at risk for cognitive decline can be identified and so that effective interventions can be implemented. The purpose of this workshop is to review the existing literature on many of the potential lower-order mediators of the relationship between physical activity and cognition with a goal of directing subsequent research that will use appropriate designs and techniques to confirm the mediational role of these variables.

EDITORS' DISCUSSION SUMMARY

Discussion Highlights

In examining the roles of mediators between exercise or activity and cognitive functions, many investigators seem to assume that physical activity or exercise plays a causative role in enhancing the cognition of older adults or, even, that this effect is unidirectional. It is equally as probable that this relationship is bidirectional. It is just as logical to propose that cognition explains the variance in physical activity as it is to say that physical activity explains a portion of the variance in cognition.

Two suggestions are made for future investigators. One, use more complex analytical methods. The multiple regression approach is less than adequate when analyzing reciprocally determining relationships, especially when the interest is in studying intraindividual changes over time. To study developmental changes in aerobic fitness and in cognition, it is necessary to acquire multiple data points. Several good models are available to handle these types of data. Latent growth curve models are one example, and other types of approaches provide very good controls for measurement error, have very reliable standard errors, and allow an analysis of the more complex relationships that clearly evolve from these types of models. Also, hierarchical linear modeling is a reasonable tool to use when you study groups within groups of subjects in communities or areas within communities, as two examples. Dave McKinnon and colleagues (Cheong, MacKinnon, & Khoo, 2003; MacKinnon, Lockwood, et al., 2002; MacKinnon, Taborga, & Morgan-Lopez, 2002) have written several articles on how to expand the use of regression techniques to more complicated models and how to use latent growth curve modeling. But these techniques have not been used very much in the arena of physical activity and cognition. Albert and colleagues' (1995) article was an early example, in which 22 variables were used as predictors of cognitive change over 2 to 2 1/2 years, but that study lacked a guiding theoretical model. Nevertheless, it was a forerunner of the way we should be heading in our studies.

Two, consider the individual differences in responses to exercise. Some individuals respond to a habitual dose of exercise with very large, positive changes in cardiorespiratory-related outcomes. Other individuals have almost no response to that same exercise dose. This is similar to the observations of genetic composition and responses to changes in diet. Jose Ordovas (2003), for example, found that there are actually people who can eat a high-cholesterol, high-fat diet and yet their cholesterol levels decline. The cholesterol levels in other people, however, remain high or increase no matter what they eat. It may very well be that exercise does in fact positively influence cognition but only in individuals with genetic compositions that include positive responses to exercise.

Research Methodology Problems

The following are four methodological suggestions that could provide a better understanding of mediating factors:

1. Test rather than control for mediators. Many potential mediators of the relationship between physical activity and cognition have been experimentally controlled rather than tested as mediators. Designs should be developed that allow for decisions to be made regarding the viability of particular variables as mediators of the relationship.

2. Use longitudinal designs. Longitudinal designs would provide information about intraindividual time-related changes that might be linked to mediators.

3. Choose an appropriate control condition. A large array of physiological, psychological, behavioral, and disease state mechanisms and their interactions could potentially explain some of the variance of cognition. Considering that an appropriate control condition differs from the treatment condition only by the independent variable, the selection and design of a control condition are actually very challenging.

4. Quantify the mediators accurately. A researcher in Great Britain was once comparing vegetarians and meat eaters on their health status and number of diseases to determine whether nutrition was a factor. Finding that these groups were not different puzzled him, and so he followed up with a much more detailed analysis of what each group actually consumed, rather than whether they categorized themselves as vegetarians or meat eaters. To his great surprise, he discovered that in addition to vegetables, the vegetarians also consumed substantial amounts of beer and chips (i.e., many fast foods that were not meat but were not healthy either). In other words, it does not make any difference how carefully the research design is selected and implemented if the potential mediator is inaccurately measured.

PART II

Exercise Effects on Mental Resources and Reserves

CHAPTER 3

Exercise, Depression, and Cognition

John B. Bartholomew, PhD, and Joseph T. Ciccolo, PhD

The University of Texas at Austin

EDITORS' OVERVIEW

Dr. Bartholomew and Dr. Ciccolo address one debilitating illness, depression, that is known to affect cognitive performance profoundly.

First, they describe how depression negatively affects cognition, and then they discuss the results from studies of exercise effects on depression. They emphasize the importance of disassociating the effects of exercise on performance state from those on functional capacity. Finally, they provide information on mechanisms by which exercise, by ameliorating depression, might enhance cognition. Examples are the psychosocial benefits that exercise provides and several physiological mechanisms such as modifications of several neurotransmitters, neurohormones, and neurotrophic factors. (Note the return arrows from Mediators, e.g., Mental resources, to Exercise in the model.)

The authors end the chapter by recommending that researchers extend the large body of research that strongly documents separate links of this model, depression and cognition, depression and exercise, and exercise and cognition, by considering all of the links simultaneously.

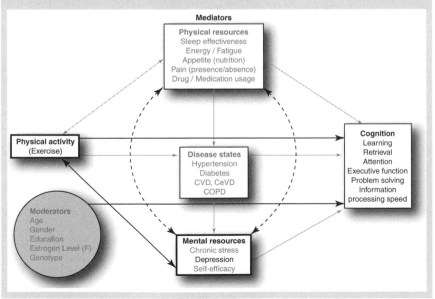

It is estimated that in any given year, 6.5% to 10.1% of the adult U.S. population suffers from depression. Depression is defined as a state of great sadness and apprehension. It is marked by symptoms of depressed mood and a loss of interest in, or the ability to experience pleasure in response to, normally stimulating, positive events. The *Diagnostic and Statistical Manual for Mental Disorders* (fourth edition, *DSM-IV;* American Psychiatric Association, 2000) criteria for major depressive disorder (MDD) are presented in table 3.1. In addition to these symptoms, high anxiety, obsessions, or panic attacks are quite common. The disorder cannot be diagnosed if the symptoms are attributable to physical illness, alcohol, medication, or street drugs. For example, although frontal lobe degeneration is associated with a loss of executive function whose symptoms can mirror those of depression, an individual with frontal lobe degeneration would not be diagnosed with depression. This issue is discussed in detail by Dr. Royall elsewhere in this volume and in the discussion that follows. Also, MDD cannot be diagnosed if symptoms last for less than 2 months after normal bereavement, among other exclusionary factors *(DSM-IV)*. Although these symptoms must be experienced for a minimum of 2 weeks, almost every day, to be considered MDD, episodes of depression can be extensive. Without treatment, an experience of MDD will last, on average, 9 months, with most episodes lasting no more than 2 years (Kapur & Mann, 1992). However, once an

Table 3.1   *DSM-IV* Symptom Criteria for Major Depression

At least one of these two	
I	Depressed mood indicated by subjective report or observation
II	Markedly diminished interest or pleasure in all, or almost all, activities

At least four of these seven	
I	Significant weight loss when not dieting or weight gain
II	Insomnia or hypersomnia
III	Psychomotor agitation or retardation that is observable by others
IV	Fatigue or loss of energy
V	Feelings of worthlessness or excessive or inappropriate guilt
VI	Diminished ability to think or concentrate
VII	Recurrent thoughts of death and suicide ideation

These must be present most of the day, nearly every day, during the same 2-week period and represent a change from previous function.

episode has subsided, there is a 50% chance that depression will return (Thase, Nierenberg, Keller, & Panagides, 2001).

The most serious consequence of depression, especially undetected depression, is increased mortality rate. For example, Caine and associates studied the postmortem records of 97 adults aged 50 and above who committed suicide. Among these individuals, 51 had seen their primary care physician within 1 month of the suicide, and of those, 45 had psychiatric symptoms. From the group of 45, only 29 physicians had recorded symptoms and only 19 patients were offered treatment, of whom only two received the recommended level of care (Caine, Lyness, & Conwell, 1996). It is clear, therefore, that MDD differs in both magnitude and pervasiveness from the common feelings of sadness that are a part of a normal response to unfortunate events.

For older individuals, U.S. prevalence rates are 5% or less (Gurland, Cross, & Katz, 1996). This would suggest that older individuals are less likely to suffer from depression than their younger adult counterparts. This finding coincides with results from psychiatric interviews of adults in the Baltimore Epidemiologic Catchment Area (ECA) that found the prevalence of major depression declining with age (Alexopoulos, 1997; Gallo & Lebowitz, 1999; Romanoski et al., 1992). However, the same study also showed an increase in depressive symptoms with age.

In fact, it has been commonly shown that older adults are less likely to be diagnosed with MDD than their younger counterparts but that they are more likely to report depressive symptoms, particularly physical symptoms (U.S. Department of Health and Human Services [USHHS], 1999). This seeming contradiction illustrates the difficulty of diagnosing depression, particularly within the older population. For instance, geriatric depression is more somatic and less ideational than depression in other age groups (Serby & Yu, 2003). Thus, older patients are more likely to report physical symptoms than psychological ones (Blazer, 1996). This is particularly problematic because primary care physicians, not mental health professionals, treat the majority of patients with symptoms of depression (Sharp & Lipsky, 2002). Because older adults are prone to numerous medical disorders, the expression of these general medical symptoms may mask the presence of physical symptoms of depression. Additionally, older individuals appear to be more likely to deny the psychological symptoms of depression or refuse to accept the diagnosis because of the stigma attached to mental illness (USHHS, 1999). This limits the usefulness of self-reported symptoms. Because both report by the individual and identification by the clinician are limited in their accuracy, the ability to recognize and properly identify depression, particularly by primary care physicians, is usually low (USHHS, 1999) and can be affected by the patient's gender (Helmes & Duggan, 2001). Despite the possibility of underdiagnosis, MDD is the most common type of clinical depressive disorder in older adults.

However, most older patients with symptoms of depression do not meet the full criteria for MDD. These individuals are instead classified as having "minor depression." Minor depression is a subsyndromal form of depression that has been proposed to characterize these patients, but it is not recognized as an official disorder. Although minor depression has not yet been standardized, it is thought to be part of a spectrum of disorders that make up MDD (Rapaport et al., 2002).

As a result, the underdiagnosis and undertreatment of depression in older adults are common problems. For example, one study found that only about 11% of depressed patients in primary care received adequate antidepressant treatment (in terms of dose and duration of pharmacotherapy), whereas 34% received inadequate treatment and 55% received no treatment (Katon et al., 1992). It has been suggested that there is an increased need to focus on older men, particularly minority men, and those who prefer treatments other than antidepressants, because these specific populations are not being adequately treated (Unutzer et al., 2003).

Both major depression and minor depression are associated with significant disability in physical, social, and role functioning (Wells et al., 1989). Although the cause of MDD is unknown, several physiological and psychological mechanisms have been cited as potential causes for depression in the aging and elderly population: biochemical changes in the aged brain causing cognitive impairments, disturbances in central metabolism of monoamines, dysfunction of the hypothalamic–pituitary–adrenal (HPA) axis, and increased psychosocial stress or isolation (Gareri, De Fazio, & De Sarro, 2002).

Major or minor depression diagnosed with first onset later than age 60 has been termed late-onset depression. Like minor depression, late-onset depression is not a diagnosis but instead refers to a subset of patients with major or minor depression who present with slightly different clinical characteristics, that is, first experiencing an episode of depression after the age of 60. Risk factors for late-onset depression, based on results of prospective studies, include widowhood (Mendes de Leon, Kasl, & Jacobs, 1994), physical illness (Bachman et al., 1992), impaired functional status (Bruce & Hoff, 1994), heavy alcohol consumption (Saunders et al., 1991), lack of joy and interest, and poor concentration (Hein et al., 2003). Other studies have indicated that late-onset depression may be caused by disorders that cause vascular damage, such as hypertension, coronary artery disease, and diabetes mellitus. It is also suggested that there is a cerebral abnormality that constitutes vulnerability for depression (Alexopoulos et al., 1997; Steffens & Krishnan, 1998). Most disturbing is that depression-related suicide is most associated with late-onset depression, and older adults (age 65 and older) have the highest rate of depression-related suicide of any group (USHHS, 1999).

Depression and Cognition

When we consider the effect of depression on cognition, it may be useful to distinguish between the transitory effects of depression on cognitive performance and the more lasting effects of depression on the cognition-related structures of the brain. As a result, we distinguish between impairments in cognition that alter functional capacity (e.g., atrophy of the hippocampus or the frontal lobe region), which affect the potential of the individual to perform cognitive tasks, and impairments in cognitive performance that reflect both the functional capacity and the transient performance state (e.g., fatigue, motivation) of the individual.

Given the list of enduring symptoms, it is not surprising that depression is linked with impaired cognitive function. This effect, however, is not limited to older adults. The reduction in cognition has been demonstrated in both younger (Fossati, Amar, Raoux, Ergis & Allilaire, 1999) and older (Adler, Bramesfeld, & Jajcevic, 1999) individuals who suffer from depression. For example, in a longitudinal study of cognitive performance among older (65-86 years old) individuals, depression scores were the best predictor of reduced performance over time (Carmelli, Swan, LaRue, & Eslinger, 1997). Cognitive impairment has been demonstrated in both measures of functional capacity and cognitive performance. Again, measures of functional capacity refer to the potential of the system and reflect changes in the structure and operation of the central nervous system. Depression-related impairments in functional capacity have been evidenced through increased encephalographic slow-wave power (Adler et al., 1999), dysfunction in the frontal lobes (Veiel, 1997), and reduced cerebral blood flow (Baker, Frith, & Dolan, 1997). In contrast, measures of cognitive performance reflect a person's ability to use his or her functional capacity, that is, a person's ability to perform cognitive tasks. Deficits in cognitive performance may be attributable to limitations in functional capacity or differences in transient performance states. Depression-related impairments in cognitive performance have been observed for selective attention and working memory (Landro, Stiles, & Sletvold, 2001), verbal (Fossati et al., 1999) and immediate memory (Lauer et al., 1994), performance on the Stroop Color Word Test (Degl'Innocenti, Agren, & Backman, 1998), vigilance tasks (Christensen, Griffiths, Mackinnon, & Jacomb, 1997), academic performance (Haines, Norris, & Kashy, 1997), and spatial processing and learning (Benedict, Dobraski, & Goldstein, 1999). In fact, the range of deficits is overwhelming and has been compared with those seen in moderately severe traumatic brain injury (Veiel, 1997).

MDD produces a number of symptoms that would be expected to compromise cognitive performance. Fatigue, a loss of energy, and an inability to concentrate are all a part of the clinical diagnosis of MDD, and each would be expected to negatively affect performance on a cognitive task. For example, it has long been recognized that depressed participants report increases in fatigue earlier in a testing session than their healthy counterparts (Byrne, 1977; Whitehead, 1973). This explanation fits well with the concepts of energetics discussed by Dr. Tomporowski elsewhere in this volume. In sum, performance on any cognitive task is based on the energy and emotional state of the individual, and performance is expected to vary with these states. As each of these states is negatively affected by depression, cognitive performance is impaired. However, these are transient states, and as the individual recovers from his or her affective disorder, cognitive performance is expected to improve. Although few studies have examined the change in cognitive performance following a remission of depression, the literature supports this interpretation. For example, there is evidence that cognitive performance improves once a depressive episode has lapsed (Burt, Zembar, & Niederehe, 1995). However, when the performance state of the individual (fatigue) was controlled before and after an episode of depression, no improvement in cognitive performance was shown following a recovery from depression (Reischies & Neu, 2000). Thus, it appears likely that depression has a transitory effect on cognitive performance that varies with the level of affective state but that some losses in cognitive function may continue regardless of the individual's affective state.

A different mechanism of action is required to explain these more lasting cognitive impairments. One possibility would be changes in cerebral milieu or atrophy of neural tissue. For example, there are clear metabolic challenges to the brain during depression that are associated with changes in cerebral blood flow (Bench, Frackowiak, & Dolan, 1995; Brody et al., 1999) and neurotransmitter function (van Broekhoven & Verkes, 2003), which have been related to impaired neurogenesis (Jacobs, 2002). In addition, hippocampal atrophy has been suggested as a direct cognitive mechanism through which depression may impair cognitive function. Specifically, lasting depression is associated with neural degradation within the hippocampus (Sapolsky, 1996, 2001). This appears to be attributable to hypersecretion of glucocorticoids that results in a volume loss that can reach as high as 20% (Sheline et al., 1999). In addition, depression appears to limit neural plasticity in the hippocampus (Gould, McEwen, Tanapat, Galea, & Fuchs, 1997), leaving the system more susceptible to challenge. Because the hippocampus is one of the primary areas associated with learning and memory, any depression-related damage to the hippocampus would be expected to compromise functional capacity of the central nervous system. Last, depression is also associated with impaired executive function, that is, the ability of the individual to integrate lower-order cognitive functions, which reflects damage to the frontal lobe region of the brain (Fossati et al., 1999).

Given the loss of brain tissue that can occur with lasting depression, lasting cognitive impairment is not surprising. Recovery from depression would be expected to halt further neuronal degradation, but it would not be expected to lead to a regeneration of lost neural tissue. Thus, impairments in cognitive performance that result from a change in functional capacity may last well beyond recovery from depression. Interestingly, recent evidence shows that treatment for depression may prevent the losses of neural tissue during the depressive episode. In an animal model of depression, control animals demonstrated a 50% increase in cortisol and a 30% decrease in hippocampal neurogenesis during a stress-induced depression model. Experimental animals were treated with the antidepressant drug tianeptine, and although they showed a similar increase in cortisol reflective of a depressive episode, they did not experience a reduction in neural proliferation (Czeh et al., 2001). Likewise, other studies have shown that antidepressants are associated with neurogenesis (Magarinos, Deslandes, & McEwan, 1999). Thus, treatment of depression may prevent or reduce the depression-related loss of functional capacity.

A vast number of effective treatments exist for depression, although patients' responses to treatment are highly variable. Treatments include both pharmacological and psychosocial interventions that may be acute or chronic in nature. Pharmacological treatments such as tricyclic antidepressants (TCAs) and selective serotonin reuptake inhibitors (SSRIs) have been widely used to treat depressed patients of all ages. There are, however, limitations to the use of these drugs. Side effects for TCAs include dry mouth or constipation or more serious effects like tachycardia or cardiac arrhythmias. TCAs may also cause central anticholinergic effects that result in acute confusional states or memory problems in the depressed older adult (Branconnier, DeVitt, Cole, & Spera, 1982). Likewise, SSRIs may cause harsh side effects, such as insomnia, anxiety, and restlessness. Finally, the time course of pharmacological treatments may exceed 6 to 8 weeks before they provide significant relief of depression (Miller, 2001). Despite these limitations, there is consistent evidence that older patients, even the very old, respond well to antidepressant medication (Reynolds & Kupfer, 1999). About 60% to 80% of older patients report reduced depression in conjunction with pharmacological treatment, whereas the placebo response rate ranges from 30% to 40% (Schneider, 1996).

Psychosocial treatments have been shown to be just as effective as pharmacological treatments. Studies cite psychotherapy as an effective treatment for late-life depression. These methods include cognitive–behavioral therapy, interpersonal psychotherapy, problem-solving therapy, brief psychodynamic psychotherapy, and reminiscence therapy, which is an intervention developed specifically for older adults on the premise that reflection on positive and negative past life experiences enables the individual to overcome feelings of depression and despair (Butler, 1974; Butler, Lewis, & Sunderland, 1991). Both group and individual formats have been used successfully with this population.

Exercise and Depression

More recently, exercise has been demonstrated as an effective tool for treating depression, particularly in older adults. Several large-scale cross-sectional studies as well as smaller community sample studies have consistently shown that individuals who repeatedly engage in physical activity are reported to have less depressive symptoms than sedentary individuals. Although the early evidence in this area was exclusively drawn from younger populations, exercise therapy has been shown to be an effective treatment for depressive symptoms in older adults (Singh, Clements, & Fiatarone, 1997; Williams & Lord, 1997), and it has been shown to normalize depressed mood (Craft & Landers, 1998). In fact, exercise therapy has been shown to be as effective as antidepressants in the older population (Babyak et al., 2000; Blumenthal et al., 1999), and it has been successful in reducing relapse of depressive episodes for older adults (Babyak et al., 2000; Singh, Clements, & Singh, 2001).

The majority of the literature has focused on aerobic exercise as a treatment. In fact, an aerobic exercise training program may be considered an alternative to antidepressants for the treatment of depression (North, McCullagh, & Tran, 1990). For example, when exercise was compared with antidepressant medication and a combination of exercise and antidepressant therapy, all groups reported similar reductions in depressive symptoms, with no clinical or statistical group differences (Blumenthal et al., 1999). Similar findings have been reported by several other researchers (Blumenthal, Williams, Needles, & Wallace, 1982; Martinsen, Medhus, & Sandvik, 1985; McNeil, LeBlanc, & Joyner, 1991).

Fewer studies have been done with resistance training; however, results are similar to those seen with aerobic exercise. Singh and colleagues (1997) asked 32 participants aged 60 to 84 with major or minor depression to complete 10 weeks of resistance training. When compared with the control group, the intervention group showed significant reductions in all depression measures as well as a significant increase in vitality and social functioning. A long-term follow-up to this study showed that 33% of the exercisers were still regularly weightlifting at 26 months postintervention and that the antidepressive effect was still detectable at 20 weeks (Singh et al., 2001). However, Pennix and colleagues (2002) compared the effects of aerobic and resistance exercise on the emotional and physical function of older adults with depressive symptoms. The authors found that compared with the control condition, aerobic exercise significantly lowered depressive symptoms over time and no effect was seen with resistance training. The resistance exercise training program was lower in intensity than that used by Singh and associates (1997). This is one of the few differences from the younger adult literature, where low- to moderate-intensity resistance training appears to be sufficient to alleviate depression (Doyne et al., 1987). The conflicting results for older adults suggest that more work is needed to determine the dose of exercise needed to reduce depression in this population.

Although there is evidence to suggest that moderate- to high-intensity exercise training can reduce symptoms of depression in older adults, no study has varied the frequency or duration of the exercise, nor has any study controlled for energy expenditure in this population. In general, all exercise programs (both aerobic and resistance) have been for 12 to 16 weeks, with participants exercising three times a week for 45 min to 1 h. Aerobic interventions in the older population have participants exercise at an intensity of 40% to 85% of heart rate reserve (Blumenthal et al., 1999; Herman et al., 2002; Pennix et al., 2002), and resistance interventions use 50% to 80% of the participants' 1-repetition maximum (1RM; Pennix et al., 2002; Singh et al., 1997; Tsutsumi, Don, Zaichkowsky, & Delizonna, 1997). Clearly, more work is needed to map the dose–response curve for both aerobic exercise and weightlifting. The lack of data with older individuals is mirrored by the lack of research with younger participants. As a result, a recent review was unable to quantify a dose–response relationship with exercise and depression (Dunn, Trivedi, & O'Neal, 2001).

One factor that determines the effectiveness of exercise as a treatment for depression is early dropout. This is particularly problematic because the fatigue associated with depression would be expected to make it difficult to adhere to an exercise regimen. Obviously, those individuals who drop out early or do not complete the prescribed protocol receive little or none of the benefits that might have been gained. Thus, it becomes important to focus on the determinants of exercise adherence within the depressed population and determine what will improve adherence to an exercise protocol among older participants. A recent study of older MDD patients revealed that baseline anxiety and life satisfaction were predictive of dropout from exercise treatment (Herman et al., 2002). It may be, therefore, that the baseline severity of the psychopathological disorder is an important factor in considering exercise as a treatment. Again, this is not surprising because the initial level of depression would be expected to correlate with feelings of fatigue and hopelessness, which would clearly serve as a barrier to regular exercise. However, additional research is needed that stratifies patients based on initial depressive symptoms to replicate this result.

It appears that in addition to ongoing exercise training, shorter training periods or even acute bouts of exercise can improve depressive symptoms among MDD patients. For example, a sample of middle-aged clinically depressed patients reported improved mood following just 10 days of aerobic exercise (Dimeo, Bauer, Varahram, Proest, & Halter, 2001). Likewise, a single bout of moderate-intensity treadmill walking was able to improve affect in a similar group of clinically depressed patients (Bartholomew, Ciccolo, & Morrison, 2003). Neither of these studies demonstrated a reduction in clinical depression. It is unlikely that any single or short-duration treatment will be successful at reducing MDD. Instead, these studies show that the transient mood of the MDD patient can be improved following a minimal application of exercise. Given the delay in effectiveness of pharmacological or psychological treatments, these data suggest that exercise may be a useful addition to other forms of treatment as a means to improve mood in the short term. Although exercise is not a means to treat the underlying clinical disorder, an improvement in mood may have implications for cognitive performance. Again, an energetics-based analysis, as described by Dr. Tomporowski elsewhere in this volume, would suggest that any intervention that enhances the energy and emotional state of the individual would be expected to benefit performance on cognitive tasks. As a result, exercise need not enhance functional capacity of the individual to improve cognitive performance. It may merely reduce those transitory effects of depression, such as fatigue, poor motivation, and poor concentration, that limit cognitive performance.

A variety of mechanisms have been proposed to explain the mediating effect of exercise on depression. For example, exercise has been shown to improve a number of self-perceptions that are related to depression in the older population: self-esteem (McAuley, Blissmer, Katula, Duncan, & Mihalko, 2000), self-efficacy (McAuley, Jerome, Marquez, Elavsky, & Blissmer, 2003), life satisfaction (Steinkamp & Kelly, 1987), social physique anxiety (McAuley, Marquez, Jerome, Blissmer, & Katula, 2002), and anxiety (Katula, Blissmer, & McAuley, 1999). Exercise has also been associated with increased social support and social functioning (Resnick, Orwig, Magaziner, & Wynne, 2002; Singh et al., 1997). In addition, a number of physiological mechanisms have been suggested. For example, exercise has been shown to modify a number of the physical markers for depression, such as serotonin (Jacobs, 1994), neuroepinephrine (Dishman, 1997), HPA axis activity (van der Pompe, Bernards, Meijman, & Heijnen, 1999), and brain-derived neurotrophic factor (BDNF; Van Hoomissen, Chambliss, Holmes, & Dishman, 2003). A more thorough review of exercise and BDNF is presented by Dr. Berchtold elsewhere in this volume.

The mechanism whereby exercise-induced increases in BDNF act as an antidepressant is particularly intriguing. For example, in animal models of depression, the injection of BDNF reduces depressive behaviors (Siuciak, Lewis, Wiegand, & Lindsay, 1997). In addition, both exercise and antidepressants have been shown to be sufficient to prevent the normal stress-induced reduction of BDNF (Russo-Neustadt, Ha, Ramirez, & Kesslak,

2001). The effect of BDNF appears to be attributable to enhanced synaptogenesis and neurogenesis in the hippocampus (Cotman & Engesser-Ceaser, 2002). As mentioned earlier, neuronal degradation of the hippocampus is a leading theory for why depression is associated with impaired cognitive functioning. Thus, increases in BDNF may be a common pathway linking the effects of exercise on depression and cognitive function (Cotman & Engesser-Ceaser, 2002).

Conclusion and Recommendations

It is clear that MDD is a debilitating disorder that is associated with a reduction in cognition. For this reason, depression is generally treated as a nuisance variable in studies of cognitive function. Either depressed people are screened from participating, or current levels of depression are controlled for statistically. We suggest an alternative approach—treating depression as an independent variable to test its role as a moderator of the relationship between exercise and cognition.

We have presented a range of data suggesting that an exercise intervention might enhance the cognition of depressed people to a greater extent than their healthy counterparts. These data are summarized in the model presented in figure 3.1. Specifically, exercise is now widely accepted as an efficacious treatment for depression, one that is on par with pharmacological or cognitive–behavioral interventions, and there is some evidence that the depression-related reductions in cognitive performance are relieved with

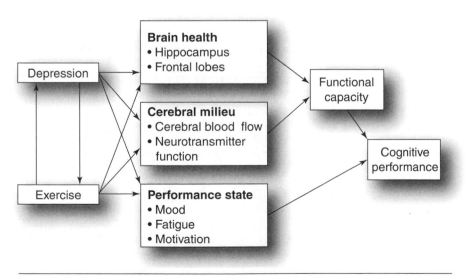

Figure 3.1 A model of exercise, depression, and cognition.

a remission in a depressive episode. This may be especially true for deficits in cognitive performance that are attributable to the transitory states that are experienced as a result of depression. Thus, at a minimum, it would be expected that an exercise-induced reduction in depression would improve cognitive performance. It is less likely that a simple reduction in depression would be associated with a regeneration of lost neural tissue. However, there is evidence that common pharmacological treatments for depression are sufficient to limit the hippocampal atrophy. In addition, exercise is associated with an increase in BDNF, which improves hippocampal plasticity. As such, an exercise-based treatment for depression may also prevent hippocampal tissue loss across a lasting depressive episode.

It is clear that exercise, depression, and cognitive function are all individually related to one another. However, no work to date has attempted to integrate these paradigms. Given the preponderance of data demonstrating the individual links, it appears that such an integration would be a useful means to extend the present work in each area. Given the numbers of older adults who are affected by depression and impaired cognitive function, the time is ripe for such an integration.

EDITORS' DISCUSSION SUMMARY

Discussion Highlights

Both substantive and methodological issues were discussed relating to the impact of depression on cognition and exercise benefits of older adults.

Eight pertinent substantive issues were noted. First, the magnitude of a depressive episode is related to cognitive impairment and exercise benefit. For example, if the primary impact of depression is a reduction in performance-related states, such as the ability to focus attention, to sustain motivation, and to resist fatigue, then *acute* bouts of exercise may sufficiently improve mood and thereby improve cognition performance. However, if the primary impact of depression is impaired brain physiology, such as hippocampal atrophy (loss of neural plasticity and brain volume) and compromised cerebral functioning (decreased blood flow, neurotransmitter dysfunction, and impaired neurogenesis), then habitual exercise may provide benefit.

Second, past depressive episodes have residual cognitive effects. A substantial number of researchers have suggested that past depressive episodes, even though not currently active, maintain persistent metabolic changes, specifically in the right hemisphere, that result in cognitive impairment. Consideration must be given to the potential of a depressive episode of 30 years ago and how it can currently impair cognition and influence the effects of exercise.

Third, identifying depression is difficult in the older population. Older adults are less likely to be diagnosed with MDD; however, they do report more depressive symptoms, particularly physical ones, and they are more likely to report these depressive symptoms to physicians, not to mental health professionals. Underdiagnosis and undertreatment of depression in older adults are common problems and increase the risk for mortality. In a study of 97 suicide cases of adults 50 years and older, 51 had seen a physician within the last month of life, 45 of them had psychiatric symptoms, and only 19 of those patients were offered treatment. Only two received the recommended level of care (Caine et al., 1996).

Fourth, symptoms of other diseases of old age may be attributed incorrectly to depression in old age. The symptoms of depression are similar to symptoms of structural frontal lobe damage or frontal system brain disease and therefore can be misattributed to depression instead of frontal lobe disease. It is possible that older adults do not report depression because it is not depressed mood but rather somatic symptoms of frontal lobe dysfunction. If this is the case, then different concerns, treatment, and expectations would be appropriate. In addition, patterns of cognitive impairment of depression are extremely difficult to differentiate from those of Huntington's disease or Parkinson's disease.

Fifth, depression is expressed differently in the young and the old and therefore creates different risk factors. Depression in older people is strongly related to frontal system vascular disease. If a person has his or her first depressive episode after the age of 60, the odds are 7:1 that a magnetic resonance image will reveal frontal system structural pathology (Alexopoulos et al., 1997). This is not true with younger people who experience depressive episodes. Depressive symptoms must be related to implications from other illnesses more common in older adults than in younger people.

Sixth, an important research question to explore is how physical activity affects depression and cognition. Is exercise a protective factor? Does physical activity (exercise) reduce depression and therefore enhance cognitive functioning, or does physical activity (exercise) protect against the cognitive impairment resulting from long-lasting depression?

Seventh, another question pertains to the types and duration of exercise that have proven to be the most effective. Resistance training and aerobic training provide similar reductions in depressive symptoms. If resistance training is used as a control group, it is usually of low intensity to prevent any change in aerobic fitness. Blumenthal and colleagues (1999) provided a much-quoted study on the effects of exercise on clinical depression in older adults. They reported that reductions in depressive symptoms were evident after 6 to 8 weeks of exercise, with the effects being greater with increased frequency (number of times per week). The effects were greater and more consistent after 12 weeks of exercise. However, recent studies have indicated that even acute bouts of exercise showed significant reduction in depressed mood in clinically depressed individuals. Exercise appears to provide a transitory effect and is not expected to have an impact on long-lasting depression or a diagnosis of MDD. Future researchers need to conduct true dose–response experimental studies to directly compare the effects.

Eighth, there may be a link between past depression and future cardiovascular disease. In addition to the link between depression and mortality, there is also a link between past depression and arteriosclerosis. Some researchers have shown that depression at age 30 can predict a fatal heart attack at age 60. A suggested mechanism for this relates to the body's use of serotonin by both the brain and the gastrointestinal tract. In other words, the depression not only affects the brain's serotonergic system but also affects the gastrointestinal system's use of serotonin. Clinical trials are under way in which antidepressants are being used to prevent stroke and heart attack.

Research Methodological Problems and Future Directions

Four methodological research problems were discussed in the depression, cognition, and exercise domain. The identification of these problems led to several recommendations for researchers. First, extant research varies in identifying the age range of older adults. Many researchers define old in their studies as age 35 and over. Future research in general, but particularly in the area of depression, should redefine the stratification by age to include a wider and more representative sample of the aging population.

Second, a potential confound exists in the literature regarding the impact of exposure to light. To date, most exercise studies have been conducted indoors, and investigators have not addressed the effects of light on depression and exercise. Some researchers have accounted for the effects of environmental factors such as location on depression. Studies are needed in which the effects of exercise on depression are analyzed under varying conditions of light.

Third, some differentiation should be made between depressive symptoms and diagnosed depression in the extant research. The difference between symptoms and diagnosis is critical, and when one is studying depression, exercise, and cognition, those differences must be clearly articulated from the onset of the study. Most researchers who study cognitive functioning and depression are referring to subclinical depression.

Fourth and finally, true dose–response experimental studies are needed on the topic of this chapter. In these studies, the effects of different amounts and types of exercise should be investigated. It will be important to determine whether exercise improves depression, cognition, or both.

A multitude of studies have been conducted to study the links between depression and exercise, depression and cognitive functioning, and exercise and cognitive function. Only recently has there been studies seeking to determine the links among depression, exercise, and cognitive functioning. This is an important research direction that should continue to be taken.

CHAPTER 4

Exercise, Stress Mechanisms, and Cognition

Nicole C. Berchtold, PhD
University of California, Irvine

EDITORS' OVERVIEW

Long-term stress exposure negatively affects general health and functioning, including cognitive function. Exercise has long been proposed to assist in stress management. In addition, evidence is accumulating that exercise benefits brain health and function, particularly in older adults. However, certain aspects of cognitive function, such as executive function and visuospatial processing, may benefit more than others from chronic aerobic exercise (Colcombe & Kramer, 2003). These cognitive functions are incidentally also the functions that reveal the most pronounced age-related performance decrements. In this chapter, Dr. Berchtold addresses formerly proposed hypotheses that exercise may support cognitive health and function throughout the aging process in part by lifetime management of the response to stress.

The purposes of this chapter are to identify stress mechanisms and how they can affect brain health and cognitive function, examine the extent to which exercise can modulate stress responses, determine whether a consensus statement can be generated based on the current literature, and recommend directions

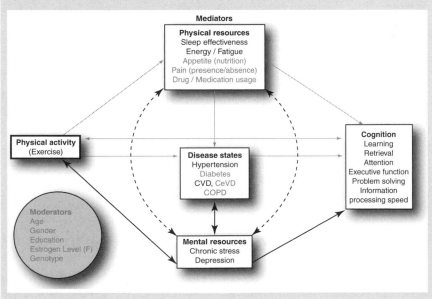

for research. We have no direct evidence for a relationship between cognitive functioning and stress management by exercise. However, there is strong indirect evidence that mediation of cognition by exercise-based stress management is both possible and likely. The indirect evidence derives from studies examining the relationship between stress and cognition and studies examining the effect of exercise on stress responses.

To assess whether stress management by exercise can mediate beneficial effects of exercise on cognitive function, Dr. Berchtold evaluates secondary consequences of chronic stress that can affect cognitive function and examines whether any of these downstream effects are managed or attenuated by exercise.

It is well established that long-term stress exposure can negatively affect general health and functioning, including cognitive function. Regular exercise is widely believed to help with stress management. In addition, there is strong evidence that exercise benefits brain health and function, particularly with aging (see Benefits of Exercise on Human Brain Health and Function, below, and Cotman & Berchtold, 2002; Cotman, Berchtold, & Christie, in press). However, certain aspects of cognitive function benefit more than others from increased aerobic fitness. The most robust enhancement is seen for executive control processes (scheduling, planning, multitasking, inhibition, working memory) and visuospatial processing (Colcombe & Kramer, 2003), which are the cognitive functions that show the most pronounced age-related performance decrements. It has been hypothesized that exercise may support cognitive health and function with aging in part through lifetime management of the response to stress. What evidences support this idea?

BENEFITS OF EXERCISE ON HUMAN BRAIN HEALTH AND FUNCTION

- Improved cognitive function (executive function, memory; Colcombe & Kramer, 2003)
- Protection from depression (DiLorenzo, Bargman, Stucky-Ropp, Brassington, Frensch, & Lafontaine, 1999; Lawlor & Hopker, 2001)
- Prevention of age-related declines in cerebral perfusion (Rogers, Meyer, & Mortel, 1990)
- Prevention of age-related brain tissue loss (Colcombe et al., 2003)
- Decreased risk and incidence of Alzheimer's disease and general dementia (Friedland et al., 2001; Laurin, Verreault, Lindsay, MacPherson, & Rockwood, 2001)

The aims of this chapter are to identify stress mechanisms and how they can affect brain health and cognitive function, examine the extent to which exercise can modulate stress responses, determine whether a consensus statement can be generated based on the current literature, and recommend directions for future research. We have no direct evidence for a relationship between cognitive functioning and stress management by exercise. However, there is strong indirect evidence that mediation of cognition by exercise-based stress management is both possible and likely. The indirect evidence derives from studies examining the relationship between stress and cognition and studies examining the effect of exercise on stress responses.

Addressing the effect of exercise on the stress response is complex because of the multifaceted repercussions of stress on the body and brain. Chronic stress has secondary effects on a number of systems, including negative consequences for the cardiovascular system, insulin sensitivity, immune function, and the brain. Suboptimal performance of any of these systems can compromise brain health and function and, by extension, cognitive function. For example, in the brain, chronic stress results in increased vulnerability of neurons to insult, atrophy of select brain regions, suppressed neurogenesis, and decreased production of neuronal growth factors. Coexisting stress-related cardiovascular dysfunction, immune suppression, or reduced insulin sensitivity can add insult to injury, further compromising brain health and function. Repercussions of these brain changes include impaired cognitive function and depression, among other manifestations.

To assess whether stress management by exercise can mediate beneficial effects of exercise on cognitive function, this chapter evaluates secondary consequences of chronic stress that can affect cognitive function and examines whether any of these downstream effects are managed or attenuated by exercise.

What Is Stress? Defining the Stress Response

Although we all know what stress is when we experience it, it is a somewhat difficult concept to define (Pacak & Palkovits, 2001). Some confusion arises because the term *stress* is used to refer to a stressor, the condition of stress, responses to stress, and long-term negative consequences of stress. For example, stress has been defined as "any condition that seriously perturbs physiological and psychological homeostasis, ranging from anxiety to posttraumatic stress disorder" (Kim & Yoon, 1998) and also "a response to aversive stimuli" (Carrasco & Van de Kar, 2003) or "the wear and tear of daily life."

In this chapter, a stressor is considered to be a condition or experience that challenges homeostasis so that stress is defined as a condition of threatened homeostasis. A stressor can be physical or psychological. In turn, stress responses are a repertoire of behavioral and physiological responses that are intended to be adaptive and to reestablish homeostasis (Chrousos, 1998). If the adaptive response is excessive or prolonged, such as in conditions of chronic stress (threatened physical or psychological homeostasis), a healthy steady state is not attained; instead prolonged stress results in secondary pathological consequences that affect not only general health and functioning but also cognitive health and function. McEwen and Seeman (1999) pointed out that "it is not just the dramatic stressful events (experienced in life) that exact their toll, but rather the many events of daily life that elevate activities of physiological systems to cause some measure of wear and tear" (p. 30). McEwen and Seeman redefined this wear and tear of stress as "allostatic load," which reflects not only the impact of life experiences but also the influence of genetic load, individual patterns of physiological reactivity, and life habits such as diet, exercise, and substance abuse. The components of McEwen and Seeman's model that are of particular relevance to this chapter are the adaptive physiological stress responses and the negative consequences of prolonged activation of these adaptive responses. For simplicity, this chapter focuses on activation of the stress response by psychological stressors as opposed to physical stressors (cold, hemorrhage, pain), with the exception of the exercise stressor. Over a lifetime, chronic (i.e., intermittent or prolonged) exposure to even moderate psychological stressors constitutes a lot of cumulative stress and wear and tear on the organism.

Positive and Negative Effects of Stress

Stress can have positive or negative consequences depending on the intensity, duration, and cumulative load of the challenges or stressors (figure 4.1). As a positive influence, stress adds excitement to life, increases productivity, and enhances cognitive functioning. Short-term exposure to the biochemical mediators of the stress response protects the body by mobilizing energy sources to maintain brain and muscle function, sharpen attention and focus on the perceived threat, optimize cardiovascular functioning for action, and mobilize immune cells, among other effects (Carrasco & Van de Kar, 2003; Chrousos, 1998; Sapolsky, Romero, & Munck, 2000). However, with prolonged exposure to elevated levels of these same biological mediators with consequent prolonged or excessive activation of the stress response, the adaptive changes become maladaptive, causing decrements in physical and mental function and even development of disease.

Drawing on the idea of beneficial and harmful effects of stress, we can envision a dose–response curve between stress and functioning (figure 4.2). The shape of the curve would differ between individuals, reflecting the variability in individual stress tolerance and stress responses. Vari-

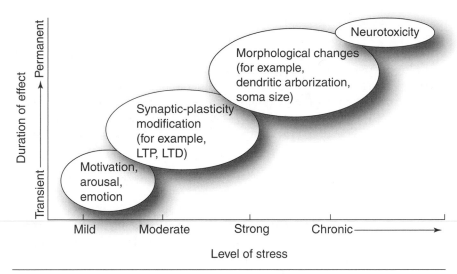

Figure 4.1 Physiological effects associated with behavioral stress. With mild stress, there are effects in motivational, arousal, and emotional systems that can influence learning and memory. As the level of stress increases (duration, intensity), adaptive and maladaptive changes are seen in the hippocampus, ranging from plasticity and process reorganization to atrophy and neurotoxicity. LTP = long-term potentation; LTD = long-term depression.

Reprinted from *Trends in Neuroscience*, Vol. 21, J.J. Kim and K.S. Yoon, Stress: Metaplastic effects in the hippocampus, pp. 505-509, Copyright 1998, with permission from Elsevier.

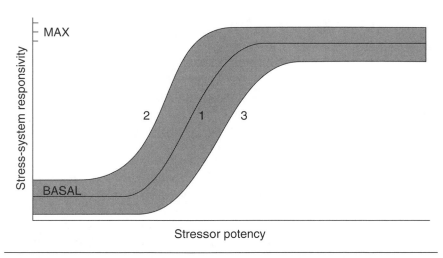

Figure 4.2 Dose–response curve: stressor potency on the x-axis and stress system responsivity on the y-axis. The middle curve (1) is a normal response, whereas (2) shows hyperresponsiveness. Management of stress reactivity by exercise could shift the curve to the right (3), effectively increasing stress tolerance.

ance in stress response is thought to be determined by inherited factors and environmental factors. Environmental factors that shape the stress system include both early life and later life events that have long-term or permanent effects (on stress sensitivity), as well as effects of lifestyle habits such as exercise or meditation. Exercise as a stress management tool is hypothesized to shift an individual's dose–response curve to increase stress tolerance (e.g., reduced responsiveness or improved feedback control). Ultimately, the goal is not to eliminate stress but to manage it so it stays in the beneficial part of the curve.

The Stress System

The stress response is subserved by the *stress system*, which is located in both the central nervous system (CNS) and peripheral organs. This stress system receives and integrates a diversity of neurosensory signals (higher cognitive and limbic feedback and sensory input from visual, auditory, olfactory, and visceral systems) and bloodborne signals (hormones, cytokines, and blood composition signals). Activation of the stress system by a physical or psychological stressor consistently leads to a cluster of physiological and behavioral changes, which constitute the *stress response* (Chrousos, 1998). These changes are an adaptive, evolutionary response that increases the chances of survival in response to an acute physical stressor (e.g., when a lion attacks a prey, the stress response helps the prey escape and ignore pain).

Neuroendocrinology of the Stress Response

The core neuroendocrine components of the stress system are the hypothalamic–pituitary–adrenocortical (HPA) axis and the sympathetic nervous system (SNS). In response to a stressor, cortisol (via HPA) and adrenaline (via SNS) are released from the adrenal gland, and noradrenaline is released from SNS terminals throughout the body. (Adrenaline and noradrenaline are respectively also known as epinephrine and norepinephrine). Noradrenaline, as well as other catecholamine neurotransmitters, is released into various parts of the brain and the spinal cord from neurons located in the brainstem. These mediators prepare the individual to cope with the demands of metabolic, physical, and psychological stressors.

As a rough sketch, neurosensory signals converge in and are processed by the paraventricular nucleus (PVN) of the hypothalamus and the locus caeruleus noradrenergic center. In response to a stressor, the PVN of the hypothalamus secretes corticotrophin-releasing hormone (CRH) and arginine–vasopressin (AVP). In turn, CRH stimulates pituitary release of adrenocorticotropic hormone (ACTH), which induces secretion of glucocorticoids from the adrenal glands. Glucocorticoids (cortisol in humans and primates, corticosterone in animals) are principal mediators of the stress response. Corelease of AVP with CRH potentiates the effect of CRH on ACTH release and thus increases glucocorticoid release. Simultaneous with HPA activation, the SNS stimulates adrenaline and noradrenaline release from the adrenal glands, noradrenaline release from sympathetic terminals throughout the body, and catecholamine release in the CNS. The catecholamine projections from the medulla and brainstem (noradrenaline from medulla and locus caeruleus neurons, adrenaline from medulla, and serotonin from brainstem raphe neurons) ascend to the forebrain where they innervate hypothalamic nuclei (including the PVN), amygdala nuclei, and limbic structures. The amygdala and limbic cortical regions (hippocampal formation and associated cortexes) are responsible for learned, motivational, and behavioral responses to stress. Note that CRH and noradrenergic neurons in the CNS reciprocally innervate and drive each other. As a result, activation of the noradrenergic pathways by CRH also stimulates noradrenaline release by the peripheral SNS, additionally driving secretion of noradrenaline and adrenaline from the adrenals.

OUTLINE OF THE BROAD FEATURES OF A TYPICAL STRESS RESPONSE (ADAPTED FROM SAPOLSKY, ROMERO, & MUNCK, 2000)

First Wave (Occurs Rapidly)

1. Within seconds—increased secretion of SNS catecholamines
2. Hypothalamic release of AVP and CRH
3. Enhanced secretion of pituitary ACTH caused by CRH stimulation (ultimately causing glucocorticoid release)
4. Decreased hypothalamic release of gonadotropin-releasing hormone (GnRH), leading to decreased secretion of gonadotropins
5. Pituitary secretion of prolactin and growth hormone (GH), leading to secretion of glucagon from pancreas

Second Wave (Within Minutes After First Wave)

1. Glucocorticoid (cortisol in humans, corticosterone in animals) release over the course of minutes in response to ACTH
2. Decline in gonadal steroid secretion

Third Wave: Genomic Effects

The first and second waves are rapid, occurring in the span of minutes, because hormones are acting via rapid second-messenger cascades. The third wave takes an hour or more until effects are initiated because the effects are principally genomic (i.e., regulation of gene activity).

Corticosteroids as the Core Mediator: Dual Role to Enhance and Limit the Stress Response

Activation of CRH and glucocorticoid release with stress is considered the core mediator of the stress response, particularly for psychological stress. The effects of glucocorticoids are widespread through the body, affecting a multitude of tissues and physiological end points (e.g., the cardiovascular profile, immune system, metabolism, appetite, glucose transport, and reproductive behavior, among others; Sapolsky, Romero, & Munck, 2000). Thus, a key aspect of the stress response is that it should be tightly controlled. An exaggerated response, or inadequate or faulty control, particularly of the glucocorticoid component, can be quite damaging to the body and can even cause illness and disease.

Interestingly, glucocorticoids both mediate and enhance the stress response as well as limit the stress response and contribute to the recovery from it. In humans, after cortisol is released in response to a stressor, it binds to receptors in the brain, particularly the hippocampus, to negatively regulate further ACTH release. In this way, cortisol provides critical negative feedback control on the HPA axis to attenuate further activation of the stress system. However, inadequate or faulty control of this negative feedback system is a risk factor for developing serious stress-related problems, including impaired cardiovascular and metabolic function, immune suppression, poor reproductive health, depression, and other cognitive effects.

Different Responsivity of the Stress System

Interestingly, it has long been noted that only a subset of the population seems to develop serious secondary effects attributable to chronic or extreme stress exposure. Why are some people more vulnerable than others to developing stress-related disorders? One angle that has been explored in the laboratory setting is that dysregulation of the stress response, including an exaggerated response or failure of the feedback mechanism to shut off the response, is a risk factor for developing stress-related problems.

Pharmacological Screening Reveals Differences in Stress System Responses

The dexamethasone suppression test, in combination with exposure to a stressor, can be used to explore individual differences in stress reactivity. This test can reveal potential dysregulation of the HPA axis, such as an exaggerated HPA response to a stressor or inadequate or faulty feedback control that would normally prevent further ACTH release.

Dexamethasone (DEX) is a glucocorticoid (type 2) receptor agonist that can be used to saturate glucocorticoid negative feedback of the HPA axis.

In a typical experiment, DEX (1 or 4 mg) is given orally, enhancing gluco-corticoid negative feedback. Four hours later, the individual is exposed to a psychological or physical stressor that normally would activate the full spectrum of HPA and sympathetic responses of the stress system. Blood levels of ACTH, cortisol, norepinephrine, and adrenaline are measured to assess the degree of HPA stressor response after dexamethasone suppression, and heart rate and blood pressure changes serve as indexes of sympathetic and adrenal activity.

In a normal population of healthy individuals, the dexamethasone suppression test reveals markedly different pituitary adrenal responses to the stressor. The population can be segregated into two discrete groups: high responders (HRs) and low responders (LRs). HRs mount a stress response (increased plasma ACTH, cortisol) after the stressor despite prior glucocorticoid (dexamethasone) administration, whereas LRs do not show a stress response (see figure 4.3). About 30% to 50% of an otherwise normal, healthy, homogeneous population of men and women are HRs, showing persistent pituitary–adrenal responsiveness to a stressor even when the negative feedback system should have shut off capacity to further respond. Baseline levels of ACTH and cortisol are equivalent between the HR and LR groups, as are other measures such as heart rate and blood pressure.

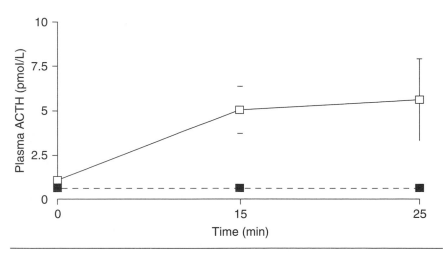

Figure 4.3 Typical stressor-induced changes in plasma adrenocorticotropic hormone (ACTH) in low responders (filled squares) and high responders (open squares) after the dexamethasone suppression test.

Reprinted, by permission, from A.B. Negrao et al., 2000, "Individual reactivity and physiology of the stress response," *Biomedicine & Pharmacotherapy* 54(3):124.

Psychological Stressors Reveal Differences in HR and LR Stress Response

Exposure to psychological stressors that mimic real-life situations can reveal different stress responses in HRs versus LRs. Psychological stressors commonly used in the lab setting include tasks like mental arithmetic, mock job interview, public speaking, and mental arithmetic performed in front of an audience (components of the Trier Social Stress Test).

In one study, exposure to psychological stressors raised heart rate, blood pressure, plasma ACTH, and cortisol in both HRs and LRs. However, HRs showed greater increases in all of the parameters (except cortisol), despite equivalent baseline measures between the groups. HRs also showed increases in heart rate and blood pressure in anticipation of the test, whereas LRs did not (as reported in Negrao, Deuster, Gold, Singh, & Chrousos, 2000). Despite the difference in degrees of stress response, both HRs and LRs reported the same subjective ratings about how they experienced the challenges.

In another paradigm, differences in habituation responses to stressors were revealed between HRs and LRs (Kirschbaum et al., 1995). In this experiment, subjects were exposed to the same psychological stressor in five consecutive sessions. Both LRs and HRs had cortisol response to session 1; however, HRs produced more cortisol. Furthermore, after the first exposure, LRs mounted no stress response in the subsequent four sessions, whereas HRs continued to mount a response throughout. The stress system in HRs, especially the cortisol output, not only appears to be overactive but also fails to habituate to a stressor.

Exercise Stressors Reveal Differences in HR and LR Stress Response

Exercise, in a given intensity range (50-100% $\dot{V}O_2$max) can activate the full spectrum of HPA and sympathetic responses of the stress system. A physical stressor that has been extensively used in the laboratory to study the stress response is graded treadmill exercise. It is a useful model to study stress responses, because in the range of 50% to 100% of $\dot{V}O_2$max, graded treadmill exercise evokes dose-dependent increases in plasma ACTH, cortisol, adrenaline, and noradrenaline. In addition, individuals with marked differences in physical fitness and training show similar neuro-endocrine and metabolic responses to the same relative exercise intensity (i.e., 90% $\dot{V}O_2$max intensity is individualized; Deuster et al., 1989; Luger et al., 1987).

Like psychological stressors, exercise stressors provoke different stress system responses in HRs versus LRs. In comparison to psychological stressors, however, exercise stressors provoke greater plasma ACTH and cortisol increases (five times greater cortisol, two times greater ACTH) in all groups.

Individuals who are HRs to psychological stress are also HRs to exercise stress. When HRs and LRs are challenged by strenuous physical exercise (90% V̇O$_2$max), HRs have higher evoked concentrations of plasma, ACTH, cortisol, AVP, lactate, and glucose than LRs, despite equivalent baseline measures. Interestingly, the response is sexually dimorphic, in that women show higher AVP, cortisol, and glucose responses to strenuous exercise challenge (90-100% V̇O$_2$max), whereas ACTH and lactate responses are comparable between men and women (Deuster et al., 1998).

Overall, adrenal cortical responses are consistently higher in HRs than in LRs in response to stressors, whether psychological or physical (figure 4.4). In addition, HRs have enhanced drive for AVP and CRH, which emerges under extreme stress conditions (90-100% V̇O$_2$max). The enhanced AVP and CRH drive may be responsible for the increase in cortisol responses measured in HRs, because AVP potentiates CRH drive on ACTH release. The basal and stress-reactive differences between HRs and LRs may represent differential risk between the groups for development of stress-related disorders. There is evidence in support of this idea from the cardiovascular field, where it was observed that atherosclerosis progression in response to stress correlated with the degree of responsiveness of the stress system (Kamarck et al., 1997; Kaplan et al., 1983; Manuck, Kaplan, & Clarkson, 1983; Sheps & Sheffield, 2001). Future studies are needed to expand knowledge on stress responsivity and later life disease susceptibility.

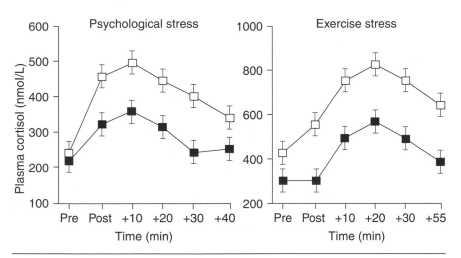

Figure 4.4 Representative stressor-induced changes in plasma cortisol in low responders (filled squares) and high responders (open squares) in response to psychological and exercise stress tests.

Reprinted, by permission, from A.B. Negrao et al., 2000, "Individual reactivity and physiology of the stress response," *Biomedicine & Pharmacotherapy* 54(3):126.

Stress-Related Pathology in the Brain and Body: What Can Exercise Do to Counter These Effects?

Chronic stress has secondary effects on a number of systems, with negative consequences for the brain, cardiovascular profile, immune response, glucose transport and insulin sensitivity, metabolism, appetite, and reproductive behavior, among others. This section explores the consequences of stress for a few of these systems and parameters that affect cognitive function, specifically the brain, cardiovascular system, and immune function. In addition, we will address whether any of these downstream effects are managed or attenuated by exercise.

Brain: Stress and Exercise

Stress and exposure to stress neuroendocrine mediators have consequences for brain anatomy and function, with effects on cognition, learning, memory, and emotional responses (Garcia, 2002; Kim & Yoon, 1998; Sapolsky, 2003). (For documentation of the effects of stress on learning and memory in a diverse array of species from fish to humans, see Maier & Seligman, 1976; Seligman, 1972). Interestingly, this relationship has an inverted U shape. Neuroendocrine stress mediators released during mild stress enhance certain aspects of cognitive function, including attention and memory consolidation. This effect is mediated in part by cortisol's facilitating synaptic plasticity in the hippocampus (a brain structure critical for learning and memory) and by adrenal steroid effects on the amygdala (involved in solidifying emotionally significant events; McEwen & Sapolosky, 1995). However, in contrast to the benefits of acute exposure to low levels of stress mediators, the effects of long-term, repeated, or extreme exposure to neuroendocrine mediators of stress are harmful to brain integrity and function, particularly the hippocampus, amygdala, and prefrontal cortex.

Stress and the Hippocampus

The damaging effects of glucocorticoids to the hippocampus are currently the focus of much attention. The hippocampus has a high concentration of corticosteroid receptors and is sensitive to modulation by stress hormones. It is an especially plastic and vulnerable region of the brain that is critical for learning and memory, and it appears to have a role in stress-related depression. In addition, the hippocampus is an important site of corticosteroid-mediated feedback to shut off the hormonal stress response in the HPA. Impaired hippocampal function attributable to stress damage could exacerbate any existing dysregulation of the stress response and perpetuate the problem.

Glucocorticoids cause anatomical, molecular, and functional changes in the hippocampus (Lee, Ogle, & Sapolsky, 2002; Gould & Tanapat, 1999; Kim & Yoon, 1998; Magarinos & McEwen, 1995). For example, they promote reorganization of nerve cells and their connections, which leads to beneficial outcomes to hippocampal function when glucocorticoids are maintained at normal low circadian levels. However, prolonged exposure to stress or high levels of glucocorticoids ultimately lead to regression of dendritic processes and hippocampal atrophy. In addition, prolonged exposure inhibits neurogenesis (the production of new neurons in the progenitor cell layer of the hippocampus) and increases neuronal vulnerability to insults such as hypoglycemia, hypoxia, and ischemia. The reduced neuronal ability to survive damage under such conditions is particularly relevant to stress conditions, considering that prolonged stress compromises cardiovascular function, glucose transport, and insulin sensitivity, making hypoxia, hypoglycemia, ischemia, and stroke likely. The resultant atrophy and damage are thought to be responsible for the decrements in cognitive performance that accompany hippocampal damage, in particular deficits in several types of memory performance, including declarative, episodic, spatial, and contextual memory. In addition, depression is associated with hippocampal atrophy and damage.

Stress, Depression, and Exercise

Depression is a consequence of stress in a subset of the population. It is accompanied by changes in hippocampal anatomy and function and has been hypothesized to be related to impaired negative feedback on the HPA axis (referred to as cortisol resistance). This theory is based on the clinical observation that patients with major depression consistently show hyperactivity of the HPA axis, and it is supported by experimental data demonstrating impaired glucocorticoid-mediated feedback in major depression. From this, it would be predicted that HRs would be at greater risk for developing depression than LRs. It is currently unclear whether HPA dysregulation is a cause or a consequence of depression. This field merits future research.

A number of cognitive parameters are impaired in depression, some of which are probably a direct result of depression-associated hippocampal atrophy. Does exercise provide a measure of protection from depression and associated hippocampal atrophy? There is strong evidence that exercise can attenuate symptoms of depression and improve cognitive parameters that are affected by depression. A number of cross-sectional and longitudinal human studies have demonstrated a positive correlation between increased physical activity and lower levels of depression (Blumenthal et al., 1999; Byrne & Byrne, 1993; Hassmen, Koivula, & Uutela, 2000; Lawlor & Hopker, 2001; Pollock, 2001). In addition, exercise has been shown to be protective against recurrent depression. In 1-, 5-, and 8-year follow-up studies, people who maintained or increased their activity levels had fewer depressive symptoms and showed more physiological and psychological benefits than those who decreased their activity levels (DiLorenzo et al., 1999; Lampinen, Heikkinen, & Ruoppila, 2000; Strawbridge, Deleger, Roberts, & Kaplan, 2002). Meta-analyses of randomized clinical trials demonstrate that, on the whole, exercise reduces symptoms of depression and has psychological benefits on mood, mental performance, concentration, and confidence (DiLorenzo et al., 1999; Lawlor & Hopker, 2001).

Some Mechanisms

Molecular changes (i.e., changes in gene activity) that are induced by glucocorticoids and other stress mediators are part of the underlying mechanisms contributing to the anatomical changes and increased neuronal vulnerability that occur after prolonged stress (for reviews, see Lee, Duan, & Mattson, 2002; McEwen, 1999). Glucocorticoids set off enormous alterations in gene and protein levels including suppressive effects on neurotrophic factors that support neuronal growth and survival. One such neurotrophin is brain-derived neurotrophic factor (BDNF). BDNF promotes neuronal health, supporting the survival and growth of many neuronal subtypes. In addition, BDNF has emerged as a key mediator of synaptic efficacy, neuronal connectivity, and use-dependent plasticity (Alonso, Vianna, Izquierdo, & Medina, 2002; McAllister, Katz, & Lo, 1999).

Recently, BDNF has attracted much attention for its putative role in depression. Decreased hippocampal BDNF levels are associated with depression in animal models of depression, especially stress-induced depression, as well as in humans. In rodents, stress and stress-induced depression rapidly reduce hippocampal BDNF messenger RNA and protein. In contrast, hippocampal infusion of BDNF protein produces antidepressant effects and protects from stress-induced depression (learned helplessness). Interestingly, major classes of antidepressants, although acting through diverse mechanisms, all converge on BDNF to increase BDNF gene expression in the hippocampus (Duman, Heninger, & Nestler, 1997; Fujimaki, Morinobu, & Duman, 2000; Nibuya, Morinobu, & Duman, 1995; Russo-Neustadt, Beard, & Cotman, 1999). In humans, serum BDNF is decreased in patients with major depression and correlates with the severity of depression (Dunn, Trivedi, Kampert, Clark, & Chambliss, 2002), whereas BDNF is up-regulated in the hippocampus of antidepressant-treated depressive patients (postmortem study; Dunn et al., 2002). These observations support the idea that BDNF regulation may be key in depression. In addition, stress-mediated suppression of hippocampal BDNF may underlie many of the negative effects of stress on brain health and function.

Note: Exercise, depression, and cognition are covered in detail by John Bartholomew.

Interventions that increase hippocampal BDNF levels may be critical for preventing stress-induced damage to the brain. Exercise is a well-established intervention that rapidly increases hippocampal BDNF gene and protein levels (for review, see Cotman & Berchtold, 2002). Exercise protects against stress-induced decreases in hippocampal BDNF. In rats, freewheel running before immobilization stress prevents the stress-induced reduction in BDNF protein (Adlard & Cotman, 2004) and also prevents learned helplessness and behavioral depression (Greenwood, Foley, Burhans, Maier, & Fleshner, 2005; Greenwood et al., 2003). Exercise and antidepressants thus have parallel effects on hippocampal BDNF and depression.

In addition to regulating BDNF, exercise regulates hippocampal expression of a number of other genes, many of which may mediate exercise benefits for depression as well as generally contribute to hippocampal health and function. Tong and colleagues demonstrated that 3 weeks of running wheel exercise altered expression of 130 genes in the rat hippocampus (Tong, Shen, Perreau, Balazs, & Cotman, 2001). These genes fell into four main categories of function: plasticity, metabolism, antiaging, and immune-related. Interestingly, the majority of the genes were associated with supporting synaptic plasticity, which is impaired by prolonged stress and glucocorticoid exposure.

Stress-Related Disorders in the Periphery

Multisystem effects of chronic stress include impaired cardiovascular profile, immune suppression, and insulin resistance. Effects on these parameters and general health can converge to affect cognitive function. Accumulating evidence documents the beneficial effects of regular exercise in preventing or ameliorating the metabolic and psychological comorbidities induced by chronic exercise. These benefits likely result both from a central (brain) effect of exercise to reduce the sensitivity to stress, as well as peripheral effects of exercise on health (e.g., improved cardiovascular, metabolic, and immune function). (For an excellent overview, see Tsatsoulis & Fountoula-kis, 2006). Exercise thus appears to provide a measure of protection from these maladaptations to sustained stress, which in turn can converge on improved brain health and preserved cognitive function (Cotman, Berchtold, & Christie, in press).

Coronary Heart Disease

One predictable component of the stress response is the effect of stress mediators on cardiovascular parameters, such as changes in heart rate, cardiac ejection fraction, and arterial blood pressure. These effects are mediated by catecholamines (sympathetic nervous system) and CRH (acting as a neurotransmitter mediating sympathetic arousal). Chronic stress demands on these cardiovascular parameters present a serious risk factor for the development of cardiac disease, such as arterial stiffening, hypertension, and atherosclerosis. It has been demonstrated in both human and nonhuman primate studies that acute or chronic psychosocial stress exacerbates the progression of atherosclerosis and impairs endothelin-mediated dilation of coronary arteries. In addition, the degree of atherosclerosis progression in response to stress appears to be correlated with the degree of responsiveness of the stress system (Kamarck et al., 1997; Manuck et al., 1983; Sheps et al., 2001), supporting the hypothesis that HRs (who have high reactivity of the stress system) are at greater risk of developing stress-related illnesses.

In contrast to alleviating psychosocial stress, exercise provides benefits to cardiovascular function, including lowered heart rate, lower blood pressure, and improved coronary artery reactivity. These cardiovascular benefits are related to improved cardiovascular profile during a stress response. In particular, exercise training has been shown to reduce blood pressure during mental stress testing as well as speed recovery after the stressor (Blumenthal et al., 1990). This is supported by cross-sectional studies showing that individuals who exercise regularly have lower blood pressure levels during psychosocial stressors and recover more quickly after the stressor, compared with controls (note that exercise combined with weight reduction has the most effect).

These findings support the idea that exercise (aerobic training) can reduce cardiovascular activity in response to psychological stress. Because increased cardiovascular stress reactivity is correlated with increased impairment of the cardiovascular system, exercise benefits long-term health by reducing the harmfulness of repeated stress responses to the cardiovascular system. Furthermore, poor cardiovascular function is a strong predictor of later cognitive impairment, suggesting that exercise-based management of stress responses is likely to benefit cognitive function in aging.

Immune System

There is an inverted U relationship between glucocorticoid level and a modulatory effect on immunological and inflammatory functions. Acute exposure to glucocorticoids leads to enhancement of the immune system, whereas chronic or prolonged stress tends to be immunosuppressive, affecting especially innate and natural resistance. SNS activation reduces T-cell responses, antiviral immune reactivity, and natural killer (NK) cell activity (Madden, 2003). In addition, CRH (through a CNS mechanism

Note: The relationships among exercise, cognition, and arterial stiffening are discussed in further detail by Hiro Tanaka and Miriam Cortez-Cooper, and the relationships among exercise, cognition, and hypertension are discussed in further detail by Charles Emery.

instead of through a direct effect on immune cells) decreases T-cell proliferation and NK cell cytotoxicity. NK activity is a major component of natural resistance. These cells constitute the first line of defense against mutant and virus-infected cells, and their specific function is to destroy infected and cancerous cells.

Stress is associated with increased illness (including cancer, tumors), which is likely to be related in part to decreased NK cell activity. In contrast, exercise is associated with improved health and has been shown to increase basal NK cell activity, particularly in the elderly population (Venjatraman & Fernandes, 1997; Yan et al., 2001). Cross-sectional comparisons also indicate an association between habitual physical activity and enhanced NK cell activity (Woods, Lowder, & Keylock, 2002). In addition, in one study endurance training in later life was associated with a lesser age-related decline in certain aspects of circulating T-cell function and related cytokine production (Shinkai, Konishi, & Shephard, 1997). Functional improvements that have been noted are reduced symptoms of upper respiratory tract infection with regular moderate physical activity. Two human studies suggest that immune function is superior in highly conditioned versus sedentary elderly subjects (see Nieman, 1997, for review).

It seems that certain immune components that are suppressed by stress are stimulated by exercise, thus exercise could counter aspects of stress-induced immune suppression. In addition to their role in general health, immune factors affect the health and function of the brain. Cytokines, previously considered to belong to the sole domain of immune function, are now understood to intimately participate in cognitive processes (Konsman, Parnet, & Dantzer, 2002). Improper immune suppression or activation may also contribute to susceptibility to certain neurodegenerative diseases or their pathological progression (Perry, 2004). Because long-term consequences of stress on the brain may be related to immune function, we need to consider whether moderate exercise can attenuate stress-mediated immune suppression or imbalance. Consistent with the literature that says that moderate exercise strengthens the immune system, recent evidence indicates that exercise improves the immune condition of the brain and can reduce damage in response to physiological stressors such as stroke or infection (Ding et al., 2005; Nickerson, Elphick, Campisi, Greenwood, & Fleshner, 2005).

Closing Thoughts

Direct evidence for a relationship between cognitive functioning as a function of stress management by exercise is absent. However, there is strong indirect evidence that mediation of cognition by exercise-based stress management is both possible and likely. Mechanisms can occur in part via direct beneficial effects of exercise on the brain as well as exercise enhancement of cardiovascular health and potentially also the immune system. An important issue to explore in future research is the role of stress response dysregulation, or poor feedback control, as a risk factor for later development of stress-related disorders. In addition, other dimensions to investigate are the effects of stress on metabolism, glucose transport, and insulin resistance, because these factors are intertwined with brain health and function. As a cautionary note, although exercise can provide a number of beneficial effects to the brain and body, the emphasis is on moderate exercise. Extreme exercise can produce many of the same symptoms seen with prolonged or excessive exposure to other stressors, including depression-like symptoms and suppressed immune function. Again, what is considered moderate will vary among individuals, depending not only on their degree of fitness but probably also on their perception of exercise as enjoyable or displeasurable.

EDITORS' DISCUSSION SUMMARY

The impact of exercise on stress as a mediator of cognitive functioning could be a productive research avenue. Nine substantive and four methodological issues were discussed.

Discussion Highlights

First, the influences of cortisol on learning should be recognized. As explained in the chapter, one aspect of the physiological stress response is the release of cortisol through the HPA axis. Cortisol plays a complex role in learning. For example, if researchers administer cortisol to human subjects before a learning task, encoding of new information improves. However, an injection of cortisol after a learning task impairs subjects' abilities to recall learned information. Further complicating the issue are the divergent roles of cortisol on procedural versus working memory, conflicting reports from animal and human data, and interactions based on subjects' gender and age. Further research is needed to elucidate the effects of cortisol in these specific situations.

Second, stem cells in the brain divide throughout life, but chronic stress impairs neurogenesis. Overturning the classic understanding of the brain as a nonregenerative organ, recent research has demonstrated that neurogenesis continues throughout life in two areas of the brain. In these areas, one of which is the hippocampus, stem cells differentiate into cell types determined by the chemical environment. New cells in the hippocampus may increase its capacity to encode new information by creating new networks. Chronic stress decreases neurogenesis by reducing expressions of growth factors. Stress also reduces the effectiveness of protective factors such as BDNF.

Third, pathologies correlate with both over- and underexpression of cortisol. Conditions associated with declines or low levels of cortisol include atypical depression, seasonal depression, and postpartum depression, as well as chronic fatigue, fibromyalgia, rheumatoid arthritis, and some symptoms of menopause. High levels of cortisol coincide with melancholic depression, panic disorder, anorexia, diabetes, malnutrition, hyperthyroidism, and childhood abuse. Of these conditions, melancholic depression, panic disorder, and anorexia respond to treatment with antidepressant drugs. Interesting questions arise from this observation and its implications for the underlying mechanisms of these disorders.

Fourth, events in early life can alter the responsiveness of the HPA axis. Animal researchers have observed that when young rats repeatedly experience a mild stressor, such as handling, the animals become more resistant to stress. One mechanism that could underlie this beneficial adaptation is remodeling of the layout of corticosteroid receptors in the brain while young animals develop. Intermittent stress could increase production of corticosteroid receptors in different brain regions, thereby enhancing feedback control of the HPA axis later in life. Human data on early life stress responses will be harder to gather because of ethical considerations.

Fifth, moderate exercise, despite acting as a mild stressor, can stimulate beneficial adaptations in the stress response system. Chronic moderate-intensity exercise activates the stress response system. However, in contrast to psychological stress, which produces harmful effects, because it continually maintains hyperactivity of both the HPA axis and the SNS, exercise provides only an intermittent stimulus to these systems followed by a period of recovery. As a result, one beneficial effect of chronic exercise is to reduce baseline levels of SNS activity, which are reflected by lower resting heart rate and resting arterial blood pressure in chronic exercisers. Baseline levels of cortisol may similarly decline after chronic exercise. Only in cases of extremely high-intensity and high-frequency exercise does the stress response produce harmful effects. Athletes who train intensely may experience immune suppression, depression, and metabolic problems. This observation suggests a dose–response curve for exercise, in which moderate levels produce the most beneficial adaptations by the stress response system.

Sixth, perceptions of exercise and feelings of self-efficacy may contribute to or detract from the beneficial effects of exercise on the stress response. Exercise can act as a psychological as well as a physical stressor, depending on the participant's perceptions of exercise. In the case of subjects who intensely dislike exercise, the psychological stress could outweigh the beneficial physical effects typical of exercise. Similarly, when older or extremely obese or unfit subjects exercise, they may interpret the soreness, shortness of breath, and other discomforts during exercise as dangerous or traumatic, thus adding a component of psychological stress to the physical challenge of the exercise. An appropriate response to such subjects would be to educate them to understand and anticipate these sensations with less anxiety.

Seventh, self-efficacy plays a role in the treatment of panic disorder and may play a similar role in reducing anxiety regarding exercise. In panic attacks, individuals feel anxiety and a loss of control that feeds forward to generate greater anxiety. Physicians treat panic disorder by inducing a controllable level of anxiety and teaching patients that they can control the situation. Patients may become comfortable with higher levels of cortisol through such treatments. The change may occur at the level of altering patients' perceptions of the controllability of the situation when cortisol levels become elevated rather than by altering their physiological responsiveness. Although a review of the literature by Dr. Berchtold did not find support for a role of self-efficacy in stress control, such a relationship is implied by the data on panic disorder and probably merits further research. In treatment of patients who have chronic obstructive pulmonary disease (COPD) but who exercise despite shortness of breath, the concept of learned self-efficacy may prove equally useful (see chapter 13).

Eighth, exercise may better relieve stress if it mimics psychological stressors. Some forms of exercise, such as boxing, mimic the physical expression of anger. Because much psychological stress arises from the suppression of anger in social settings, such behavior-modeling forms of exercise may relieve psychological stress more effectively than purely physical forms such as running or lifting weights.

Ninth, the relationship of HPA axis hyperactivity to subclinical Alzheimer's disease needs to be better defined. Alzheimer's disease and subclinical Alzheimer's pathology sufficient to affect the hippocampus in nondemented older people may arise as a manifestation of HPA axis hyperactivity with age (see chapter 10 by Dr. Vitiello for more on the HPA axis hyperactivity theory of aging). Hence, HPA axis hyperactivity may represent a tool for diagnosis of mild cognitive impairment.

Methodological Research Problems

Five methodological problems are noted in the extant research. One, most research in this area does not use population-based samples. Volunteers may not be representative of the population of interest, especially if they are college students. Most studies incorporate young people as subjects, but they are not representative of the older population. Subjects also differ greatly in individual stress reactivity (differential stress sensitivity and response), so stress sensitivity should be a covariate when comparing experimental conditions in clinical studies (see Negrao, Deuster, Gold, Singh, & Chrousos, 2000, for discussion).

Two, the social context has not been controlled in studies of exercise and mood or anxiety. The nonspecific effects of attention or human contact on mood and anxiety have been ignored in many previous studies. When exercise is evaluated against nonexercise conditions, subjects in the nonexercise group must be involved in some structured and supervised activity that does not involve exertion so that they will have the same attention and exposure to the investigators as the exercise group has. Also, the effects of exercise undertaken within a social context should be compared with those arising from self-initiated exercise undertaken as a solitary activity. Are beneficial changes in mood attributable to the exercise or simply to the social contact associated with exercise programs?

Three, participants' subjective perceptions of exercise may be an important factor to control in studies of stress reduction. Does exercise constitute an additional stressor for people who find exercise unpleasant? Put another way, is exercise as beneficial for stress reduction and mood elevation for the people who hate it?

Four, experimental, rather than correlative, data are needed to assign a direction of causality, if any, between dysregulation of the HPA axis and depression. Most previous studies have used regression, descriptive, and cross-sectional methods. True experimental designs should be strongly considered in the future.

Future Directions

Eight potential fruitful research directions were discussed. One, identify the relative importance of secondary effects of stress. Stress has many secondary effects on health, all of which contribute to brain health and cognitive function. Which secondary effect of stress is the most important to modulate to preserve long-term brain health and cognitive function?

Two, examine the impact of anxiety reduction medications in comparison with exercise. Is exercise an effective way to contain stress response? Or would antianxiety medication be more effective to contain the stress response, reserving exercise as a supplement to benefit brain health through other mechanisms? A future study might use exercise as a supplement to medication interventions, such as antidepressants or anxiolytics, that are commonly used to control stress.

Three, determine how exercise effects might be altered by the response sensitivity of individuals. Analyzing HRs and LRs to stress is an important direction that can probably provide some insight into who is vulnerable to developing the severe outcomes of stress (e.g., depression, coronary disease, immune issues). Following are some very interesting questions:

- Do HRs develop more secondary stress-related disorders in later life? That is, test early in life to identify HRs or LRs, then assess periodically over life (e.g., every 10 years) for health, to determine if the HRs have a higher incidence of stress-related disorders over time.
- Would HRs and LRs receive the same long-term benefit from exercise? Could it potentially be bad for either group?
- What is the effect of exercise on sensitivity of the feedback regulation system of the HPA? Can habitual exercise help prevent dysregulation or at least assist in it functioning better?

Four, determine what types of exercise and which types of stressor are beneficial to stress reduction. Exercise is a stressor and activates the same stress systems as psychological stress does, perhaps even to a greater degree. What is different about exercise stress that makes it generally good for us? Is it a matter of degree of stress activation?

Five, investigate the roles of cortisol in learning. What are the roles of cortisol in encoding of new information and in different types of memory? Studies could be conducted that compare the effects of elevated cortisol on animals versus humans, on males versus females, and on young versus older subjects.

Six, investigate the mechanisms of hypercortisolic disorders. What mechanisms are common among melancholic depression, panic disorder, and anorexia? What are their relationships to cortisol? Because all three conditions respond favorably to treatment with antidepressants, and both antidepressants and exercise raise levels of BDNF, could exercise be used as a therapy for these conditions?

Finally, determine the role, if any, of self-efficacy in exercise used to attenuate stress. Does adherence attenuate stress? If we compare identical absolute or relative quantities of exercise, does self-efficacy improve the effectiveness of exercise in attenuating stress?

CHAPTER 5

Self-Efficacy, Physical Activity, and Cognitive Function

Edward McAuley, PhD
University of Illinois at Urbana-Champaign

Steriani Elavsky, MS
The Pennsylvania State University

EDITORS' OVERVIEW

In this chapter, Edward McAuley and Steriani Elavsky explore how self-efficacy might fit in the model of physical activity and cognition, but they also suggest that self-efficacy plays a role at points in the model other than that proposed.

Their strongest emphasis is that social cognitive theory, on which their study of physical activity, self-efficacy, cognition, and several other variables is based, takes the perspective that behavior, cognition, physiology, and environment all operate as interacting determinants of each other. Thus the model, which is unidirectional, must have arrows returning to exercise and physical activity, not only from cognition but from most of the mediators as well. *(Note the return arrows from Mediators, e.g., Mental resources, to Exercise in the model.)*

Thus, the authors suggest that self-efficacy is bidirectional in this model. Self-efficacy influences the initiation and the continuance of physical activity, so that it should be viewed as preceding physical activity *(added box in the model is boldfaced)*. Conversely, self-efficacy is an outcome of the physical activity experience, which would enhance adherence to exercise and thus would indirectly

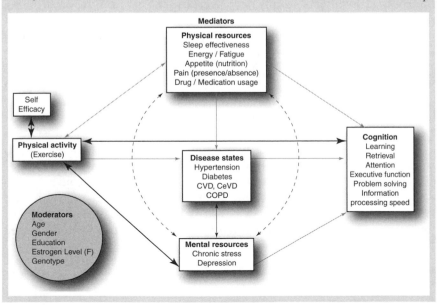

influence cognitive function via the beneficial effects of exercise on the various mediators such as physical resources, disease states, and mental resources.

In this chapter, the authors suggest that self-efficacy plays a potential mediating role in physical activity effects on anxiety, stress responses, and depression. *(These Mental resources are boldfaced in the model.)*

The authors conclude the chapter by proposing that one of the exciting directions of research on this topic will be teasing out the extent of these reciprocal relationships and the conditions under which they operate: exercise, self-efficacy, and cognition.

Introduction: Aging and Self-Efficacy

Perceived choice or control over one's life has consistently covaried with elements of psychological and physical well-being (Bandura, 1997; Rodin, 1986; Skinner, 1996). As one ages, control is diminished in multiple domains of functioning. For example, stereotyping of old age influences feelings of control and leads to reduced coping abilities and beliefs of personal incompetence (Bandura, 1997; McAuley & Katula, 1998). As one grows older, there is a tendency for others to provide assistance, whether required or not, subsequently undermining one's sense of control and capabilities (Avorn & Langer, 1982). Enhanced perceptions of control have been shown to influence memory, satisfaction, and physical health (Bandura, 1997); are essential to one's overall judgment of competence; and are therefore fundamental to human functioning (Rodin, 1986). Although more than 100 different terms have been used to capture the construct of control (Skinner, 1996), we have elected to focus on one aspect of control that has met with considerable success in the understanding of human behavior: self-efficacy (Bandura, 1977, 1986, 1997).

Skinner (1996) classified self-efficacy as an agent–means type of control in which the necessary means (capabilities) to exercise control over a particular behavior or situation are available to a specified agent, usually the self. Social cognitive theory (Bandura, 1986) takes a more complex view of self-efficacy, noting that to effectively exert control one must bring together knowledge structures, appropriate levels and hierarchies of skills, and the capabilities to deal with varying conditions (Bandura, 1997). Self-efficacy is concerned with the individual's beliefs in his or her capabilities to execute necessary courses of action to satisfy situational demands (Bandura, 1986). By definition, self-efficacy is a situation-specific sense of control or confidence. In the case of physical activity, self-efficacy may be represented

Acknowledgment: The authors were supported by grants from the National Institute on Aging while writing this chapter (grants AG 12113 and AG 20118).

by the individual's beliefs in his or her capabilities to exercise on 5 or more days of the week for 30 min or more in the face of commonly reported barriers to activity such as time management, bad weather, and lack of an exercise partner. In the case of cognitive performance, for example memory, self-efficacy judgments might be based on the individual's beliefs relative to remembering incrementally more difficult numbers of names, directions, and locations. Thus, at the outset, we must keep in mind this distinction between control (efficacy) in particular domains and a more general sense of control across broader domains of functioning.

Self-efficacy is a crucial element of social cognitive theory (Bandura, 1986, 1997). The social cognitive perspective views human behavior, the environment, cognition, and physiology as interacting determinants of each other. Underlying this reciprocal causation are the individual's basic human capabilities and beliefs regarding what one can do with those capabilities. Indeed, Bandura (1997) noted that individual motivation levels and affective responses are driven more by their belief systems than by reality. Efficacy beliefs are therefore central to human function and influence behavior in a variety of ways. Specifically, more efficacious individuals approach more challenging and varied tasks. They expend greater effort in such activities and persist longer at tasks in the face of failure or aversive stimuli. In addition, efficacy cognitions also influence thought processes and affective reactions (Bandura, 1986). A growing body of literature identifies self-efficacy as influential in multiple domains of healthy functioning (Bandura, 1997).

Self-efficacy beliefs are based on four primary sources of information: mastery experiences (performance accomplishments), social modeling or vicarious experiences, verbal and social persuasion, and the interpretation of physiological and emotional states. Mastery experiences are the most potent source of efficacy information, often providing objective evidence relative to what constitutes a success or failure. Success enhances efficacy, whereas failure, in particular early and frequent failure, can severely undermine perceived efficacy. Of course, success does not always facilitate efficacy and failure does not always debilitate it. How the information is processed by the individual plays an important role in how mastery information is translated into perceptions of capabilities (Bandura, 1997). Appraisals of both performance and nonperformance information such as task difficulty, level of effort expended in the task, whether assistance is provided by others, and the sequencing of successes and failures all come in to play in the formation of efficacy expectations.

Social modeling is often considered an important source of efficacy expectations when one has not necessarily garnered personal experience in a particular domain or task. In these cases, one must gauge one's efficacy for a particular task as a function of the relative success or failure of others. Studies that have provided false normative feedback relative to physiological capacity have successfully demonstrated that such feedback can effectively influence efficacy expectations and associated psychosocial responses (Jerome et al., 2002; Marquez, Jerome, McAuley, Snook, & Canaklisova, 2002; McAuley, Talbot, & Martinez, 1999). Typically, efficacy expectations are raised when we view others with similar characteristics, experience, and capabilities successfully performing the task in question. Social persuasion is a common source of efficacy information used by individuals to enhance the efficacy of other people. The encouraging verbal support of important others is useful in persuading individuals to put forth more effort in the belief that they possess the capabilities necessary for the task to be accomplished. Such verbal persuasion is likely to be most successful when the persuader is considered to be knowledgeable and credible and when the discrepancy between what the individual believes she can do and what she is being encouraged to do is moderate (Bandura, 1997).

A final information source, the interpretation of emotional and physiological states, can also effectively bolster or debilitate personal efficacy. In the context of physical activity participation in older adults, this source of information may be particularly potent. Older, sedentary adults beginning an exercise program are likely to experience fatigue, muscular pain, and increased respiratory distress. Such somatic disturbances can quite easily be interpreted negatively. Instead of translating these signs as the body's natural responses to stress on the physiological system, subjects cognitively process these signs as evidence of declines in capabilities and possible indicants of impending trauma. How one perceives somatic information, regardless of its intensity, is what determines one's judgments of capabilities (Bandura, 1997; Cioffi, 1991). Affective states can similarly influence self-efficacy. Being in a bad mood during a physical activity session can set the stage for any slight physical setback during activity to be interpreted negatively and construed as inefficacy. This lack of efficacy can, in turn, influence subsequent affective responses to activity (McAuley, Talbot, & Martinez, 1999). In sum, the cognitive processing of information from a variety of sources forms the basis of efficacy beliefs and their effects on human functioning.

Self-Efficacy Relationships With Physical Activity

Social cognitive theory (Bandura, 1986) has been one of the most commonly applied theoretical approaches to understanding correlates and determinants of physical activity behavior across multiple populations (McAuley & Blissmer, 2000). It is fair to say, however, that self-efficacy, as the primary variable of interest in this theory of motivation, has attracted the most interest. Efficacy cognitions are postulated to influence thought processes and affective reactions and have consistently been shown to be important determinants of physical activity and exercise behavior, as well as social, clinical, and health-related behaviors (Bandura, 1997; McAuley & Blissmer, 2000). In keeping with the reciprocal deterministic basis of social cognitive theory, there is evidence in the physical activity domain to suggest that self-efficacy can act as both a determinant and a consequence of physical activity participation. In addition, efficacy expectations are theorized to mediate or moderate the effects of physical activity on a number of psychosocial responses including anxiety, depression, self-esteem, and affect (Bandura, 1997). Thus, self-efficacy's role in the guiding model proposed in this book has implications for other constructs, such as depression and stress responses, reviewed in this volume (see John Bartholomew & Joseph Ciccolo and Nicole Berchtold, this volume). In subsequent sections, we briefly examine the reciprocal nature of self-efficacy and exercise behavior and interventions that have attempted to directly influence or manipulate self-efficacy.

Self-Efficacy as a Determinant of Exercise Behavior

A number of studies, in populations ranging from adolescent to elderly and healthy to symptomatic, have shown self-efficacy to be a significant predictor of exercise adherence (King, Haskell, Young, Oka, & Stefanick, 1995; McAuley, Jerome, Marquez, Canaklisova, & Blissmer, 2003; Oman & King, 1998; Sallis et al., 1986). Early studies using community samples adopted the perspective that exercise is a dynamic and complex process and were able to demonstrate that self-efficacy was related to different types of activity at different stages of the exercise process (Sallis et al., 1986). Additionally, changes in efficacy over time were related to changes in exercise behavior over time. Subsequent exercise trials have shown that self-efficacy typically plays a more prominent role in the prediction of exercise behavior in the early adoption and adaptation stages of exercise programs but is less potent in the maintenance phases (e.g., McAuley, 1992). Additionally, when activity is measured at long-term follow-up to postprogram termination, self-efficacy has been shown to be a significant determinant of activity (McAuley, 1993; McAuley, Jerome, Marquez, et al., 2003).

Oman and King (1998) supported previous findings that self-efficacy has differential effects across the time course of exercise, noting that self-efficacy was a significant predictor of exercise adoption and played a lesser role during exercise maintenance. This supports the social cognitive perspective that the challenges associated with beginning an exercise regimen offer a greater opportunity for mediation by cognitive control than when exercise becomes more habitual. Similarly, self-efficacy's role in the exercise process takes on importance once again when structured exercise programs are terminated and the individual must rely heavily on cognitive and social strategies to develop his own program of exercise. For example, maintaining a program of vigorous activity over a prolonged period of time is certainly more challenging than maintaining a regimen of light or moderate activities. Indeed, self-efficacy has been shown to be predictive of both the adoption and maintenance of vigorous activity in community-dwelling adults (Sallis et al., 1986). Moreover, McAuley, Jerome, Marquez, and colleagues (2003) reported evidence to support that self-efficacy is a significant determinant of 18-month physical activity follow-up in older adults.

Much of the research examining self-efficacy as a determinant of exercise behavior has involved formal supervised activity programs; however, self-efficacy has also proved to be a significant correlate of home-based physical activity for older adults. For example, King and colleagues (1995) conducted a randomized controlled trial contrasting home-based and formal exercise programs of varying intensity. Results suggested that self-efficacy was a significant predictor of long-term exercise adherence in older adults. However, self-efficacy is but one determinant of physical activity behavior, and its contribution should be examined in conjunction with other personal, social, and environmental variables (see Satariano & McAuley, 2003). Bandura (1997) carefully articulated how social cognitive theory subsumes such variables that are the mainstays of other theoretical models. At any rate, systematic investigation of the role of self-efficacy across stages of behavior and within various theoretical frameworks should help provide essential information needed to develop effective exercise interventions.

Given the proposed model of the relationship between physical activity and cognitive function that originally guided the workshop on which this book is based, it would seem quite plausible and theoretically correct to view self-efficacy's first appearance in the model as occurring prior to physical activity. As previously noted, self-efficacy can be viewed as a potential moderator of initial engagement in physical activity.

Physical Activity Effects on Self-Efficacy

Although most often considered as determinants of behavior, efficacy expectations are also considered as important outcomes of acute and chronic exercise experiences that can be considered inactive mastery sources of efficacy information. Early studies typically showed that significant increases in efficacy occur with exposure to acute bouts of physical activity and that chronic exercise interventions result in still more dramatic effects (McAuley, Lox, & Duncan, 1993). Few efforts have been directed at examining the development of self-efficacy across exercise trials and follow-up. McAuley, Katula, and colleagues (1999) reported self-efficacy to follow a curvilinear function with efficacy increasing from baseline to the end of a 6-month exercise program followed by significant declines at postprogram follow-up.

However, assessments of efficacy in this study were limited to beliefs relative to acute bouts of activity. In a recent study, McAuley and his colleagues (McAuley, Jerome, Elavsky, Marquez, & Ramsey, 2003) assessed beliefs in capabilities to continue prescribed exercise over the course of subsequent months and in the face of barriers to activity bimonthly over a 6-month period. Latent growth curve models indicate significant declines in efficacy. The authors argued that although such findings might appear counter-intuitive, they are in fact to be expected given the temporal sequence of measurement. For example, the sharpest declines in efficacy to continue prescribed exercise came at 4 and 6 months with efficacy declining about 20% from baseline, a period when participants were coming to the end of the trial and were faced with the prospect of continuing to exercise on their own. In addition, McAuley, Jerome, Elavsky, and colleagues (2003) confirmed the veracity of mastery experience, social support, and affective responses as reliable sources of efficacy information.

Other researchers have reported similar influences of exercise interventions on self-efficacy in populations with diseases, including osteoarthritis (Rejeski, Ettinger, Martin, & Morgan, 1998), cardiovascular disease (Taylor, Bandura, Ewart, Miller, & DeBusk, 1985), and chronic obstructive pulmonary disease (COPD; Kaplan, Reis, Prewitt, & Eakin, 1994). For example, a 12-week outpatient, pulmonary rehabilitation program resulted in significant increases in self-efficacy in COPD patients, and these changes were associated with enhancements in health-related quality of life and exercise tolerance (Lox & Freehill, 1999). Similar longitudinal work with COPD patients has shown that efficacy increases as a result of physical activity–based interventions and gradually erodes following the intervention (Kaplan et al., 1994). More important, Kaplan and colleagues reported that exercise self-efficacy was a significant predictor of long-term survival compared with standard physiological indicators.

Manipulating Self-Efficacy Information

Despite a considerable literature examining the reciprocal relationship between self-efficacy expectations and physical activity, until recently few empirical efforts had been directed at structuring exercise environments to more thoroughly understand this relationship. Turner, Rejeski, and Brawley (1997) contrasted the effects of a socially enriched instructional environment with a bland social environment on both efficacy and affective responses in a physical activity setting. The enriched social environment resulted in increased positive affect and self-efficacy. The manipulation of efficacy through the provision of false normative physiological feedback has been shown to result in enhanced self-efficacy following the manipulation and before subsequent exercise bouts (Jerome et al., 2002; Marquez et al., 2002; McAuley, Talbot, et al., 1999). Additionally, successful manipulation of efficacy expectations had implications for subsequent psychosocial responses typically associated with acute activity. For example, levels of state anxiety following exercise were lower in the high-efficacy condition than in the low-efficacy condition (Marquez et al., 2002), and high-efficacy subjects reported greater perceptions of well-being and lower psychological distress and fatigue than low-efficacy participants (Jerome et al., 2002). These differences occurred under conditions in which subjective (ratings of perceived exertion) and objective (exercise heart rate) indexes of exercise intensity were identical throughout the exercise bout. Thus, it appears that preexisting levels of self-efficacy not only determine subsequent physical activity but also moderate other psychosocial constructs known to be influenced by physical activity and integral parts of the working model.

These previous studies focused on shaping the environment to influence self-efficacy. However, it has also been demonstrated that self-efficacy-based interventions can be used to influence exercise behavior. In a randomized controlled trial, an efficacy information–based exercise program was contrasted with an attentional control exercise program (McAuley, Courneya, Rudolph, & Lox, 1994) in a study of exercise adherence in older adults. Significant differences in activity patterns were demonstrated over a 5-month period, with the intervention group adhering at a significantly greater rate than the control group over the 5-month period. Efficacy was also significantly related to patterns of adherence. Taken together, the findings from these experimental and intervention studies offer promising evidence to suggest that the exercise environment plays an important role in shaping efficacy cognitions and that efficacy-based programs can significantly influence exercise adherence and associated psychosocial states.

Such conclusions have further implications for our working model. Specifically, we can now consider that self-efficacy mediates the effects of physical activity on such outcomes as fatigue and energy, depression, anxiety, and stress responses. If indeed these latter variables play some influential role in cognitive function, then providing an exercise environment that maximizes self-efficacy and, in turn, influences these other potential mediators of cognitive function would appear to be crucial.

Thus far, we have presented evidence to support the reciprocal relationship that exists between physical activity and self-efficacy and recent work that has attempted to manipulate sources of efficacy information. Although the self-efficacy and physical activity relationship appears to be quite consistent in the literature, the nature of this relationship is quite complex. That is, efficacy does not predict activity patterns at all times nor do all physical activity stimuli have equal effects on self-efficacy. These relationships can vary according to the action in question, the context under which exposure to activity is experienced, the individual's perception of the task, and the temporal nature of the exercise exposure. This is quite in keeping with Bandura's (1997) theorizing about sources of efficacy information. For example, given the situation-specific nature of self-efficacy, one would expect participation in aerobic exercise and nonaerobic activity to have differential impact on efficacy for walking incremental distances but to have little differential effect on more general measures of physical efficacy (McAuley, Katula, et al., 1999). This, of course, has important ramifications for predictions about the ability of self-efficacy to mediate physical activity effects on cognition. That is not to say that self-efficacy is unrelated to psychobiological responses. Efficacy expectations have been shown to influence how individuals perceive and process potential threats (Sanderson, Rapee, & Barlow, 1989) and to be related to autonomic responses and plasma catecholamines (Bandura, Reese, & Adams, 1982; Bandura, Taylor, Williams, Mefford, & Barchas, 1985). Moreover, a sense of personal efficacy has been demonstrated to mediate the effects of social support mechanisms on depression (Mueller & Major, 1989) and physical activity (Duncan & McAuley, 1993) and has been reported to be instrumental in increasing immunocompetence responses to stressors (Wiedenfeld et al., 1990). Clearly, self-efficacy appears to be an important self-regulatory mechanism for exercising personal control over the life course (Bandura, 1997).

Self-Efficacy, Cognitive Function, and Aging

Although the focus of this volume is on the ability of physical activity to effectively maintain late life cognitive function and to attenuate those declines in cognitive function that have accrued with aging, it is useful to consider both the biological and social cognitive explanations of the aging process. As we age and witness losses in stamina, declines in functional capabilities, and losses of strength, the temptation is to attribute all of these functional declines to the biological aging process. The social cognitive interpretation of these declines is that they may have more to do with misperceptions about what one can do rather than with the actual skills and abilities that one possesses (Bandura, 1997). The same is true of cognitive function. As has been argued elsewhere (Kramer, Hahn, & McAuley, 2000; McAuley, Kramer, & Colcombe, 2004), the brain does not age uniformly and brain functions do not decline uniformly. It is clear from both cross-sectional and longitudinal studies that deficits in a variety of perceptual, cognitive, and motor functions can be observed with some of these changes beginning during young adulthood and others not being realized until the 60s or even 70s (Park et al., 2002; Schaie, 2000). Indeed, one of the most striking findings from longitudinal studies is the vast individual differences in the timing and pattern of decline. As Bandura (1997) noted, intellectual development and decline coexist.

Memory performance appears to be the most common type of change in intellectual function associated with aging. Bandura (1997) argued that the memory lapses that older adults experience, are concerned with, and attribute to age-related declines are often ignored by younger adults. Some adults believe that memory is a controllable cognitive attribute that can be maintained with effort, whereas others see it as a basic biological aptitude that will eventually decline with age (Lachman, Bandura, Weaver, & Elliott, 1995). The former approach suggests that one can enhance one's confidence in cognitive performance with training, strategy, and effort (i.e., improve one's memory efficacy). The biological capacity perspective is likely to be accompanied by beliefs that one cannot control this aspect of cognitive function and to interpret lapses as cognitive decline (i.e., low memory efficacy). Older adults who believe memory lapses to be caused by aging and who fail to make appropriate comparisons of their performance with that of their peers are more likely to experience declines in efficacy (Bandura, 1997; Berry, 1999; Welch & West, 1995).

The literature linking self-efficacy and cognitive function focuses almost entirely on the development of memory efficacy and its relationship with memory performance. Briefly stated, memory self-efficacy has been viewed as a "dynamic, self-evaluative system of beliefs and judgments regarding one's memory competence and confidence (Berry, 1999, p. 70). The memory self-efficacy construct is typically measured in the literature in one of two ways. One approach is to assess degrees of confidence in hierarchically arranged items reflecting specific types of memory skill (e.g., beliefs in capabilities to remember names, directions, faces, words, numbers), an approach that accurately reflects social cognitive recommendations for the measurement of self-efficacy (Bandura, 1986). An alternative approach has been to assess attitudes and beliefs in a more global fashion by assessing beliefs in general competencies across a variety of different memory tasks. The Metamemory in Adulthood questionnaire (MIA; Dixon, Hultsch, & Hertzog, 1988) is typical of such measurement. Although both methodological approaches have been used to examine self-efficacy and memory performance relationships, the former taps situational specific beliefs, whereas the latter assesses both dispositional and variable aspects of memory confidence.

Although consistent support has been provided for the position that self-efficacy is related to memory performance (Berry, West, & Dennehy, 1989; Cavanaugh & Poon, 1989), there appears to be little reason to believe that participation in physical activity is likely to have any effect on memory efficacy as a possible mediator of cognitive function improvements. By virtue of the situation-specific nature of self-efficacy, physical activity is likely to enhance beliefs in capabilities related to endurance, strength, skill, and ability to overcome barriers to physical activity (McAuley & Mihalko, 1998) but not beliefs about remembering grocery lists or being able to switch attention between tasks on the appearance of stimuli. However, a few studies have established links between physical performance, efficacy beliefs, and cognitive performance.

These studies report data from the MacArthur Studies of Successful Aging, a longitudinal, three-site cohort study of high-functioning older adults aged 70 to 79 years in 1988 (e.g., Albert et al., 1995; Seeman, McAvay, Merrill, Albert, & Rodin, 1996; Tabbarah, Crimmins, & Seeman, 2002). Albert and colleagues (1995) used structural equation modeling to predict cognitive performance and cognitive change over a 2- to 2.5-year period using 22 demographic, physical, and psychosocial variables as predictors. Cognitive performance was based on the combined scores from a battery of neurocognitive tests. The self-efficacy measure assessed perceptions relative to capabilities to perform instrumental activities such as transportation, relationships, productivity, and living arrangements (Rodin & McAvay, 1992). A series of cross-validation analyses indicated that education, peak expiratory flow rate, current level of strenuous activity (energy expenditure in daily activities such as cleaning and yard work), and self-efficacy were all direct predictors of cognitive change. With respect to the role played by physical activity, Albert and colleagues (1995) contended that their findings support the position that more vigorous activity is needed for effects on brain function, a position that has been contested by results from recent studies (e.g., Kramer et al., 1999; Colcombe et al., 2004). The role played by self-efficacy in these data suggests that confidence across a broad array of instrumental activities (i.e., a more generalized sense of control) may be related to cognitive change. Interestingly, Albert and colleagues viewed self-efficacy as a personality disposition implying stability over time, a perspective that is entirely at odds with social cognitive theory (Bandura, 1986). Whether assessments of efficacy relative to memory, attention, and physical activity might underlie a latent, more global construct of self-regulatory control has yet to be determined.

Seeman and colleagues (1996) focused exclusively on the potential of self-efficacy to contribute to successful cognitive aging and thereby serve as a target for interventions. They argued that a weaker sense of self-efficacy might result in declines in participation in challenging cognitive activities as well as reductions in effort and persistence in such tasks. Lower self-efficacy can also lead to declines in performance of cognitive activities because of increases in anxiety and debilitating thought patterns that can weaken motivation and negatively affect performance. Seeman, Rodin, and Albert (1993) had previously reported cross-sectional associations between efficacy and cognitive function and were attempting in a longitudinal fashion to determine whether changes in efficacy were related to changes in cognitive function in older adults. In essence, these analyses were a more sophisticated and thorough examination of relationships among contructs previously reported by Albert and colleagues (1995). In this study, two types of efficacy were assessed: instrumental efficacy (e.g., beliefs regarding ability to perform instrumental tasks such as arranging transport, being productive, and maintaining safety) and interpersonal efficacy (e.g., beliefs regarding abilities to deal with relationships among family members, spouse, and friends). Assessment of cognitive function involved measures of abstraction, verbal memory, nonverbal memory, and spatial ability. In the earlier cross-sectional study, Seeman and colleagues (1993) had reported verbal memory and instrumental self-efficacy to be related in men. Consequently, in the more recent analyses, separate structural equation models were conducted for males and females and for each of the four areas of cognitive function to determine the contribution of baseline and change in efficacy to changes in cognition. These data indicated that baseline instrumental efficacy and changes in instrumental efficacy were significantly related to changes in verbal memory (e.g., naming recall, story tasks) but only in the male sample. Thus, there was evidence to support the position that one aspect of effective cognitive function (verbal memory) was associated with self-efficacy and that gender differences in self-efficacy exist. For example, when efficacious men fail, they increase their efforts and persist longer than low efficacious males. Conversely, in women, regardless of self-efficacy level, failure has been reported to result in reduced effort (Bandura, 1989). These data support perhaps a tenuous link between physical activity, self-efficacy, and cognitive function in that efficacy for instrumental activities was a predictor of change in verbal memory. Without more precise and specific assessment of efficacy and appropriate mediator and moderator analyses, it is unclear what role physical self-efficacy plays in the physical activity–cognitive function relationship.

However, some speculation on this role might be advanced in the context of findings from Tabbarah and colleagues' (2002) examination of relationships between cognitive performance and physical performance. Again, these data were based on longitudinal assessment in the MacArthur Study of Successful Aging. Tabbarah and her colleagues hypothesized that physical performance measures that reflected novel and attention-demanding tasks (e.g., standing on one leg, standing with tandem foot placement) would be related to cognitive function whereas routine physical tasks such as chair stands, walking at a normal pace, and gripping with one's dominant hand would not. Over a 7-year period, participants ($N = 223$-438) demonstrated significant declines in cognitive and routine and novel physical performance. After the authors controlled for a host of covariates known to be associated with the variables of interest, regression analyses indicated that changes in cognitive performance were associated with changes in all six novel physical performance measures and all five routine physical performance measures. Greater declines in cognitive function were associated with greater declines in physical performance, although these relationships were not particularly strong (range of .04-.17 units of change). The importance of these findings may lie in determining how to most effectively assess self-efficacy in studies of physical activity and cognitive function. Certainly, one would not expect a physical activity intervention to result in changes in memory self-efficacy. From a theoretical perspective this would make little sense. However, physical activity interventions would be expected to influence self-efficacy relative to control of balance, gait, falling, and enhanced physical function in general. The extent to which such changes in these types of self-efficacy play a role in any physical activity effects on cognitive function is worthy of pursuit. Certainly, there is recent evidence to suggest that fitness training enhances cognitive function (McAuley, Kramer, & Colcombe, 2004; Colcombe & Kramer, 2003; Kramer et al., 1999). However, it is unclear whether improvements in other aspects of fitness (e.g., functional fitness) may contribute further to improvements in cognitive performance and whether self-efficacy relative to such functional change may explain additional variance in the prediction of cognitive function.

Further Research Directions and Concluding Remarks

The role played by self-efficacy in effective human function is well established (Bandura, 1997). Moreover, there is a considerable literature to support the reciprocal deterministic relationship of physical activity and self-efficacy and the role played by self-efficacy in mediating and moderating the effects of physical activity on other psychosocial outcomes associated with physical activity participation (McAuley & Blissmer, 2000). Self-efficacy specific to memory performance has been associated with improved memory function (Berry, 1999), as have assessments of efficacy relative to taking care of instrumental activities (Seeman et al., 1996). Physical exercise has been reported to maintain and improve cognitive function in both humans and animals (Churchill et al., 2002). Moreover, Kramer and colleagues (1999) reported that physical fitness training interventions resulted in improvements in cognitive functions that were specific to frontal and prefrontal areas of the brain (i.e., executive control function). In addition, Colcombe and Kramer's (2003) meta-analysis of randomized controlled trials of fitness training effects on cognitive function reached the conclusion that improved fitness is associated with improved cognitive performance. Recent data would appear to support such a conclusion. For example, Colcombe and colleagues (2003) presented cross-sectional human data derived from magnetic resonance imaging to show that higher levels of fitness were associated with preservation of gray and white matter tissues in the frontal, parietal, and temporal cortexes. In a more recent study reporting both cross-sectional and intervention data (Colcombe et al., 2004), older aerobically trained individuals showed significantly less behavioral interference after the 6-month training protocol, whereas control participants showed no such benefit. Additionally, aerobically trained individuals showed an increase in the recruitment of attentional circuitry and a reduction in activity in the dorsal anterior cingulate after the 6-month training protocol, compared to control participants.

If indeed fitness training or fitness improvements help restore and maintain cognitive function, does self-efficacy play a role in this relationship? Any such determination will require appropriate assessment of self-efficacy and potentially assessments of multiple aspects of self-efficacy to determine whether a latent efficacy construct plays a more prominent role in this relationship than more specific measures. Alternatively, different types of self-efficacy may play different roles at varying points in the process during which physical activity influences cognitive function. Certainly, the specificity of efficacy measures might suggest this to be the case. For example, self-efficacy might antedate physical activity as a moderator of who is likely to begin exercise initially. There is also evidence to suggest that efficacy expectations mediate the relationship between physical activity participation and such outcomes as fear (McAuley, Mihalko, & Rosengren, 1997) and anxiety (Katula, Blissmer, & McAuley, 1999). Thus, it might be hypothesized that efficacy may play a mediating role in the relationship between physical activity and fitness and cognitive function inasmuch as fitter, more active, and more efficacious older adults are likely to demonstrate less anxiety in challenging cognitive situations, thereby performing better than their less active, less fit, and less efficacious counterparts. Additionally, whether the restoration and maintenance of cognitive health are more effectively achieved through physical activity or cognitive training programs has yet to be effectively determined. Whether such interventions might provide independent or additive effects on cognitive function can only be determined through randomized controlled trials examining the comparative effectiveness of the two interventions.

Finally, we would be remiss to conclude without mentioning once again the importance of considering the prospective reciprocally determining nature of our model. As it currently stands, the major outcome of the model is cognitive function. However, Dr. Royall (this volume) has stated the case that cognitive decline leads to reduced physical function and activity rather than the case that inactivity leads eventually to compromised cognitive function. To reiterate, the social cognitive perspective views behavior, the environment, cognition, and physiology as interacting determinants of each other. Thus, in a very simple sense, more active individuals might be hypothesized to have better cognitive function, which might lead them to explore and engage in further physical activity. Naturally, multiple other factors will come into play along this feedback loop. A major challenge will be to tease out the extent to which such relationships exist, under which circumstances they operate, and how to effectively maximize them to enhance the quality of life of older adults.

EDITORS' DISCUSSION SUMMARY

Discussion Highlights

The impact of self-efficacy on cognition has received a significant amount of attention in the last decade. Four substantive issues could be further highlighted in this research. One, it is noted that self-efficacy influences behavior choice, effort expended, and persistence over adversity. For older adults who are engaging in physical exercise for the first time, these elements of behavior are particularly important in initial stages of an exercise program. Self-efficacy serves, therefore, as a potential moderator in exercise participation and may lead to cognitive function changes.

Two, the sources of self-efficacy could be further noted. Beyond mastery, modeling, and social persuasion, there are other sources of self-efficacy information: *physical symptoms* and *emotional symptoms*. Sedentary older adults engaging in physical activity initially can experience fatigue, discomfort, and increased respiration. Their interpretation of that physiological feedback indicates their level of exercise self-efficacy. For example, if the symptoms are interpreted as an impending heart attack, then their exercise self-efficacy will diminish. However, if these symptoms are recognized as signs of natural physiological responses to new stressors, the individual will experience an enhanced exercise self-efficacy. In the same way, emotional symptoms also influence exercise self-efficacy. Moods set the tone for the interpretations of exercise self-efficacy. A bad mood will exaggerate any slight inability to perform; however, a positive mood can help an individual accept challenges to successful performance. In both cases, interpretation of symptoms influences exercise self-efficacy.

Three, self-efficacy, exercise, and cognition could form a reciprocally determining relationship. Social cognitive theory emphasizes that the individual's information level, behavior, physiological responses, and environment together influence the potential for future behavior. Dr. McAuley and Dr. Elavsky suggest that the most obvious role for self-efficacy in the model (demonstrating the reciprocity of determinants) is as a moderator of physical activity initiation and as a potential mediator of subsequent adherence. For example, self-efficacy determines exercise behavior, which in turn influences self-efficacy. If a person appraises himself as successful, his level of self-efficacy increases and subsequently increases the motivation to continue. This in turn has the potential to improve the exercise behavior itself and promote adherence to exercise.

Four, exercise self-efficacy is a dynamic variable. Self-efficacy changes with conditions: exercise experience, knowledge, health status, and perceived barriers. In addition, the accuracy of the reported self-efficacy differs depending on when the assessment is made. For example, sedentary adults will typically report high self-efficacy before the onset of a walking program when they do not have actual experience. However, within a few weeks of walking, they will report a more accurate level of self-efficacy as they encounter barriers.

Research Methodological Problems

A primary methodological problem in the extant research is that precise and specific assessment of efficacy and appropriate mediator and moderator analyses must be developed. Without these, it is unclear what role physical self-efficacy plays in the physical activity–cognitive function relationship. A next step should be to consider the prospective reciprocally determining nature of the fitness–cognition model used as a framework in this volume. As it currently stands, the major outcome of the model is cognitive function. However, Dr. Royall (this volume) has postulated the case for cognitive decline leading to reduced physical function and activity rather than inactivity leading eventually to compromised cognitive function.

Future Directions

Three potential research directions are noted. The first focuses on the interpretation of physical and emotional symptoms of physical activity. Little research has been reported that explains the influence of perceived symptoms resulting from physical exercise on older adults. Misinterpretation of such symptoms affects self-efficacy and, in turn, the potential for adherence.

Second, research on generalization of self-efficacy would be informative. How is self-efficacy in one area generalized or transferred to other areas, such as self-esteem? Some evidence suggests that self-efficacy predicts behavior over the construct of dispositional optimism; however, not much research has been conducted regarding its relationship to physical activity.

Third, the investigation of gender and cultural influences on self-efficacy could further elucidate potential mechanisms. Some investigators have reported gender differences in exercise self-efficacy; that is, at baseline males estimate greater exercise efficacy than do females. However, as a study progresses, further assessment of self-efficacy for females equals if not exceeds that of the males, and researchers conclude that self-efficacy predicts as well for both. Dr. McAuley and Dr. Elavsky suggest that those initial differences may be attributable to sociocultural differences more than to gender, because the cohort studied were of the generation when physical activity was not encouraged for women. Further research is needed to examine whether gender differences actually exist regardless of the cultural aspects of the cohort.

CHAPTER 6

Cognitive Energetics and Aging

Phillip D. Tomporowski, PhD

University of Georgia

EDITORS' OVERVIEW

Dr. Tomporowski has tackled perhaps one of the most difficult mediators in this model, the concept of mental energy and fatigue. We know that cognition requires mental energy and that undergoing a task that requires considerable mental energy for a long period of time induces mental fatigue. We also know that sleep, relaxation techniques, and the consumption of some types of food or drink seem to be able to replenish cognition. The question Dr. Tomporowski addresses in this chapter is whether physical activity or exercise also has restorative powers on cognition and whether these effects are short term, long term, or both.

It would be of great benefit for adults of any age if systematic exercise could counteract the loss of energy and inability to concentrate that occur following long-term, intense cognition and at the end of the day.

Dr. Tomporowski grounds his review on energetics theory and systematically explains how behavior may be explained by this approach, physiological resources

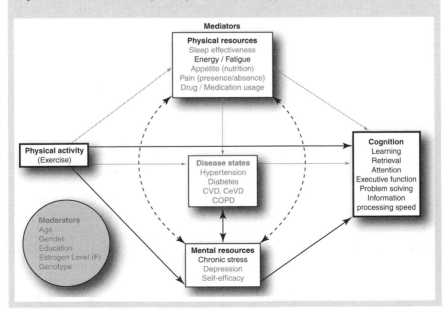

may influence cognitive resources, and physical activity may affect energetic resources. He completes the chapter by assessing the extent to which energetical constructs can explain age-related changes in task persistence and drive.

Older adults often report an inability to muster the level of energy that they once had. Such reduced energy levels are frequently used to explain why an individual may either avoid activities that were at one time considered pleasurable or demonstrate an inability to complete a once-routine daily task. Psychologists are interested in identifying and understanding factors that contribute to an individual's decision to stop making the effort required to complete a task. Aging is clearly associated with significant changes in a host of physiological systems. However, can older adults' decisions to stop participating be explained entirely in terms of declines in physical resources? Clearly, at any given moment an individual's choices are guided by more than an appraisal of his or her current physiological status; volitional action is a dynamic interaction between biological resources and psychological resources.

Numerous theories have been developed over the past century to explain factors that govern an individual's willingness to expend physical or mental effort. Contemporary energetics theory attempts to explain how people regulate goal-directed behaviors and the interrelationship between such psychological processes as will, desire, and intentions and such physiological states as arousal, fatigue, and activation. Older adults' performance can be degraded when physical health is impaired by declines in functional capacity, disease, injury, and the side effects of some medications. Physical activity has been viewed as a means of maintaining or improving older adults' functional capacity. Older adults' perceptions of the state of their physiological resources would be expected to play an important role in decisions that center on the initiation, regulation, and maintenance of behavior. Energetics theory provides a conceptual framework to examine the regulation of behavior in terms of both physiological and psychological resources.

Cognitive energetics draws on and incorporates themes that have long histories in psychological research. The models developed under the rubric of cognitive energetics are based on the assumption that people consciously attempt to optimize their performance by controlling and regulating their physical and mental states. The regulation of these states can be understood in terms of cybernetic principles, which describe how an individual reduces discrepancies that exist between the psychophysiological state he or she expects to experience and the actual state he or she is experiencing.

Energetics theory provides a conceptual framework for evaluating the multifaceted nature of people's mental processes and how those processes influence learning and performance. Historically, mental processes have been described in terms of three properties: (1) cognition, reflecting the knowledge and skills that an individual brings to a performance environment; (2) affection, reflecting the feelings and emotions that are interjected into the performance situation; and (3) conation, reflecting an individual's willingness, or motivation, to expend physical and mental effort to perform (Hilgard, 1980).

The longstanding philosophical conception of the mind as a trilogy of mental processes had an impact on early American psychologists. The rise of behaviorism in the first half of the 20th century, however, later suppressed discussion of mental phenomena for several decades. The advent of cognitive science in the 1970s was spurred by a resurgence of interest in the mind's properties, and, once again, researchers focused their efforts on understanding cognition, affection, and conation. Research conducted within each domain has provided a wealth of information that has a direct bearing on developmental, life span issues. However, relatively few attempts have been made to integrate the data obtained from these three research domains. Cognitive energetics theory was developed as a general theoretical framework that promotes a synergy among the interests of researchers who study cognition, neurophysiology, and conation.

The goals of this chapter are to describe energetical approaches to the study of behavior, evaluate the role of physiological resources on optimal cognitive performance, assess the impact of physical activity on energetic resources, and assess the extent to which energetical constructs can explain age-related changes in task persistence and drive.

Cognitive Energetics: Basic Assumptions

Energetics theory (e.g., Hockey, Gaillard, & Coles, 1986; Sanders, 1983, 1998) came about in response to the perceived limitations of contemporary computer-based information-processing theories that have come to dominate much psychological research today. Many science historians consider the publication of the Miller, Galanter, and Pribram text, *Plans and the Structure of Behavior* (1960), to be a milestone in the emergence of cognitive psychology. The model of learning and performance proposed stressed the roles of mental structures and their operations. The fundamental building block of their theory was the test–operate–test–exit (TOTE) unit, a cybernetic mental construct that functioned to analyze environmental information and to assess the degree to which one's present environment matched a desired environment. The TOTE unit was hypothesized to guide an individual's behavior action plan. A plan was conceptualized as a list of tests, arranged sequentially and designed to attain a desired outcome or goal. The TOTE unit was thought to underlie a broad range of human activities. A case was made for the role of the TOTE unit in skill learning, language, memory, personality, and motives.

Theoretical conceptualization of the operation of the human information-processing system has become increasingly more complex since the introduction of the TOTE unit. The introduction of the additive factors method (Sternberg, 1969) did much to advance the development of computer models of information processing. Analysis of the pattern of individuals' reaction times under various experimental conditions provided evidence for the operations of specific stages of mental operation. Likewise, Atkinson and Shiffrin's (1971) conceptualization of memory storage led researchers to consider that mental operations function analogously to those of hardware computer systems. The view that the human mind can be conceptualized in terms of computer-like neurological hard wiring has been central to several influential theories of human cognition (e.g., Anderson, 1983; Rummelhart & McClelland, 1986).

Much of contemporary information-processing theory has evolved into what Koelega (1996) referred to as "dry" cognition. That is, the regulation of human behavior is viewed as the end result of a calculation of the relative weight of individual bits of stored information (filtering, expectancy matching, probability matching, automatic and controlled processing). The roles of such constructs as planning and goal setting and their impact on behavior, which were central to the work of Miller, Galanter, and Pribram, were either reduced or abandoned entirely. As a result, dry information-processing theories place relatively little emphasis on individual differences factors and how behavior can be affected by internal states such as mood, emotion, drug effects, or stress. Energetics theory focuses on the dynamic interaction between biological processes and psychological processes that govern human action and behavior. It focuses on interfaces that exist between physiological structures and psychological structures and how those systems are energized into action.

Energetics theory is an extension of previous theories and research that focused on "wet" cognition, that is, the "intensive aspects of behavior, the energy, or degree of vigor" (Koelega, 1996, p. 309). The concepts that are central to cognitive energetics can be traced to early research and theorizing about the concept of arousal and its role as a mechanism underling adaptive behavior (Hebb, 1955). The construct of arousal and the study of its impact on human performance have a long and somewhat controversial history (Robbins & Everitt, 1995). Although there has been some debate regarding the construct of arousal, it has played a role in several theories that reflect wet cognition.

Every activity performed, whether physical or mental, involves both action and reaction to demands. The human body has the capacity to monitor and sense discrepancies that exist between its expected state and its current state and, if necessary, to take action to decrease the discrepancy.

The body is equipped with a multitude of regulatory systems that function with and without conscious awareness. Attention is considered to be an agent that controls and regulates these systems.

Daniel Kahneman's (1973) theory of attention and effort was grounded in neurophysiology and provided a major contribution to biologically based, wet explanations of human thought and action. As described in greater detail subsequently, he conceived attention as a limited-capacity resource that is drawn upon to perform specific tasks. More recently, multiple capacity theories of attention have been proposed. These theories focus on organismic factors rather than computer-based metaphors and, as such, provide a conceptual framework that serves as the underpinning for contemporary energetics theory. Energetics theory assumes that human behavior can be conceptualized in terms of physiological and psychological states that can be self-regulated, human behavior is directed toward particular goal states, and the regulatory processes drawn upon to direct behavior involve costs to other regulatory processes.

State Regulation

The term *energetics* is used to denote all constructs that are used to describe the state of an organism (e.g., activation, arousal, fatigue) (Hockey et al., 1986). The regulation of an individual's state has been hypothesized to be controlled via three sources of processing: computation, emotion, and mental effort (Gaillard & Wientjes, 1994). Cognitive control that is exerted via *computation* uses structures and functions of the information-processing system. Information flowing from sensory systems is perceived, stored, and manipulated according to formal and logical rules. The frontal lobes of the neocortex are implicated as key neurological structures involved in the process of computation and the initiation of action. Cognitive control that is exerted via *emotion* does not follow formal rules of logic or reason. The limbic system initiates regulatory responses by way of structures of the autonomic nervous system. Discrepant environmental conditions lead to changes in physiological arousal (heart rate, respiration) that are linked to subjective feelings (such as anxiety and fear). Cognitive control that is exerted via *mental effort* reflects goal-oriented motivation that expresses itself in terms of trying harder (increased concentration and attentional focus) and the willingness to expend physical and mental resources. It is assumed that people use all three sources of processing daily activities. The source that dominates state regulation at any moment is determined by a variety of experiential, ability, developmental, and situational factors.

Goal States

Conation has been defined as an "aspect of personality characterized by a conscious willing, strong, and purposive action" (Wolman, 1989, p. 68). It reflects an intrinsic unrest that is opposite that of homeostasis (English & English, 1958). The natural unrest of human action is thought to reflect a genetically linked characteristic of the functions of the brain. Fluctuations in the processes of the central nervous system are conjectured to have important implications for adaptation to environmental demands and, as a result, important evolutionary significance. Indeed, Ursin (1986) suggested that the unrest (e.g., tension, restlessness, impatience) or conation exhibited by humans reflects biological mechanisms that are built into the brain. Thus, a state of tension leads to cognitive and behavioral activation that resolves the condition. The resolution of tension can be attained via a variety of strategies.

The strategies that are used to regulate behavior directed toward achieving a goal state are central to the study of volitional behavior. They underlie the dynamic interaction between cognitive processes (e.g., will, desire, intentions) and physiological processes (e.g., central and peripheral fatigue, muscular strength, chronic pain, medications). Attainment of a desired goal state is not always possible; thus, an individual who is attempting to alter or resolve his or her state condition is constantly involved in reevaluating the relation between present and desired goal states. The individual's behaviors will be moderated by variables that have their basis in both physiological resources and psychological resources. The fundamental issue for the individual revolves around the availability and utilization of resources.

Regulatory Costs

State-regulatory behaviors are assumed to consume available physiological and psychological resources. Specific brain processes are engaged to address and reconcile discrepancies between actual and desired goal states. The manner in which brain processes are selected and used differs as a function of environmental task conditions faced by the individual. The concept of resource utilization has been addressed extensively by theorists over the past 3 decades. Sanders' (1998) overview of issues of cognitive resources led him to conclude that theorists tend to conceptualize cognitive resources in one of two ways: Proponents of resource volume models envision the brain as possessing multiple systems whose operating capacity is diminished as a function of available computational resources, and proponents of resource strategy models suggest that energetical resources remain constant and that performance reflects differences in the operational efficiency of specific cognitive systems.

Cognitive energetics theory (Hockey & Hamilton, 1983) addresses how both resource volume utilization and resource strategy utilization may play roles in explaining intensive, goal-directed human behavior. Central to the theory is the assumption that there are two levels of processing. A lower-level system of processes reflects the activation of well-learned behaviors that are engaged automatically and require little or no conscious control.

Automatic processes are assumed to occur with minimal associated costs. An upper-level system of processes involves active monitoring of the success or failure of automatic processes to achieve goal-state conditions. Perceptions of discrepancy between present and desired goal states lead to active, strategic, and conscious selection, or effort monitoring, that is involved in selecting specific processes that, when put into action, attempt to regulate state conditions. An individual's upper-level regulation is assumed to be driven via negative feedback and directed by both short-term and long-term goals.

The operations of upper-level regulatory system are believed to be particularly sensitive to individual differences in the value of particular goals, the person's willingness to meet challenges, and his or her associated levels of physical and psychological demand. These operations are also predicted to be affected by such short-term factors as fatigue and emotional states and also by the presence of illness or chronic stress (Hockey, Payne, & Terry, 1996).

Summary

Energetics theory addresses topics that have direct relevance to the study of life span development and aging. The theory explores relationships that exist among cognition and age-related changes in information processing, neurophysiology and age-related changes in biological processes (involving both the central and peripheral nervous systems), and motivation and individual differences in behavioral effort and drive. Specific predictions concerning the impact of various mediators on behavior can be drawn from the theory. The theory, however, relies heavily on a number of constructs that have been difficult for researchers to operationalize and to evaluate empirically.

Energetics Theory: Linking Constructs to Physiological Resources

The overriding goal of energetics theory is to evaluate interrelationships between mental resources and physiological resources and to determine how the utilization of these resources affects the intensity of goal-directed behavior. Resources, and their use, are thought to affect the manner in which individuals approach and overcome the challenges of everyday life (e.g., learning new skills, adapting to environmental changes).

Two issues are of central interest for this presentation: the degree to which energetic resources (particularly physical resources) mediate optimal cognitive functioning and adaptive behavior, and the impact that exercise and physical activity have on these energetic resources (figure 6.1). To that end, several physiologically based constructs that reflect energetical

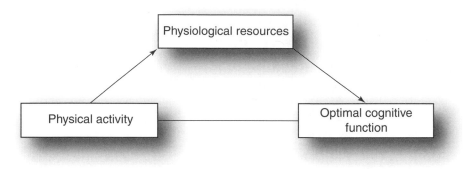

Figure 6.1 Potential mediators between physical activity and cognition.

characteristics have been drawn from extant theories. These constructs are evaluated first in terms of their relation to optimal cognitive functioning and second in terms of the degree to which they are influenced by physical activity and exercise.

Energetic Constructs

Scientists employ constructs to explain empirical observations. Hypothetical constructs are often used as heuristics that tie together relations seen in nature. Several constructs have been employed to explain how human behavior is activated and energized.

Arousal

Daniel Kahneman's (1973) theory of attention and effort provides researchers with a model that describes how an individual's actions are regulated by an allocation policy. The effort directed toward task performance was proposed to be determined by four factors: enduring dispositions, evaluation demand, momentary intentions, and arousal. Of these constructs, arousal is taken to reflect a physiological process that mediates an individual's allocation policy and behavior. Indeed, Kahneman (1973) suggested that measures of heart rate (e.g., sinus arrhythmia, cardiac variability) and sympathetic activity (e.g., pupillary dilation, skin conductance) could be used as indexes of effort (1973, p.18). According to Kahneman's theory, an individual's level of arousal is the result of two factors: the demand characteristics of the task to be performed (i.e., the challenge inherent in preparing for and performing a given task) and miscellaneous determinants not directly related to the task (e.g., intensity of stimulation, drug effects, or stressors). Thus, an individual's level of arousal is in a constant state of flux that is attributable either to the moment-to-moment demands of the task being performed or to the stress that the individual is experiencing.

Andries Sanders (1983, 1998) conceptualized attention in terms of three energy stores, each of which is controlled by an executive process (see figure 6.2). This model emphasizes the relationships between three levels of mental operations: a computational level, an executive control level, and an energy pool level. Computational processes include stimulus encoding, the storage and retrieval of information from interconnected memory structures, response selection, and response programming. The mechanistic activities of computational processes and resultant behavior are guided by processes taking place at the executive control level, where goal-directed, purposeful actions are formulated. The executive function addresses discrepancies that may exist between an organism's desired state and actual state. The executive processor evaluates discrepancies in terms of goals that can be attained via action. The direction and intensity of those actions are determined by the allocation of resources that are present in three pools of energy: the effort pool, which determines the overall motivational state of the organism; the energy pool, which determines the resources that will be allowed to meet the demands encountered in the process of attaining specific goals; and the arousal pool, which is activated both by the effort pool and by stimulus input factors. The arousal pool responds in a phasic manner to variations in the quantity and quality of incoming sensory information. The allocation of energy from the arousal pool is reflected behaviorally through the speed at which an organism responds to novel stimuli or warning cues. The activation pool is affected by the allocation of effort resources and by motor programming and the execution of actions. The activation pool responds in a tonic manner and is reflected behaviorally to the extent to which actions are sustained over time.

Sanders did not explicitly link the energy pools in his model to underlying physiological structures. However, physiological brain structures associated with the energy constructs of arousal, effort, and activation have been proposed. Early neurophysiological research by Pribram and McGuinness (1975) led them to conclude that arousal was linked to processes within the amygdala, effort was associated with functions within the hippocampus, and activation was regulated via activity cycles within the basal ganglia. More recently, arousal mechanisms have been described in terms of specific neurotransmitter system activity. Catecholamines function to enhance stimulus processing. Norepinephrine neurons originating from the locus coeruleus appear to promote brain changes that help maintain selective attention (discriminability) during stressful conditions. Dopamine neurons play a role in the activation of motoric or cognitive output. Serotonin neurons dampen cortical functions (see Robbins & Everitt, 1995).

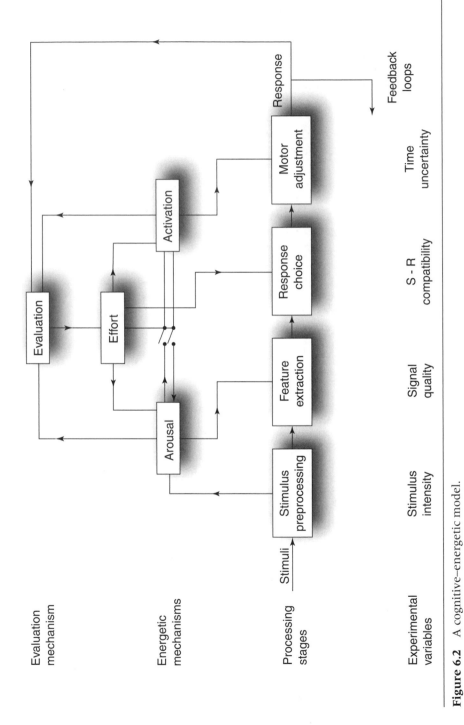

Figure 6.2 A cognitive–energetic model.

This article was published in *Acta Psychologica*, Vol. 53, A.F. Sanders, Toward a model of stress and human performance, pp. 61-97, Copyright Elsevier, 1983.

Workload and Stress

Distinctions between the constructs of workload (mental load) and stress have been made by several researchers interested in energetics (Gaillard & Wientjes, 1994; Kramer & Weber, 2000). Several key differences between workload and stress are summarized in Mental Load vs. Stress.

First, task-induced stress and mental load both disrupt an individual's physiological and psychological state and both result in the mobilization of resources directed toward state regulation. The onset of a stressor, however, elicits a defensive coping response, which is directed toward reducing or avoiding a threat. The onset of a mental load elicits an active coping response, which is directed toward an analysis of the task at

MENTAL LOAD VS. STRESS

1. Coping Strategy
- Mental Load: Coping is oriented toward the execution of the task. Actions are taken to solve the problems.
- Stress: Self-protection is a defensive style of palliative reactions aimed at reducing the negative effects of (potential) threats.

2. Emotions
- Mental Load: The situation is experienced as challenging (positive emotions).
- Stress: The situation is experienced as threatening (negative emotions).

3. Regulation
- Mental Load: The load is limited to the period during which the task has to be executed.
- Stress: Activation persists outside the task situation and inhibits recovery.

4. Error Detection and Mobilization
- Mental Load: The mind is tuned by the demands of the task and aimed at improving or maintaining performance efficiency by focusing attention.
- Stress: Activation is dysfunctional.

Adapted from Gaillard & Wientjes (1994).

hand in terms of a problem in need of solving. Second, when stressed, people typically report feelings of threat or being strained. When under increased mental load, they report positive feelings and increased energy. The distinction made between the emotional states produced by stress and mental load is similar to Selye's distinction between distress, which is destructive to health, and eustress, which is beneficial to health (Selye, 1974), and to the distinction made by contemporary researchers who distinguish stress in terms of its threat, potential for harm or loss, or potential for growth and challenge (Folkman & Lazarus, 1985; Lazarus, 1993a, 1993b). Third, stress results in generalized and pervasive arousal that continues to elicit coping responses even after the source of the stress has terminated. The stress syndrome is characterized as a sequence of stages during which the activity of entire physiological systems heightens over time and leads to irreversible wear and tear. The arousal that is associated with mental load is more circumscribed than that produced by stress. Although physiological and psychological arousal is experienced during a mental load, the arousal is maintained only until the problem is solved or terminated. Fourth, proponents of stress models suggest that the inefficient coping responses (errors) people make while attempting to reduce stress perpetuate a downward spiral of task avoidance and decreased motivation to perform the actions that are essential for success. Workload theorists suggest that people do not dwell on the errors that they make; rather, they use the information as objective feedback that can be used to improve their future performance. Task-relevant feedback motivates the performer to engage in off-task problem analysis that, in turn, motivates him or her to reengage the task.

Fatigue

To most individuals, reductions in human performance are typically explained in terms of the buildup of fatigue, that is, a feeling of lack of energy, weariness, and aversion to further effort (Pandorf, 1982). However, the construct of fatigue is seldom emphasized in energetic models of performance. Fatigue is widely experienced and serves as a convenient explanation for changes in performance; however, it is a vague and difficult construct to operationalize (Wessely, Hotopt, & Sharpe, 1998). Most theorists use the term but tend to place it in a miscellaneous category (e.g., Kahneman, 1973).

Numerous studies have examined the aftereffects of physical activity both on motor performance and on cognitive performance. The results of these studies have been difficult to interpret, however, because human performance tends to be quite unaffected by moderate levels of peripheral fatigue. Performance decrements tend to be seen only when strenuous physical activities are required; this observation has led some to speculate that central (psychological) factors play a very large role in maintaining performance (Holding, 1983).

The mechanisms that underlie central fatigue have only recently begun to be explored (see Davis, 1995). The results of research studies conducted thus far are intriguing because they focus on the roles of neurotransmitter systems that are implicated in arousal (norepinephrine, dopamine, and serotonin). Furthermore, the data obtained suggest that these transmitter systems are influenced both by exercise and by diet and nutritional supplements.

Summary

The energetic constructs found in theories of Kahneman, Sanders, and Hockey depend heavily on the role of physiologically based processes to explain individual differences in the availability of resources that are required for intensive and sustained goal-directed behavior. Regulation of behavior is explained in terms of brain structures and neurotransmitter systems and in terms of the regulation of the autonomic nervous system. Optimal behavioral regulation and performance are assumed to be degraded when these physiological systems are impaired. The impairment of these physiological systems can come from two sources: by the workload engendered by the preparation and actual performance of a given task and by stressors that are not directly related to the task to be performed.

Physical Activity and Resources

There is sufficient empirical evidence that physiologically linked energetical resources play important roles in optimizing cognitive processes that are essential for adaptive human behavior. Open to question, however, is the degree to which exercise and physical activity influence these resources. As discussed by Baron and Kenny (1986), a mediating variable must meet three criteria: (1) There must be a significant relationship between the mediator variable (e.g., energetic resources) and the outcome variable (e.g., adaptive cognitive function), (2) there must also be a significant relationship between an intervention (e.g., physical activity or exercise) and the mediator variable (e.g., energetic resources), and (3) the effects of the intervention on the outcome variable should not be significant when one controls for the relationships between exercise and energetic resources and between energetic resources and adaptive cognitive function.

Physical Activity and Brain Function

Attempts to understand the physiological basis of mental processes have led researchers to focus their attention on structures of the brain, particularly the neocortex and its control of subcortical structures. Of central importance is the study of the organization of the brain and how brain systems work together to control sensation, perception, thought, and action. New knowledge about the brain is accumulating at an extremely rapid pace. Many of these findings reinforce the view that the brain follows a pattern of hierarchical organization. Areas of the brain perform very restricted mental operations that are carried out in a very specific manner. Operations proposed in basic models of the brain are controlled by higher-level modules that are, in turn, controlled by even higher-level modules (see Posner & Raichle, 1997). The activation of brain structures is controlled by neurotransmitter systems. Several of these transmitters (norepinephrine, dopamine, and serotonin) were described previously and have been implicated as central determinants of arousal. The mechanisms that guide the actions of these neuronal systems are complex, and they are presently the focal point of considerable experimental research.

A review of research that examined the acute effects of exercise on cognitive function led Tomporowski (2003a) to speculate that aerobic exercise facilitates cognitive functioning. Acute bouts of moderately intense exercise were hypothesized to function in a manner similar to that of psychostimulant drugs. Using Sanders' (1983) model as a conceptual framework, Tomporowski proposed that exercise selectively affects the activation of specific pools of attentional resources. Physical activity may lead to the allocation of resources that adjusts or fine-tunes the capacity of sensory systems to pick up specific environmental information and prepares the individual to mobilize and initiate motor activity. Exercise-linked changes in arousal, activation, and effort energy pools may be the result of physiological changes that accompany aerobic activity. Exercise is known to produce increased plasma levels of neurohormonal substances such as epinephrine and norepinephrine, which have been linked to cognitive function.

Chronic exercise training may produce long-term changes in the brain and structures that underlie arousal states. A recent review of studies that examined the effect of chronic physical activity on brain functions in animals suggested that improvements in the integrity of brain function may be attributable to changes in synaptogenesis and neuronal architecture, neurogenesis and growth of new neurons, glial plasticity of nonneuronal cells of the brain, or vascular plasticity and blood flow (Churchill et al., 2002).

Physical activity is speculated to enhance the integrity of brain function; however, support for this contention is hampered by the methodological and procedural difficulties of measuring neurotransmitter functions in the human brain (see Buckworth & Dishman, 2002). Nevertheless, the advances that have been made in understanding brain function over the past 10 years have been striking. Findings from a number of research areas provide converging evidence for the link between physiological brain function and cognition.

Physical Activity and Autonomic Nervous System Regulation

The human body responds in extremely predictable ways to changes in environmental conditions. Decades of research have clearly mapped out how the autonomic nervous system (ANS) responds to environmental and psychological perturbations. Researchers who study the impact of physical activity on ANS regulation have paid particular attention to two interrelated neural–hormonal systems. First, the hypothalamic–pituitary–adrenocortical system (HPA) links the release of adrenocorticotropic hormone (ACTH) from the anterior area of the pituitary gland to the cortex of the adrenal gland. When the adrenal cortex is stimulated by ACTH, it varies the amount of glucocorticoids released into the bloodstream, which have the capacity to enter cells and direct their nuclei to increase protein production and energy supplies. Second, the sympathetic–adrenal–medullary (SAM) system releases adrenaline and noradrenaline into the bloodstream. These substances play a critical role in quickly preparing the body to meet environmental challenges. Circulating adrenaline stimulates the release of glucose into the bloodstream and increases the amount of blood that flows to the brain. The brain, a major consumer of energy, benefits from the increased availability of energy supplies, particularly when its structures are responding to threatening or stressful environmental situations. At the same time that circulating adrenaline benefits the brain, the body's muscle tissue is benefiting from circulating noradrenaline. When faced with a potential threat, the muscle system increases its activity. The mobilization of the body for rapid action draws on available energy supplies. Noradrenaline helps skeletal muscle tissue by increasing blood flow to muscles and aiding in the release of free fatty acids, which are broken down and used by muscle cells.

Several researchers have hypothesized that physical activity changes the manner in which HPA and SAM systems function under stressor conditions (Dienstbier, 1989, 1991; Sothmann et al., 1996; Van Doornen & De Geus, 1993). An early meta-analytical evaluation of 25 research studies concluded that chronic exercise training programs had an impact on physiological reactivity to stressors equal to approximately one half of a standard deviation (Crews & Landers, 1987). However, authors of a recent systematic review of studies in this area suggested that the relationship between chronic exercise training and physiological reactivity is complex and that there is insufficient evidence to support a causal relation between physical activity and ANS functions (Dishman & Jackson, 2000).

There is support for a relationship between exercise and changes in those energetic variables hypothesized to serve as moderators of adaptive cognitive functioning. However, this support should be viewed with caution because the research on these topics conducted in the field of exercise psychology suffers from a number of methodological and conceptual weaknesses. The early views of generalized HPA and SAM system responses to all stressors have been challenged. The pattern of ANS activation to stressors appears to vary as a function of the type and intensity of the event (Dishman & Jackson, 2000).

Aging and Energetical States

Many older adults report an inability to muster the level of activity that they once had, or they describe their general energy level as low. The data obtained that describe the functions of the cardiorespiratory system (Shephard, 1999), muscular system (Faulkner, Brooks, & Zerba, 1990), and neurohormonal system (Roth, 1990) corroborate the feelings experienced by older adults (see Spirduso, 1995). Older adults also describe noticeable changes in memory and mental quickness. The data obtained that describe neural changes in the brain and their impact on learning, memory, and information-processing speed (Woodruff-Pak, Coffin, & Sasse, 1991; Woodruff-Pak & Papka, 1999) also corroborate many older adults' subjective reports of their mental capabilities.

Aging is clearly associated with significant changes in a host of physiological systems. The two primary interests of this chapter, however, are the relationship between age-related changes in physiological systems and constructs that are central to energetic theory (arousal, stress, mental load, and fatigue) and the degree to which physical activity affects these states and ultimately affects older adults' adaptive cognitive functioning.

Aging and Arousal

Aging is accompanied by both changes in brain structure and declines in neurochemistry. Early electroencephalographic research, combined with observations of age-related decreases in gross brain weight and volume, led to the development of competing ideas about the consequences of these changes on arousal. One early neurological theory of aging posited that changes in brain structure lead to a state of underarousal. James Birren (1960, pp. 326-327) stated, "There is the possibility that the well-established psychomotor slowing of advancing age is a consequence of reduced physiological activation. This agrees with what limited literature exists on age differences in activity and drive levels. Assuming a less energized or activated organism with age, in any unit of time there will be less interaction between the individual and his environment. This reduces the opportunity for all psychological processes to take place; e.g., perception, acquisition, manipulation of symbols, and storage." However, Alan Welford (1965, p. 14) suggested that age-related changes in brain function lead to a state of overarousal. He stated, "Both clinical and everyday observations of middle aged and older people point rather to over-activation resulting in unduly heightened activity and anxiety."

Contemporary research on age-related declines in brain structures purported to affect older adults' cognitive function has targeted the prefrontal cortex, which has been implicated in a wide array of executive processes believed to be critical for controlled mental processing (e.g., decision making, self-monitoring, and behavioral inhibition (Woodruff-Pak & Papka, 1999). There is substantial evidence for age-related declines in cognitive functions that are believed to be controlled by frontal lobe executive processes (Kramer & Willis, 2002; West, 1996).

Age-related changes in cognitive function have been explained in terms of decreased integrity of brain structures, changes in blood flow and glucose availability, and the integrity of neurotransmitter systems, in particular those with acetylcholine, norepinephrine, and serotonin neurons. Neurotransmitter system efficiency can be compromised by a variety of mechanisms (see Woodruff-Pak et al., 1991). The net effect of these changes is alteration of both excitatory and inhibitory synapses.

A recent review of reviews published before 2002 concluded that results of studies that assessed the impact of physical activity on older adults' cognitive performance have been equivocal (see Tomporowski, 2006). However, a recent series of publications by Arthur Kramer and his colleagues (Churchill et al., 2002; Colcombe & Kramer, 2003; Kramer et al., 1999, Kramer & Willis, 2002) provides compelling evidence for benefits of chronic exercise on older adults' cognitive functioning. In one of their studies, the cognitive performance of 58 older adults (mean age = 66.0 years) who participated in an exercise program was compared with 66 older adults (mean age = 67.3 years) who participated in a toning program. Those who exercised improved on several tasks hypothesized to reflect executive-control processes (e.g., stopping, task switching, and response compatibility). The strongest fitness effects were associated with tasks that emphasized response speed more than response accuracy. The exercise program promoted improvement in tasks that required rapid identification and selection of information and mobilization of action. The increase in older adults' efficiency of stimulus extraction and movement mobilization is not unlike that observed in young adults following acute bouts of exercise (Tomporowski, 2003a). This comparison is speculative, however, because no studies have been published that examine the effects of acute exercise bouts on older adults' cognitive function. Nevertheless, the results of empirical research support predictions derived from energetical models that describe how information processing is regulated both by an arousal energy pool and by an activation energy pool (e.g., Sanders, 1983).

Kramer and his colleagues have amassed considerable evidence that physical activity has salutary effects on the aging brain. Churchill and colleagues (2002) provide an excellent review of research on aging. Their review of cross-sectional, prospective, and retrospective epidemiological studies of older humans led them to conclude that there is indeed a link between fitness level and brain vitality and, furthermore, that the link is particularly strong when the effects of exercise training are evaluated through the use of cognitive tasks that tap into executive processing. Their review of studies that examined physical activity and animal brain function led them to speculate about possible mechanisms by which exercise produces its effects on brain functions (i.e., synaptogensis, neurogenesis, glial plasticity, vascular plasticity, and angiogenesis).

Aging and Stress

A general theory of mental health proposed by Dienstbier (1989, 1991) suggests that aging is linked to reduced β-receptor sensitivity and reduced levels of peripheral catecholamines. The decreased neurological integrity associated with advancing chronological age leads to declines in physical health, cognitive functioning, and affect. Dienstbier evaluated data obtained from both animal and human research and assessed the role of neurotransmitter and neurohormonal patterns that occur during and following stressful events. First, he observed that test subjects who show a rapid rise and then a rapid decline in catecholamine production following a stressor also show good performance on laboratory tests with low anxiety. Second, he observed that test subjects who show increases in HPA axis functioning following a stressor show poor test performance and evidence psychological distress. More recent reviews of research on age-related changes in the patterns of HPA functions corroborate these observations (Finch & Seeman, 1999). Recent research has strengthened the view that HPA dysregulation has negative effects on cognitive function. Evidence points to the negative impact of circulating glucocorticoids on the hippocampus, a structure that plays a particularly important role in learning and memory. The hippocampus is located in an area of the brain that is rich in adrenal steroid receptors, which are sensitive to adrenal steroids that cross the blood–brain barrier. Finch and Seeman (1999) proposed that age-related individual differences in HPA resiliency are a function of lifelong, cumulative exposures to glucocorticoids. The accumulation of stress experiences and circulation of cortisol lead to a gradually less resilient pattern of HPA activation. The decline in resiliency promotes the onset of risks of diseases associated with aging.

Dienstbier (1989) concluded from his review that an individual's responses to stress are affected by his or her history. Repeated challenge (either physical or mental) was hypothesized to lead to a buildup of the resources needed to meet environmental demands and cope with the stresses of life. Dienstbier characterized challenging situations as those that are demanding but yield positive outcomes; stressful situations are characterized as threatening, with potential negative outcomes or loss.

There is evidence that systematic physical activity improves older adults' HPA responses to stressors; however, as discussed previously, the relationships between physical activity and functions of the autonomic nervous system are complex. Substantial individual differences exist among individuals' stress responses. Furthermore, HPA stress patterns may reflect the end result of years of experiences. It would appear unlikely that participation in a relatively brief physical activity program would result in much of a change in HPA resiliency. Significant gains, in all likelihood, will accrue only with long-term lifestyle change that occurs in the context of daily activities.

Emotional responsiveness is a key component of the energetic state regulation. It would be expected that the negative feelings associated with HPA dysfunction would interact both with the way in which an individual processes information and with the level of mental effort the individual elects to expend.

Aging and Mental Workload

Mental workload reflects the task-generated demands on an operator. The mental load engendered by a task is determined by such factors as stimulus presentation rate, stimulus quality, and the degree of interactivity among task elements. Considerable research in the human factors field has evaluated the mental processes that govern people's rational decision making regarding whether to expend mental effort to learn a skill or to perform a task. Central to energetical theory is the assumption that state regulation is critical to human performance. The demands of a task lead a person to attempt to decrease discrepancies that exist between a desired state and an actual state by engaging in rational cost–benefit judgments and by allocating the physical and mental effort that is required to attain state regulation. An individual is assumed to enter into novel learning or operational situations with a priori expectations concerning the level of performance that will be required to achieve specified target goals. Individuals use task-produced feedback to verify the veracity of their expectations and to establish performance criteria that will lead to a desired goal state. Tasks judged as either more demanding (overload) or less demanding (underload) than expected typically lead people to respond to the task with one of two strategies. One strategy is to modify targeted goals and adjust ongoing performance criteria. This strategy typically results in declines in the individual's motivation and effort, particularly when she perceives a large discrepancy between her actual and desired level of performance and the amount of effort and practice that will be required to attain a goal. The alternative strategy is to exert additional mental effort. Those who use this strategy recognize that their behavior may in the short run produce episodes of frustration and anxiety but that in the long run, the increased effort they expend will lead them to acquire high levels of terminal performance and to attain desired goal states.

Task performance is known to be affected by such factors as past experience, perceptions of skill level, and age. Older adults are known to respond to novel learning situations differently than do younger adults

(Griffiths, 1997; Tomporowski, 2003b; Van Gerven, Paas, Van Merrienboer, & Schmidt, 2000). Older adults are believed to exhibit more trepidation about engaging in a novel task than younger individuals, particularly if the task involves a new technology or demands effortful information processing. Older adults are described as less likely than younger adults to initiate the learning of new skills, and they display less motivation to persist in learning the skill.

Stones and Kozma (1988) hypothesized that chronic exercise training offset age-related declines in cognitive function in two ways: (1) Exercise influences physiological systems that have a beneficial influence on older adults' functional capacity, and (2) exercise results in overpracticing skills. Older adults' cognitive performance benefits from both physical training and mental training programs (see Kramer et al., 2002; Tomporowski, 1997). These improvements in older adults' cognitive functioning may be mediated by their perception of competence, task mastery, and skill level. The impact of task-related knowledge on the use of response strategies is a key component of energetical models of human performance. It predicts that the effort exerted during the planning and execution of a task will depend on cost–benefit analyses during which the individual assesses the match between the demands of the task and his or her skill level.

Aging and Fatigue

Epidemiological research has assessed age-related differences in reports of general fatigue. The results are conflicting, however. Two Swedish population studies reported declines in fatigue from middle age to older age (Essen-Moller, 1956; Tibblin, Bengtsson, Furunes, & Lapidus, 1990), but one American study reported a steady increase in reports of general fatigue from middle age to older age (Hammond, 1964). These conflicting reports have been interpreted as indicating the difficulty of assessing the construct of general fatigue and indicating that reports of fatigue in older adults are influenced by the prevalence of disease and mood disorders (Wessely et al., 1998).

There is clear evidence that reductions in physical activity, whether attributable to injury, immobilization, or simple disuse, increase sensations of fatigue and prompt an overall reduction in the desire to exercise. Furthermore, reduction in activity alters people's perceptions of their level of effort during exercise. A systematic overview of the research conducted on general fatigue and chronic fatigue syndrome suggested that exercise may lead to reductions in reports of fatigue (Wessely et al., 1998). However, the evidence obtained thus far is difficult to interpret because of the significant dropout rates of individuals from these studies. One of the impediments to research on the effects of physical activity on fatigue is that most individuals accept on face value the general belief that the most effective treatment for fatigue is rest, rather than activity.

Summary

There is clear evidence for age-related physiological changes in specific structures that underlie the constructs of arousal, stress, and mental load. The construct of fatigue appears to be a nonspecific response to multiple physiological processes. Variations in states of arousal, stress, and mental load influence older adults' cognitive performance, and physical activity appears to influence some of the physiological systems that underlie these states. It has been speculated that the effects of physical activity are selective and that these selective changes in physiological integrity have significant and long-lasting effects on older adults' cognitive function.

Energetical Theory Within the Broader Context of Resource Theory

Contemporary theories of conation have common descriptions concerning pathways of human behavior. Humans are assumed to be driven to engage in actions that will permit them to attain goals. The notion of conation and restless behavior activity can be traced historically to early European Gestalt psychologists. Members of this group were influenced by developments in quantum physics and the study of force fields in the early 20th century; they elected to model processes of the brain and human behavior on the notion of interrelated natural forces and events. The assumption that human thought and behavior were dynamic forces diverged greatly from the assumptions of early 20th century American psychologists who fashioned mechanistic theories in terms of Newtonian physics (Hergenhahn, 1992). The theoretic work of Kurt Lewin provided the underpinnings that are central to many contemporary theories of motivation, drive, and energy. Biological and psychological needs, according to Lewin, cause tension, which results in behavioral movement and action. An individual's actions were dictated, however, by valences that either pulled him or her toward the goal or pushed him or her away from the goal. Contemporary field theories address how various factors (e.g., resources) affect an individual as he or she proceeds down a pathway.

Limitations of Energetical Theory

Energetics theories focus only on part of the action pathway. As described in figure 6.3, for instance, Kahneman's (1973) theory focused primarily on moment-to-moment changes that affected an individual's allocation policy. Theories developed by Sanders and Hockey tended to incorporate more of the pathway; they focused on variables that regulate both an individual's preparations to act and changes in her actions during the performance of a task. Other resource theories focus on variables that affect thought

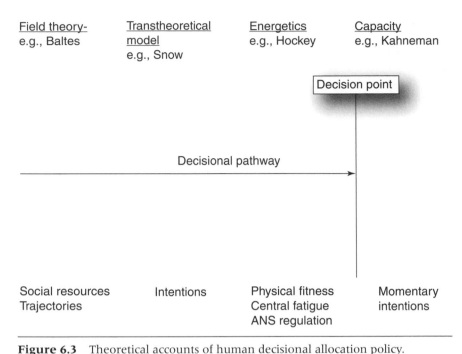

Figure 6.3 Theoretical accounts of human decisional allocation policy.

Reprinted, by permission, from D. Kahneman, 1973, *Attention and effort* (Englewood Cliffs, NJ: Prentice-Hall, Inc.).

and behavior that occur more remotely from a desired goal state than do energetics theory. Snow and Jackson (1994), for instance, examined the contribution of personality variables and intelligence variables on the development of people's wishes, intentions, and actions. Baltes and his colleagues (Baltes, Staudinger, & Lindenberger, 1999; Staudinger, Marsiske, & Baltes, 1993) used a multilevel approach to human development that focuses on gains and losses that accrue within and across functional domains of behavior. The resources drawn upon at these more remote points of the action pathway tend to differ from the resources that are more proximal to the behavioral decision point. Gaillard and Wientjes (1994) pointed out that energetical theories target the effects of such factors as workload, sleep loss, fatigue, drugs, and noise on operational performance, whereas transtheoretical models (e.g., Snow, Baltes) target the effects of such factors as psychosocial factors and health risks on psychological well-being.

Advantages of Energetical Theories

The interrelations among physiological, cognitive, and subjective factors that contribute to human behavior are indeed complex. Nevertheless, progress in understanding conation and the factors that motivate human behavior ultimately depends on multidomain approaches such as those proposed in energetical theory. Constructs such as arousal, stress, and fatigue have been part of the history of psychological research, and energetics theory may advance our understanding of these constructs through the following:

1. Improving methods of objective psychophysiological measurement of such constructs as arousal, stress, workload, and fatigue.

2. Integrating rapidly growing research data pools. Advances are being made in a number of research domains that span from cellular biology to environmental systems.

3. Targeting the impact of individual differences in motivation and human behavior.

Conclusions and Recommendations for Future Research

Energetics theory has been presented here as a conceptual framework for understanding the interrelationship between physiological and psychological resources. The value of theory, however, is determined by the extent to which specific predictions can be verified through experimentation and observation. Historically, energetics theories have been criticized for using terms such as *drive*, *effort*, or *resources* because the constructs were difficult to operationalize and lacked measurement procedures necessary to define the constructs (Hockey et al., 1986). Advances in cognitive neuroscience over the past few decades, however, have provided the means to measure brain systems that are central to cognitive energetics. Recommendations can now be made for empirical research that can offer directs tests of predictions made by cognitive energetic theory.

EDITORS' DISCUSSION SUMMARY

Discussion Highlights

The discussion of this chapter focused on whether researchers ask the correct questions regarding the impact of exercise on cognition. Perhaps one of the failings in the search for an exercise–cognition relationship in earlier research was that the researchers did not use the right task or ask the right questions. True progress in understanding the relationship between physical activity and energetical states will come about through systematic theory-based research. Much of the early research in the study of exercise and cognition was atheoretical. Most of these studies used test batteries designed to assess global indexes of mental functioning. Furthermore, exercise interventions varied considerably among research studies. Thus, the results obtained from early research studies were difficult to interpret. Advances in cognitive neuroscience have provided contemporary researchers a unique opportunity to evaluate the interrelationships among brain systems, behavior, and subjective reports. Advances in cognitive theory development are leading researchers to posit specific hypotheses concerning the impact of physical activity on older adults' cognitive function. It may be the case that physical activity affects only a subset of mental processes; however, this subset of mental processes may be critical for successful aging.

For example, now there is intriguing literature that associates activation of the anterior cingulate region with effort on mental tasks, in conjunction with literature that associates anterior cingulate activation with the distribution of mental resources that are recruited to accomplish a task. Some of these studies have shown that after frontal head injury, brain regions are activated during tasks such as letter cancellation, but it is a different pattern of activation than you see in persons who have not had brain trauma, although the performance may be the same. After the head injury, more parts of the brain are recruited to accomplish the task. Even more interesting, the anterior cingulate's metabolism is related to which parts are recruited. Some researchers have shown that the anterior cingulate is activated temporally when the new area is recruited, so the anterior cingulate fires and then one region is activated, followed by activation of the anterior cingulate again, followed by activation of another area. In old age the pattern of activation that is observed looks very much like frontal head injury. In other words, older people actively recruit more parts of the brain to accomplish these tasks. Their performance is not different necessarily, but the pattern of activation is different and the anterior cingulate's activity is related to their subjective reports of effort. So the concept that old people apply more energy to accomplish a task that they think is important actually has an imitable correlate.

How might recent findings apply to exercise and cognitive function? It has long been thought that environmental experiences and challenges might alter brain structures in ways that would enhance adaptive functioning. Recent advances in life span developmental neuropsychology provide evidence to suggest that chronic physical activity has an impact on the structure and functions of the central nervous system. It is clear that the neurological circuitry that underlies cognitive function is malleable. An examination of the processes that are involved in cognitive rehabilitation following brain injury may help us to understand how physiological systems come to be reorganized and lead to the allocation of mental resources. Brain mapping techniques such as quantitative electroencephalography, positron emission tomography, and functional magnetic resonance imaging have been used to evaluate changes that occur during recovery from brain trauma. Similar approaches could be used to assess changes in brain functions that accompany exercise training.

Research Methodological Problems

Two methodological challenges were noted. One, the challenge for researchers who explore the construct of energetics will be to conduct well-controlled experiments to evaluate the covariation of multiple measures that are obtained while an individual is performing a challenging task. Hockey et al.'s regulatory control model (1996) provides a broad framework for analysis of performance changes under workload demands. An individual's regulation of his or her mental and physical effort is required as task demands increase. Maintenance of task performance requires the selection of compensatory strategies. Although compensatory strategies may result in the maintenance of task performance, it comes at a cost to the individual and a latent degradation of energetical resources.

Two, empirical research is needed that directly tests predictions made by cognitive energetic theory. Advances in cognitive neuroscience over the past few decades have provided the means to measure brain systems that are central to cognitive energetics.

Future Directions

Six fruitful research directions were discussed. One, researchers should find a way to integrate subjective reports of workload derived from valid instruments into theory development. Subjective reports (e.g., arousal, fatigue, or effort) provide insight into general underlying state of awareness.

Two, an important thrust of the future will be evaluating the impact of moderators and mediators (e.g., physical activity, drugs, aging) on resource utilization.

Three, greatly needed are techniques to assess individual differences in resource utilization. The critical test of any theory is the degree to which it can account for variability in human performance (Underwood, 1975).

Four, the assumption that physiological processes play an important role in the overall regulation of human information processing needs to be tested. Theory development is now at a point where physiological principles can provide some useful constraints for cognitive theory.

Five, brain structures and their functions must be mapped onto specific cognitive processes. It would be expected that select measures of brain processes would be related to performance of specific cognitive tasks.

Six, the assumption that objective test performance measurements provide indexes of energetical states must be tested. Laboratory-based tests designed to measure reaction time, error rates, and response variability can be used to describe changes within specific components of the information-processing system.

CHAPTER 7

Exercise and Mental Resources: Methodological Problems

Timothy A. Salthouse, PhD, Moderator and Discussion Leader
University of Virginia

EDITORS' OVERVIEW

Dr. Salthouse served as a consultant on cognition throughout the Advanced Research Workshop. This chapter is a summary of his reactions to the papers and discussions of the morning session, which was titled *Exercise Effects on Mental Resources and Reserves*.

The first few paragraphs in the discussion focus on issues that he suggested all researchers interested in this topic should heed. This is followed by a synthesis of the group discussion about the global topics of mental resources, exercise, and cognition.

The papers and discussions of exercise and mental resources have been very interesting, but one observation I would like to make is that in our discussions, we have all acted as though our brains work perfectly for most of our lives and then suddenly at age 60 there is a dramatic decline. In reality, age-related deficits begin very early and continue throughout most of adulthood. These trends are apparent in many studies using convenience samples, such as those in my laboratory, but are also apparent in different measures of fluid intelligence obtained from nationally representative samples used as norms for a variety of different cognitive test batteries such as the Wechsler, Woodcock–Johnson, and Kaufman test batteries. In fact, if the scores are expressed in terms of proportion of the maximum, it is apparent that half or more of the decline from the peak level of performance has already occurred by age 60, a fact that should be considered when we design interventions to prevent cognitive decline.

Aging is a continuous process. It starts at about age 18, not age 65, and much of the cognitive decrement that researchers are interested in has already occurred by the time their subjects are 65.

What Do We Mean by Cognition?

Another issue that strikes me as very important is what we mean by cognition. We can look at this from two different perspectives. The first of these is that many people focus on a single variable and use that single variable as though it exhaustively and exclusively represents a particular theoretical construct. For example, clinicians who focus primarily on older adults might use the Mini-Mental Status Examination, the EXIT25 test, or the CLOX test. However, these instruments tend to have a lot of measurement error, and they tend to be influenced by many different factors. One solution to this problem is to focus on the variance that several variables share and see whether the intervention (exercise, in this case) has an effect at that level. Relying on subjective categorizations of the variables will always result in different investigators producing different results. We have to have some empirical basis for categorizing variables.

Using higher-order cognition factors derived from factor analyses would allow the effects of exercise, age, or any other variable to be studied in terms of its effects on different levels in this hierarchy. Of all the levels in this type of cognitive hierarchy, the *least* informative is at the level of the observed variable, because it is a weaker relationship attributable to the specific unique variances associated with the methods, the materials, the context, and the measures of that particular variable.

The use of only one or two indicators of cognition has been a shortcoming of most large-scale population studies. Because of the large number of variables being measured, many times over the telephone or via one-shot interviews, the investigators want an assessment of cognition that takes only a few minutes, because they only have limited time with each subject. Thus, huge compromises in research measurements are made. But progress will be slow on this research question until we insist on multiple indicators of cognition.

What Is Executive Function?

In recent years it has become popular to use the term *executive function* in place of terms such as *controlled cognition* or *resource demanding cognition*. I'd like to briefly describe a study that we conducted recently where we questioned whether there is meaningful covariation among variables that are purported to represent executive function. That is, is executive function distinct from existing cognitive ability constructs? All the subjects in our study were administered all the tests to establish reference abilities, and then we used two different approaches to assess cognitive functioning, or executive functioning. The first approach used a neuropsychological perspective using very familiar types of tests such as the Wisconsin Card Sorting Test, the Tower of Hanoi test, the difference between Trail Making Parts A and B, and some tests of verbal fluency and figure fluency. The goal in one of our sets of analyses was to see whether those variables hang together and if so how they differ from these other constructs.

Another perspective on executive functioning emphasizes executive control processes from the cognitive psychology perspective. We investigated aspects of executive control related to updating (or working memory), time sharing, and inhibition of prepotent responses. What amazed me is that when we analyzed the relationships of these measures of executive function to other cognitive variables, the executive functioning construct from the neuropsychological perspective correlated .94 with a construct representing fluid intelligence. This means that essentially the same dimension of individual differences is captured by quite different types of tests, and thus we have to be careful about using a term such as *executive functioning* as though it represents something that is really distinct from other dimensions of cognitive functioning that we have known about for a long time.

Now I have a question that I would like to raise with all of you. In the study that I just described, we also administered a questionnaire in which we asked people to list their physical activities and their leisure activities and to rate the frequency, intensity, and duration of them so that we could estimate the subjects' metabolic expenditures per month. We also believed that it is very desirable in this kind of study to have a wide age range to see whether the age-related effects or the exercise interventions are just parallel or are differential. One of you suggested that they were differential, which would be more consistent with sedentariness contributing to some of the age-related declines. But the answer to that requires having a wider age range and a long-term follow-up to see what happens after the intervention. We expect to have an immediate short-term effect, but the real question is what happens after that. Does the intervention change the person's lifestyle?

I used a measure of physical activity based on a questionnaire about physical activity, and we found that this measure was unrelated to any of our cognitive constructs. This seems to be inconsistent with the idea that there is a relationship in cross-sectional data, and we also did not find any evidence of moderating relationships. I would therefore welcome any suggestions for why we did not find a relationship between physical activity and cognition.

EDITORS' DISCUSSION SUMMARY

The first response that immediately comes to mind is the well-known observation that most subjects' ability to recall their physical activities is poor. Some people are very regimented and can remember or reconstruct from their calendars over a considerable time period in the past, whereas most individuals are not able to do this. Self-report, unless it is scrupulously monitored, is notoriously unreliable. Older subjects are usually not as familiar with exercise or physical activity testing as younger people are and have to be provided explicit instructions on how to respond on a self-report form. The interviewer has to be very skilled and attentive to acquire accurate data. But a much more complicated and difficult problem for everyone, and probably for you in your study, is the issue of quantifying physical activity.

What Do We Mean by Physical Activity?

In your study described previously you used multiple indicators and higher-order factors to quantify cognition but only one self-report scale to assess physical activity. The entire field of researchers who study the relationship of physical activity to any other variable set is hampered by the ambiguity and variation of definitions of physical activity. What do we mean by physical activity? Do we mean any type of physical activity? Do we mean exercise? How much physical activity is necessary to improve or maintain cognitive function? Are individual differences in responses to exercise important? Do individuals respond to different types of exercise differentially?

What Is the Best Measure of Physical Activity?

Is $\dot{V}O_2$max the best measure of physical activity or exercise? This has been used many times, but Dr. Etnier suggested in chapter 2 that levels of $\dot{V}O_2$ are not related to levels of cognition. Many researchers now are reporting that it really does not take very high intensity exercise or activity levels to make a significant difference in variables such as self-efficacy, well-being, or some cognitive functions. Several have reported that little additional effect is gained by increasing work intensity above 40% or 50% of $\dot{V}O_2$max. A corollary observation was made many years ago in a study of cerebral blood flow changes and work intensity in humans. Cerebral blood flow increased with supine pedaling up to 40% of $\dot{V}O_2$max, but blood flow increases reached a plateau above that workload. So it may not be surprising that $\dot{V}O_2$max is not linearly correlated or related to cognitive function improvements in older adults. There may be, however, some type of threshold improvement that is necessary before cognitive gains can be observed. These are important questions that need to be answered.

Many investigators use the length of time that an individual is physically active, but the physical activity of an 18- or 20-year-old is not at the same intensity as that of a 65-year-old. Asking subjects how long they were active only provides an absolute measure, not one that is relative to each individual's maximum capacity. In other words, an absolute activity level of 5 metabolic equivalents (METs) might be a considerable stress for a 65-year-old, whereas 5 METs of activity might produce almost no stress for a 20-year-old. Therefore, if young and old individuals self-report equal activity time, these times do not represent the same relative stress. If duration and frequency of physical activity are quantified, they should probably be relative to an individual's estimated maximum capacity.

Are Some Individuals More Responsive to Increases in Physical Activity or Exercise?

It is possible that some subgroups of the population may be more likely to benefit from physical activity than others. People who are living with chronic disease, those who appear to be biologically older, or those who have lifestyle behaviors that are associated with biologically older or younger persons might be appropriate subgroups with which to study this issue. For example, diabetics look and behave physiologically very much like people 10 years older than they are chronologically. Other subgroups that might provide useful information would be those with comorbidities, or at the other end of the continuum, health and exercise fanatics. A potential model of this type of investigation would be studies in which researchers recorded and analyzed the waxing and waning planes of insomnia and sleep disturbance and found that insomnia essentially appeared or disappeared with the increase or decrease in medical burden experienced by the person. Findings such as this emphasize the interactions of sleep and potential medical burden and could be identified better in a subgroup of insomniacs than in those whose sleep difficulties did not approach pathological insomnia. Long-term study of cognitive function in special populations undergoing exercise programs that followed this type of model might be very instructive.

Another possibility would be to study the physical activity of subgroups based on cognitive activity. The physical activity–cognition relationship might be better clarified by comparing groups who were homogeneous in their cognitive activities (i.e., mentally active: those who write or work crossword puzzles, versus mentally passive: those who watch TV or listen to the radio) but who differ in their physical activity. If physical activity affects brain neurosubstrate, it might be more visible if variability in cognitive activity (active vs. passive), which would also affect neurosubstrate, could be reduced.

Clustering these different individuals with different types of outcomes and risk factors and analyzing their responses to physical activity might lead to a better isolation of the effects of exercise and, ultimately, better understanding of its effects on cognition. Positive results from studies like these would also provide a rationale for targeting some individuals more than others for exercise intervention.

Some of this clustering strategy is already happening with genotyping. Some investigators are suggesting that physical activity is very beneficial for people who carry the genotype ApoE-4 but has relatively little effect on people who are noncarriers. The implication is that the ApoE-4 factor creates variance that is unaccounted for in most studies of physical activity and cognition. If we studied only a group of ApoE-4 carriers (who have many negative health outcomes), we might find a big exercise effect. Individual differences in exercise responses have been shown in many other variables, such as blood pressure, $\dot{V}O_2$max, and muscular endurance changes. It is possible that some earlier failures to find beneficial effects on cognition from exercise interventions could be attributed to the nature of the samples that we select.

In fact, if considering individual differences in *physiological* responses to physical activity would clarify the exercise and cognition link, we should also consider the individuality and uniqueness of different people's *psychological* responses to exercise. Some people respond to stress aggressively, but they have had to learn to suppress this aggression. Other people respond to stress in a different way, maybe very quietly. People might be grouped by these different responses and undergo exercise programs specifically designed for them. The more aggressive people might respond to karate or some other combatant activity. The less aggressive ones who are more suppressive might respond to a more rhythmic physical activity, such as jogging or rowing. Physical activity programs could be tailor-made for groups of individuals differing in some personality variables. This way all experimental groups would have a positive exercise response from everyone in the exercise groups, rather than having half of the exercise group not responding to the intervention because it does not suit them. Perhaps a major reason why some exercise intervention studies do not have beneficial effects on cognition is that, depending on the way researchers obtain their samples, different proportions of the intervention groups are receiving different doses of exercise.

What Types of Research Designs Are Appropriate?

Another important issue is the type of study designs that we should use. Some of you have recommended structural linear equation modeling, using multiple first-order constructs so that we can get to second- or third-order constructs to model. That method has some constraints, one of which is that it requires 6 to 8 h of the subject's and the researcher's time. The reality is that when we are conducting a repeated-measures intervention study over time, this strategy is not practical at all. One possible way to simplify this issue might be to abandon trying to analyze the full model that we have been thinking about and turn to submodels. We might factor analyze different clusters of people and then in detail, in terms of the physical exercise, fitness, and cognition dimension, group them into different clusters and determine what similarities and differences would differentiate each cluster. Perhaps this may be a backdoor way of answering some of these questions.

In summary, many questions remain unanswered concerning the nature, extent, and time course of the relationship between physical activity and cognitive functioning across the life span. It is clear that to answer these questions, significant additional research is needed. Future research needs to include more careful assessment and evaluation of both the exercise and cognition constructs than have occurred in most research studies. Recent advances in brain imaging and genetic analysis have the potential to provide provocative new insights into these important relationships.

Implications for Public Policy

Dr. Salthouse made a plea in his opening statements for researchers to study cognitive decline at several different points in the aging cognitive trajectory rather than measure just the differences between 20-year-old and 65-year-old adults. He pointed out that a very large amount of decline in cognition has already occurred by age 65. Rather, we must identify the shape of the aging decline trajectory so that interventions can be developed to flatten that trajectory, or maintain cognition for a much longer time. This suggests that for physical activity to be effective in preserving cognitive functioning, activity should be integrated into everyday life throughout the life span and not simply initiated upon reaching old age. This perspective is consistent with recent findings from other areas of preventive medicine strongly suggesting that to prevent the development of chronic conditions, physical activity must be undertaken at all stages of the life span.

PART III

Exercise and Physical Resources and Reserves Influencing Cognition

CHAPTER 8

Diet, Motor Behavior, and Cognition

James Joseph, PhD
Tufts University

EDITORS' OVERVIEW

Oxidative stress and inflammation are contributing factors to the behavioral decrements seen in aging. A major focus of Dr. Joseph's research is concerned with the possible benefits of dietary supplementation of antioxidants and anti-inflammatories in reducing the deleterious effects of reactive oxygen species (ROS) and inflammation when their levels overwhelm the organism's defense capacities and damage cellular macromolecules such as lipids, proteins, and DNA.

In this chapter, Dr. Joseph provides evidence that the combinations of antioxidant and anti-inflammatory polyphenolics found in fruits and vegetables, which are particularly concentrated in blueberries, may postpone cognitive aging. Indeed, in supplementation studies, Joseph and others (Joseph et al., 1999; Youdim, Shukitt-Hale, et al., 2000) found that the significant effects of blueberries on both motor and cognitive behavior were attributable to many actions, in addition to those involving antioxidant and anti-inflammatory activity. Thus, it may be possible to reverse or forestall the motor behavior deficits in aging via diets containing combinations of antioxidants such as those found in

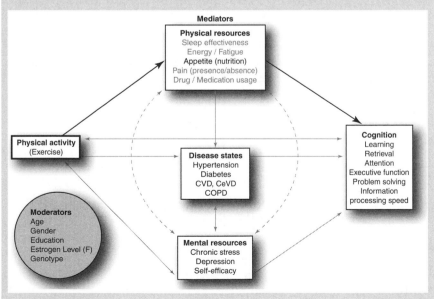

blueberries. Dr. Joseph suggests additional mechanisms involved in these effects that he and his colleagues are pursuing. He proposes that these mechanisms may involve direct or indirect effects on cell signaling, particularly with respect to mitogen-activated protein kinase (MAPK) (e.g., extracellular signal-related kinase [ERK]) activation, striatal carbachol-stimulated guanosine triphosphatase (GTPase), and various isoforms of protein kinase.

As the U.S. population continues to age, there will be increases in age-associated diseases (e.g., cancer, cardiovascular disease) including the most devastating of these that involve the nervous system (e.g., Alzheimer's and Parkinson's diseases). By the year 2050, 30% of the total population will be older than 65 years, and there is a high probability that they will be exhibiting the most common correlative motor and cognitive behavioral changes that occur in aging. Notably, these changes occur even in the absence of specific age-related neurodegenerative diseases but could interact to exacerbate the behavioral aberrations exhibited in these conditions, especially by providing a suitable environment for the development of these conditions. In these cases, and possibly as a function of normal aging as well, it is likely that in cases of severe deficits in memory or motor function, hospitalization or custodial care would be a likely outcome. This means that unless some means are found to reduce these age-related decrements in neuronal function, health care costs will continue to rise exponentially, especially as the baby boomers reach senior citizen status. Thus, in both financial and human terms, it is extremely important to explore methods to retard or reverse the age-related neuronal deficits as well as their subsequent behavioral manifestations. In this review I describe motor and cognitive deficits and behavior, show how these deficits are related to increased vulnerability to oxidative stress and inflammation, and describe the possible role of nutritional supplementation with antioxidants in reversing or forestalling these deficits.

Aging and Cognitive and Motor Deficits

Aging is associated with both cognitive and motor deficits, which are expressed behaviorally. Two major mechanisms that are involved in these deficits are oxidative stress and inflammatory events. These are discussed below, with the final section discussing the interactions among oxidative stress and inflammatory event responses and behavior.

Behavioral Decrements

A plethora of research indicates the occurrence of numerous neuronal and behavioral deficits during aging, even in the absence of neurodegenerative disease. These changes may include decrements in calcium homeostasis (Landfield & Eldridge, 1994) and in the sensitivity of several receptor systems, most notably (a) adrenergic (Gould & Bickford, 1997), (b) dopaminergic (Joseph, Berger, Engel, & Roth, 1978; Levine & Cepeda, 1998), (c) muscarinic (Egashira, Takayama, & Yamanaka, 1996; Joseph, Kowatch, Maki, & Roth, 1990), and (d) opioid (Kornhuber, Schoppmeyer, Bendig, & Riederer, 1996). These decrements can be expressed, ultimately, as alterations in both motor (Joseph et al., 1983; Kluger et al., 1997) and cognitive behaviors (Bartus, 1990). The alterations in motor function may include decreases in balance, muscle strength, and coordination (Joseph et al., 1983), whereas memory deficits are seen on cognitive tasks that require the use of spatial learning and memory (Ingram, Jucker, & Spangler, 1994; Shukitt-Hale, Mouzakis, & Joseph, 1998). Indeed, these characterizations have been supported by a great deal of research in both animals (Bartus, 1990; Ingram et al., 1994; Shukitt-Hale, Mouzakis, & Joseph, 1998) and humans (Muir, 1997; West, 1996). Age-related deficits in motor performance are thought to be the result of alterations in the striatal dopamine (DA) system, because the striatum shows marked neurodegenerative changes with age (Joseph, 1992), or in the cerebellum, which also shows age-related alterations (Bickford, 1993; Bickford, Heron, Young, Gerhardt, & De La Garza, 1992). Memory alterations appear to occur primarily in secondary memory systems and are reflected in the storage of newly acquired information (Bartus, Dean, Beer, & Lippa, 1982; Joseph, 1992). It is thought that the hippocampus mediates allocentric spatial navigation (i.e., place learning) and that the prefrontal cortex is critical to acquiring the rules that govern performance in particular tasks (i.e., procedural knowledge), whereas the dorsomedial striatum mediates egocentric spatial orientation (i.e., response and cue learning; Devan, Goad, & Petri, 1996; McDonald and White, 1994; Oliveira, Bueno, Pomarico, & Gugliano, 1997; Zyzak, Otto, Eichenbaum, & Gallagher, 1995). It appears that oxidative stress (Shukitt-Hale, 1999) and inflammation (Hauss-Wegrzyniak, Vannucchi, & Wenk, 2000; Hauss-Wegrzyniak, Vraniak, & Wenk, 1999) are contributing factors to the behavioral decrements seen in aging.

In animal models of aging, motor function is measured by using a battery of different psychomotor tests, whereas cognitive function is usually measured in a maze. Maze procedures can be used to assess learning (acquisition) and memory functions, the latter of which include working (short-term) and reference (long-term) memory. Reference memory is believed to reflect learning the trial-independent procedural aspects of the task (spatial cue locations), that is, information that is relevant for many trials, often for the entire experiment (Frick, Baxter, Markowska, Olton, & Price, 1995; Luine, Richards, Wu, & Beck, 1998). Reference memory is consistent from trial to trial and is required to learn the general rules of any task (e.g., swim to a platform; Frick et al., 1995). In contrast, working memory is trial dependent and describes the ability of the subject to hold this trial-dependent information (places previously visited) in memory (Frick et al., 1995; Luine et al., 1998). Working memory involves the retention of trial-specific or trial-unique information for short periods of time, and it is necessary to remember both the type of stimulus presented and the time of stimulus presentation (Frick et al., 1995). Maze procedures that have been developed to measure working memory include within-trial reentries in the radial arm maze (RAM) or the radial arm water maze (RAWM), alternation in the Y-maze, and delayed matching-to-position in the Morris water maze (MWM). Reference memory is memory for the learned aspects of the task, such as knowing that the object is to find the platform in the MWM (measured as latency to find the platform when the platform remains stationary over trials) or to obtain the food reward by visiting each arm only once in the RAM. Old rats have previously been shown to have decrements in both reference and working memory in the MWM (for review, see Brandeis, Brandys, & Yehuda, 1989; Ingram et al., 1994; Shukitt-Hale, 1999), RAM (for review, see Ingram et al., 1994), and RAWM (Shukitt-Hale, McEwen, Szprengiel, & Joseph, 2004).

Oxidative Stress

A major focus of our research is concerned with the possible beneficial effects of dietary supplementation of antioxidants and anti-inflammatories in reducing the deleterious effects of reactive oxygen species (ROS) and inflammation when their levels overwhelm the organism's defense capacities and damage cellular macromolecules such as lipids, proteins, and DNA. Data are accumulating to suggest that one of the most important factors mediating the deleterious effects of aging on behavior and neuronal function is oxidative stress (OS) (see Floyd, 1999, for review). The central nervous system (CNS) appears to be especially vulnerable to OS effects, partially as a result of additional factors such as increases in the ratio of oxidized to total glutathione (Olanow, 1992), significant lipofuscin accumulation (Gilissen, Jacobs, & Allman, 1999) with bcl-2 increases (Sadoul, 1998), increases in membrane lipid peroxidation (Yu, 1994), reduced glutamine synthetase (Carney, Smith, Carney, & Butterfield, 1994), reductions in redox active iron (Gilissen et al., 1999; Savory, Rao, Huang, Letada, & Herman, 1999), and alterations in membrane lipids (Denisova, Erat, Kelly, & Roth, 1998). In addition to these considerations, it has been shown that not only is the CNS particularly vulnerable to OS but this vulnerability increases during aging (see Joseph, Denisova, Fisher, Bickford, et al., 1998; Joseph, Denisova, Fisher, Shukitt-Hale, et al., 1998 for review). With respect to aging, we (Cantuti-Castelvetri, Shukitt-Hale, & Joseph, 2003) have shown that senescent rats exhibited significantly greater motor behavioral deficits and reduced tyrosine hydroxylase immunoreactivity (in pars compacta) than young rats following intranigral applications of DA. Research has also shown that besides the factors discussed previously (e.g., reductions in glutathione levels; Olanow, 1992), OS vulnerability in aging may be the result of three additional factors: alterations in the membrane microenvironment, alterations in calcium buffering ability, and differential vulnerability of neurotransmitter receptors. The latter two of these are discussed in more detail in a later section, but in the case of membranes and aging, indications are that age-related changes in the neuronal plasma membrane molecular structure and physical properties (e.g., increased rigidity) may increase vulnerability to oxidative stress and inflammation (Joseph, Denisova, Fisher, Bickford, et al., 1998; Joseph et al., 2001).

Calcium buffering has been shown to be significantly reduced in senescence (Joseph et al., 1999; Landfield & Eldridge, 1994). The consequences of such long-lasting increases in cytosolic calcium may involve cell death induced by several mechanisms (e.g., xanthine oxidase activation; Cheng, Wixom, James-Kracke, & Sun, 1994) with subsequent pro-oxidant generation and loss of functional capacity of the cell. However, we have demonstrated that blueberry (BB) supplementations may, in fact, increase hippocampal and striatal calcium[45] buffering capacities following KCl-induced depolarization in synaptosomes derived from these areas. Therefore, it will be of extreme importance, mechanistically, to determine if the polyphenolics found in the various brain regions in the BB-supplemented rats will have similar effects on calcium[45] flux.

Inflammation

Recent evidence also suggests that, as I discussed previously with respect to OS, inflammatory events in the central nervous system play an important role in aging. For example, by middle age there is an increased glial fibrillary acid protein expression (Rozovsky, Finch, & Morgan, 1998) that later, in the elderly, even occurs in the absence of an inflammatory stimulus (McGeer & McGeer, 1995). In conjunction with this observation, it has also been reported that tumor necrosis factor (TNF)-α is produced in higher amounts during cytotoxic reactions in the elderly (Chang et al., 1996) and that neuronal inhibition of glial activities may be lost during aging (Chang et al., 2001). Other studies have reported increases in TNF-α and interleukin (IL)-6 in the sera of aged mice and humans (Spaulding, Walford, & Effros, 1997; Volpato et al., 2001). In fact, it has been suggested that the up-regulation of C-reactive protein may be one factor in biological aging (Kushner, 2001).

There may be important interactions of ROS-generating agents and cytokines. For example, ROS-independent activation of nuclear factor-κB by IL-1β in epithelial cells appears to involve the acidic sphingomyelinase–ceramide transduction pathway (Piette et al., 1997). There is also evidence for flavoenzyme-generated ROS in the induction of c-*fos* and collagenase expression by IL-1 in chondrocytes (Lo, Conquer, Grinstein, & Cruz, 1998). In fact, most growth factors and cytokines appear to generate ROS at or near the plasma membrane.

Also paralleling the results seen with respect to oxidative stress are increases in sensitivity to inflammatory mediators with aging. For example, Manev and Uz (1999) showed that old rats were more sensitive to kainate-induced excitotoxic brain injuries and enhanced 5-lipoxygenase expression in limbic structures. The results of such increases in inflammatory reactions involving such factors as cytokines, complement proteins, and adhesion molecules may be extracellular signals that act in concert with OS to initiate decrements in neuronal function or glial neuronal interactions (Rosenman, Shrikant, Dubb, Benveniste, & Ransohoff, 1995; Schipper, 1996; Steffen, Breier, Butcher, Schulz, & Engelhardt, 1996; Stella et al., 1997; Woodroofe, 1995). Thus, it appears that the increases in sensitivity that are seen with respect to OS and inflammation in senescence and as discussed subsequently may play a role in mediating the deficits in behavior that have been observed in aging.

Behavior, Oxidative Stress, and Inflammation

As I pointed out previously, several decrements are seen in behavior as a function of aging. Interestingly, there are changes in behavior with increases in oxidative stress and inflammation that parallel those seen in aging (for review, see Hauss-Wegrzyniak et al., 2000; Hauss-Wegrzyniak, Vraniak, & Wenk, 1999; Shukitt-Hale, 1999). In this respect, we have shown that exposing young rats to radiation particles of high energy and charge (high-ionizing high energy [HZE] particles) disrupts the functioning of the dopaminergic system and dopamine-mediated behaviors, similar to the adverse behavioral and neuronal effects seen in aged animals (Joseph, Erat, & Rabin, 1998; Joseph, Shukitt-Hale, McEwen, & Rabin, 2000). In one set of these experiments, we showed that whole-body exposure of rats to HZE particles, primarily 600 MeV (millions of electron volts) or 1 GeV ^{56}Fe (Giga-electron volts), impairs motor behavior (Joseph, Hunt, Rabin, & Dalton, 1992), spatial learning and memory behavior (Shukitt-Hale, Casadesus, McEwen, Rabin, & Joseph, 2000), and amphetamine-induced conditioned taste aversion (Rabin, Joseph, & Erat, 1998). Associated with these findings were deficits in oxotremorine-enhancement of K^+-evoked DA release and carbachol stimulated GTPase activity that paralleled those seen in aging (Joseph et al., 2000) and that are dependent on the integrity of the central dopaminergic system (Rabin, Joseph, Shukitt-Hale, & McEwen, 2000). Therefore, the deficits induced by radiation are similar to those that occur during aging, are associated with free radical damage, and support the hypothesis that these changes may share a common chemical or biological mechanism (Joseph et al., 1992). Another model used to produce oxidative stress involves exposing young rats to a normobaric hyperoxia environment of 100% oxygen at 760 mmHg (sea-level pressure). We have shown that motor function, as measured by accelerating RotaRod, wire suspension, small rod walk, and large rod walk, is impaired following 48 h of 100% oxygen (Shukitt-Hale, 1999), as is cerebellar β-adrenergic and striatal muscarinic receptor functioning (Bickford et al., 1999). Again, these effects are similar to those seen in aging. An additional treatment that also produces OS similar to that seen in aged rats involves decreasing OS protection by administering a glutathione-depleting drug, buthionine sulfoximine (BSO), and then increasing the OS with an injection of DA. BSO given before DA administration selectively impaired psychomotor (rod walking, wire suspension, and plank walking; Shukitt-Hale, Denisova, Strain, & Joseph, 1997) and cognitive performance (spatial learning and memory measured by the Morris water maze; Shukitt-Hale, Erat, & Joseph, 1998); however, in the reverse condition (DA + BSO), no decrements in performance were observed relative to vehicle administration. Additionally, neither BSO alone nor DA alone had detrimental effects on behavior. Therefore, decreasing OS protection with BSO and then increasing the OS with DA injections lowered protection, produced OS, and altered behavioral performance in rats, similar to that seen in aging.

In the case of inflammation, increases in inflammatory mediators (e.g., cytokines) known to be involved in the activation of glia cells and perivascular–parenchymal macrophages, as well as increased mobilization and infiltration of peripheral inflammatory cells into the brain, have also been shown to produce deficits in behavior similar to those observed during aging (Hauss-Wegrzyniak et al., 2000). One model to induce neuronal inflammation is via central administration of lipopolysaccharide (LPS), a bacterial toxin that is a potent inflammatory agent. Previous studies (Hauss-Wegrzyniak et al., 2000; Hauss-Wegrzyniak, Dobrzanski, Stoehr, & Wenk, 1998; Hauss-Wegrzyniak, Vraniak, & Wenk, 1999; Hauss-Wegrzyniak, Willard, Del Soldato, Pepeu, & Wenk, 1999; Yamada et al., 1999) showed that chronic (28-37 days) infusion of LPS into the ventricle of young rats can reproduce many of the behavioral, inflammatory, neurochemical, and neuropathological changes seen in the brains of Alzheimer's disease patients in some similar regions (e.g., cingulate cortex) as well as produce changes in spatial learning and memory behavior (Hauss-Wegrzyniak et al., 1998; Hauss-Wegrzyniak et al., 2000; Hauss-Wegrzyniak, Vraniak, & Wenk, 1999; Yamada et al., 1999). These changes include, but are not limited to, increased activated astrocytes; increased number and density of activated microglia, particularly within the hippocampus, cingulate cortex, and basal forebrain; increased levels of cytokines; degeneration of hippocampal pyramidal neurons; and an impairment in working memory (Hauss-Wegrzyniak et al., 1998; Hauss-Wegrzyniak et al., 2000;

Hauss-Wegrzyniak, Vraniak, & Wenk, 1999; Hauss-Wegrzyniak, Willard, et al., 1999). Use of a chronic injection directly into the brain restricts the inflammation-induced changes to the CNS; the rats do not develop fever, and plasma cytokine levels are not elevated (Hauss-Wegrzyniak, Vraniak, & Wenk, 1999). It has been shown that nonsteroidal anti-inflammatory drugs (NSAIDs) can attenuate the neuroinflammatory reaction and reduce the inflammation-induced memory deficit associated with this model. However, it was also shown that the effects of NSAIDs are age dependent; that is, daily peripheral administration of an NSAID significantly attenuated the memory deficit produced by chronic LPS in young (3 months) rats and reduced the degree of inflammation in both young and adult rats (9 months) but did not improve water maze performance in either adult or old (23 months) rats (Hauss-Wegrzyniak, Vraniak, & Wenk, 1999).

Fruit and Vegetable Supplementation— Why Blueberries?

Numerous studies have examined antioxidants with respect to reducing the deleterious effects of brain aging, with mixed results (discussed subsequently). However, our research (also discussed subsequently) suggests that the combinations of antioxidant and anti-inflammatory polyphenolics found in fruits and vegetables may show efficacy in aging. Plants, including food plants (fruits and vegetables), synthesize a vast array of chemical compounds that are not involved in their primary metabolism. These secondary compounds instead serve a variety of ecological functions, ultimately to enhance the plant's survivability. Interestingly, these compounds may be responsible for the multitude of beneficial effects of fruits and vegetables on an array of health-related bioactivities, two of the most important of which may be their antioxidant and anti-inflammatory properties. Because OS appears to be involved in the signaling and behavioral losses seen in senescence, an important question is whether increasing antioxidant intake would forestall or prevent these changes. The literature is replete with studies that have used a large variety of dietary agents to alter behavioral and neuronal deficits with aging. These studies have included such nutritional supplements as vitamin C or E, garlic (Youdim & Joseph, 2001), herbals (e.g., ginseng, ginkgo biloba, ding lang; see Cantuti-Castelvetri, Shukitt-Hale, & Joseph, 2000), and dietary fatty acids (reviewed by Youdim, Martin, & Joseph, 2000).

As alluded to previously, we believed that given the considerable antioxidant and anti-inflammatory potential of fruits and vegetables, they might show considerable efficacy in reducing the deleterious effects of aging. In our first study we used fruits and vegetables identified as being high in antioxidant activity via the oxygen radical absorbance capacity assay (ORAC; Cao, Sofic, & Prior, 1996; Prior et al., 1998; Wang, Cao, & Prior, 1996) and showed that long-term (from 6 to 15 months of age; F344 rats) feeding with a supplemented AIN-93 diet (strawberry extract or spinach extract [1-2% of the diet] or vitamin E [500 IU]) retarded age-related decrements in cognitive or neuronal function. Results indicated that the supplemented diets could prevent the onset of age-related deficits on several indexes (e.g., cognitive behavior, Morris water maze performance; Joseph, Shukitt-Hale, et al., 1998).

In a subsequent experiment (Joseph et al., 1999) we found that dietary supplementation (for 8 weeks) with spinach, strawberry, or BB extracts in an AIN-93 diet was effective in reversing age-related deficits in neuronal and behavioral (cognitive) function in aged (19 months) F344 rats. However, only the BB-supplemented group exhibited improved performance on tests of motor function. Specifically, the BB-supplemented group displayed improved performance on two motor tests that rely on balance and coordination, rod walking and the accelerating RotaRod, whereas none of the other supplemented groups differed from control on these tasks. Note that the beneficial effects of BB on motor performance seen in rodents have also been observed in aged humans (mean age 65). Preliminary results from a study in which reaction speed was examined in response to a stimulus indicated that as the daily intake of blueberries was increased from 0 to 2 cups per day over 12 weeks, the BB-supplemented group significantly reduced their reaction time by 6% (unpublished data).

In the study by Joseph and colleagues (1999), the rodents in all diet groups, but not the control group, showed improved working memory (short-term memory) performance in the Morris water maze, demonstrated as one-trial learning following the 10 min retention interval. We also observed significant increases in several indexes of neuronal signaling (e.g., muscarinic acetylcholine receptors sensitivity) and found that BB diet reversed age-related dysregulation in Ca^{45} buffering capacity. Examinations of ROS production in the brain tissue obtained from animals in the various diet groups indicated that the striata obtained from all of the supplemented groups exhibited significantly less ROS levels (by assaying 2',7'-dichlorofluorescein diacetate) than the controls. A subsequent study using a BB-supplemented NIH-31 diet replicated the previous findings (Youdim, Shukitt-Hale, et al., 2000). However, it was clear from these supplementation studies (Joseph et al., 1999; Youdim, Shukitt-Hale, et al., 2000) that the significant effects of BBs on both motor and cognitive behavior were attributable to a multiplicity of actions, in addition to those involving antioxidant and anti-inflammatory activity. Thus, given these findings and those described previously, it might be possible to reverse or forestall the motor behavior deficits in aging via diets containing combinations of antioxidants such as those found in blueberries. We are currently exploring additional mechanisms involved in these effects, and this research suggests that they involve direct or indirect effects on cell signaling, particularly with respect to MAPK (e.g., ERK) activation, striatal carbachol-stimulated GTPase, and various isoforms of protein kinase. The results thus far indicate that blueberry supplementation can enhance the activity of the MAPKs as well as the other molecules described. At least part of the efficacy of the blueberry supplementation may be in strengthening areas of the brain that are showing the ravages of time, allowing them to communicate more effectively with other brain regions involved in both motor and memory performance.

EDITORS' DISCUSSION SUMMARY

Discussion Highlights

Evidence is accumulating that many age-related decrements in motor and cognitive behavior are related to increased vulnerability of the CNS to oxidative stress and inflammation. Dietary supplementation with antioxidants and anti-inflammatories may play an important role in reducing the deleterious effects of oxidative stress and inflammation in old age.

Animal researchers have provided substantial evidence suggesting that the CNS appears to be especially vulnerable to OS and that this vulnerability increases with advancing age. The increased vulnerability of older rats appears to be attributable to a variety of factors including reductions in glutathione levels, alterations in the membrane microenvironment, alterations in calcium buffering ability, and differential vulnerability of neurotransmitter receptors. Recent evidence suggests that inflammatory events in the CNS also play an important role in age-related changes in behavior. Older animals appear to be differentially sensitive to inflammatory reactions involving such factors as cytokines, complement proteins, and adhesion molecules that act in concert with oxidative stress to initiate decrements in neuronal function. The behavioral consequences of increased oxidative stress and inflammation in experimental animals include impaired psychomotor (rod walking, wire suspension, and plank walking) and cognitive performance (spatial learning and memory measured by the Morris water maze).

Dr. Joseph's previous research results suggest that combinations of antioxidant and anti-inflammatory polyphenolics found in fruits and vegetables may provide protective effects against many of the degenerative effects of oxidative stress and inflammation observed in the aging nervous system. Animals fed diets high in natural antioxidants had significantly fewer age-related decrements in cognitive or neuronal function than animals fed a standard laboratory diet.

Although beneficial neuronal and cognitive effects have been shown for a variety of antioxidants (spinach, strawberry, and blueberry extracts), the most reliable improvements in motor performance have been found in animals supplemented with blueberry extract. Examinations of ROS production in the brain tissue obtained from animals in these experiments suggest that animals fed antioxidant supplements exhibit significantly lower ROS levels than normal diet controls. The overall conclusion from these animal studies is that it may be possible to reverse or forestall the motor behavior deficits in aging via diets containing combinations of antioxidants such as those found in blueberries. That is, blueberry supplementation may strengthen areas of the brain that may be showing the ravages of time, allowing them to communicate more effectively with other brain regions involved in both motor and memory performance.

Research Methodological Problems

One methodological problem in this area of research is that the timing and protocols used as indicators of oxidative and inflammatory stress should be normalized. Contradictory results arise when researchers report stress measured by different methods at different stages in the course of damage. Oxidative stress is particularly hard to measure consistently, because levels of ROS change quickly and are highly localized. Similarly, but to a lesser degree, inflammatory response occurs in a series of distinct steps, such that events that result in inflammatory damage may not produce visible effects until days later.

Future Directions

Five future directions are promising in this line of inquiry. First, isolate the pathways and mediators of action of high ORAC foods, particularly berries. Second, compare beneficial effects of caloric *selection* compared with caloric *restriction*. Decades of research support the role of caloric restriction in increasing health and longevity. Blueberry supplementation studies suggest that caloric selection may be as important as caloric restriction. However, this claim remains unsubstantiated and requires further research to be validated. Third, study potential differential effects of dietary supplementation on young versus old adults. Fourth, identify the chemical agents in spinach and berries that protect the brain from aging effects. Why does spinach work better for long-term supplementation, whereas berries work best for psychomotor improvement with acute supplementation?

Fifth, define the dose–response curve, that is, the amount and duration of food supplementation necessary to achieve a given level of improvement. Preliminary data suggest that increasing the dose of blueberries in humans from 0 to 2 cups per day over a period of 12 weeks was associated with measurable differences in central processing speed. However, further research could clarify the relative benefit of intermediate quantities or durations of blueberry supplementation more representative of normal dietary patterns.

CHAPTER 9

Exercise and Sleep Quality

Martita Lopez, PhD
The University of Texas at Austin

EDITORS' OVERVIEW

Research studies that address the indirect effects of exercise on cognition through the mediator of sleep are almost nonexistent. In this chapter, Dr. Lopez lays the groundwork for understanding the structure of sleep, the deleterious effects of aging on sleep, the profound impact that sleep deprivation has on general well-being, and the evidence supporting the hypothesis that exercise enhances sleep. In chapter 10, Dr. Vitiello discusses physiological mechanisms that may explain aging and exercise effects on sleep and then addresses the interactions of exercise, sleep, health, and cognition.

Dr. Lopez begins by explaining the structure of sleep, that is, sleep architecture, and shows how and where in the structure aging decrements occur. A primary alteration in sleep with age is change in the circadian rhythm. She describes the known causes of sleep disturbance and shows how they are associated with many age-related medical conditions.

Epidemiological studies of the acute and chronic effects of exercise on sleep are discussed. Although acute exercise confers no clinically significant sleep benefit, chronic exercise seems more promising. Finally, Dr. Lopez points out

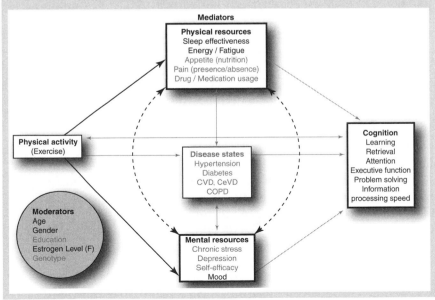

methodological issues that reduce the generalizability of many of these results: (1) lack of objective sleep quality measures in addition to self-report measures, (2) the confounding effect of light exposure with exercise, (3) the confounding effect of the mood-altering function of exercise with other exercise effects, and (4) expectancy or other effects attributable to the lack of an attention control or wait-list control group.

Several areas of research exploring the mechanisms of the relationship between exercise and sleep merit further attention. Perhaps the most important are light exposure and the circadian rhythm.

Older adults commonly report disturbances in sleep quality and related daytime impairment (Foley, Monjan, Brown, & Simonsick, 1995). Recent research has increasingly demonstrated that sleep disorders correlate with marked decreases in quality of life (Kubitz, Landers, Petruzzello, & Han, 1996). Disturbances include insomnia, changes in the structure of sleep, and changes in circadian rhythm. This chapter reviews the causes of sleep problems, the effect of exercise on sleep, and sleep models that predict exercise effects. The results of epidemiological studies of both acute and chronic effects of exercise are also reviewed.

The prevalence of insomnia generally increases with age (Ohayon, 2002). For example, the number of older adults with insomnia in a primary care setting was found to be 23% in one study (Hohagen et al., 1994) compared with only 10% of younger adults in a primary care population (Simon & VonKorff, 1997). In a community survey of 9,000 subjects who were older than 65, 52% reported having inadequate sleep or daytime alertness most of the time (Foley et al., 1995). However, these higher rates may occur primarily among older adults with comorbid chronic illness rather than those who are otherwise healthy. The Foley survey found that sleep complaints were significantly associated with respiratory symptoms, physical disabilities, and lower self-perceived health. Other studies have shown that when older adults with significant medical problems are excluded, reported rates of insomnia are the same or close to those reported in younger populations (Ohayon, 2002; Vitiello, Moe, & Prinz, 2002).

Poor sleep quality negatively affects daytime cognitive performance and motor function (Dinges et al., 1997; Stepanski, Lamphere, Badia, Zorick, & Roth, 1984). These symptoms of sleep disruption underlie the higher rate of automobile and other accidents of people with chronic insomnia, as well as memory impairment, failure to accomplish daily tasks, diminished ability to concentrate, and interpersonal difficulties (The Gallop Organization, 1991). Untreated sleep problems strongly predict nursing home placement in the elderly (Pollak, Perlick, Linsner, Wenston, & Hsieh, 1990).

Compared with those with normal sleep, people with insomnia also use medical services significantly more (Johnson & Spinweber, 1983) and have more health problems (Dement & Mitler, 1993; Mellinger, Balter, & Uhlenhuth, 1985). A recent study showed that the insomnia reported by 10% of 1,962 HMO patients predicted greater functional disability and higher health care utilization after the researchers controlled for depression (Simon & Von Korff, 1997). Insomnia has been shown to be an independent predictor of decreased quality of life among those with chronic illness, almost to the same extent as depression and the chronic illness itself (Katz & McHorney, 1988). Insomnia has also been causally linked to the development of clinical depression (Ohayon, 2002), itself a predictor of more health problems and increased use of services.

Structural Changes in Sleep

Sleep structure is measured with the polysomnogram (PSG). Polysomnography consists of overnight monitoring of 12 or more channels of physiological data, including recordings of brain waves (electroencephalogram), eye movements (electro-oculogram), and chin muscle tone (electromyogram). In addition, respiratory airflow, oxygen saturation, electrocardiogram, and limb movements are monitored. PSG data indicate that human sleep may be divided into four stages of non–rapid eye movement (NREM) sleep and one stage of rapid eye movement (REM) sleep. These stages start with drowsiness in stage 1, proceed to light sleep in stage 2, and continue to deep, slow-wave sleep in stages 3 and 4. REM sleep typically occurs after the other stages and is accompanied by episodic rapid eye movements and a deep relaxation of the muscles. REM sleep is highly associated with dreaming. With increasing age, changes occur in sleep structure that greatly affect subjective sleep quality.

One of the changes in sleep structure is in the continuity of sleep. Older adults report more awakenings during the night, and PSG data indicate more shifts between sleep stages, compared with younger adults (Bosselli, Parrino, Smerieri, & Terzano, 1998). The duration of sleep also decreases steadily with age as does sleep efficiency, the time asleep divided by the time in bed. In addition, stage 3 and 4 sleep consistently declines with age (Prinz et al., 1982). As a result, compared with younger adults, older adults experience more stage 1 and 2 sleep, characterized as structurally lighter. These changes are associated with lower subjective sleep quality (Riedel & Lichstein, 1998).

Changes in Circadian Rhythm

The aging process also affects the circadian system (Youngstedt, Kripke, Elliott, & Klauber, 2001). The circadian rhythm allows sleepiness and alertness to cycle across a 24-h period. Circadian rhythm is regulated by a combination of internal biological regulators and environmental time cues. The internal pacemaker is located in the suprachiasmatic nucleus and maintains the sleep–wake schedule through active promotion of both sleep and wakefulness. Environmental time markers that help regulate the biological clock include mealtimes, work schedules, and especially the light–dark cycle. It is generally agreed that light exposure is the most important regulator of human circadian rhythm.

A variety of biological functions are controlled by the circadian system, including body temperature and the secretion of growth hormone, melatonin, and cortisol. Body temperature is the most important of these for understanding disorders such as insomnia. The daily rhythm in body temperature is very consistent and is closely tied to alertness and sleepiness (Monk, Leng, Folkard, & Weitzman, 1983). Alertness is linked to rising temperature and drowsiness to falling temperature. Under laboratory conditions with no time constraints or time cues, sleeping correlates with temperature falling, whereas waking correlates with temperature rising (Monk & Moline, 1989).

Some researchers posit that the primary alteration in sleep with age is the decreased amplitude of the circadian rhythm (Djik, Duffy, & Czeisler, 2000). This argument would help explain the finding that older adults are more wakeful at night and drowsier during the day than younger adults. Youngstedt, Kripke, Elliot, and Klauber (2001) concluded that circadian malsynchronization might be a common and significant cause of disturbed sleep among older adults. Generally accepted effects of circadian rhythm disturbance have centered on loss of flexibility and adaptability. For example, workers over the age of 50 have increased difficulty adapting to shift work (Brugere, Barrit, Butat, Cosset, & Volkoff, 1997). Older adults report more difficulty sleeping, as well as increased fatigue, when sleeping on irregular schedules than do younger workers. Older adults also have more difficulty than younger adults in adjusting to transmeridian jet travel (Dement, Seidel, Cohen, Bliwise, & Carskadon, 1986) and to sleep deprivation (Webb, 1981). Common circadian rhythm problems in older adults are shown in figure 9.1.

Causes of Sleep Disturbance in Older Adults

Major risk factors for disturbed sleep in older adults can be divided into two categories: (a) those unique to older adults and associated with aging and (b) those that occur more commonly in older adults but cause poor sleep in people of all ages. Most risk factors are similar for all adults. Examples of conditions that often contribute to sleep disturbance include pain, primary sleep disorders, medical conditions that decrease respiratory stability, neurodegenerative disorders, medication effects, depression, anxiety,

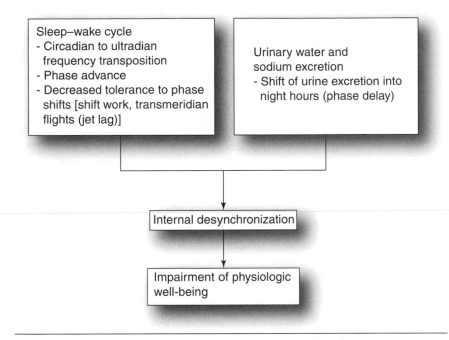

Figure 9.1 Common circadian rhythm problems in older adults.

cardiopulmonary disorders, and congestive heart failure. Older adults are at higher risk for poor sleep primarily because of the increased prevalence of these well-documented causes of poor sleep. In fact, many older adults have multiple risk factors.

Although there is a consensus on those factors that cause poor sleep in young and old alike, identifying causes of poor sleep that are unique to the aging process is more controversial (Stepanski, Rybarczyk, Lopez, & Stevens, 2003). As mentioned previously, most older adults experience decreases in the continuity, duration, and depth of sleep. Changes in the physiology of the circadian rhythm with aging and a decrease in stage 3 and 4 sleep are examples of the causal factors that have been implicated. Several other probable factors in age-specific sleep disruption include primary sleep disorders, circadian rhythm sleep disorders, and parasomnias.

1. *Primary sleep disorders.* These disorders originate from abnormalities of sleep physiology. The prevalence of sleep-disordered breathing, central sleep apnea, restless legs syndrome, and periodic limb movement disorder increases dramatically with age (Phillips & Ancoli-Israel, 2001). These disorders can decrease total sleep time and lead to deterioration of sleep quality and daytime impairment.

2. *Circadian rhythm sleep disorders*. Some researchers have hypothesized that older adults are at increased risk for advanced sleep phase syndrome (Weitzman, Moline, Czeisler, & Zimmerman, 1982). In this disorder, the biological clock is programmed to initiate sleep at a time earlier than is desired, and individuals will awaken at an earlier time than is desired.

3. *Parasomnias*. REM behavior disorder is characterized by a lack of the muscle atonia that is usually present during REM sleep (Schenck, Bundlie, Ettinger, & Mahowald, 1986). Left untreated, this disorder can result in injurious behavior associated with an individual physically acting out dreams.

Sleep Disorders Associated With Age-Related Medical Conditions

Neurodegenerative diseases often present with a variety of sleep complaints, ranging from insomnia to hypersomnia, abnormal motor activity during sleep, snoring, apneas, and changes in circadian rhythm. Some sleep disturbance may arise from direct degeneration of structures responsible for the sleep–wake cycle, such as the suprachiasmatic nucleus of the hypothalamus.

In *Alzheimer's disease*, nocturnal episodes of confusion and disorientation can reverse the sleep schedule, leading to sleeping during the day and wakefulness at night. In *Parkinson's disease*, patients commonly report difficulty initiating or maintaining sleep and consequent daytime sleepiness. Additional sleep symptoms include periodic limb movements of sleep and restless legs syndrome, as well as REM behavior disorder.

Stroke can result in sleep disruption for a variety of reasons. Many stroke patients develop obstructive sleep apnea (Bassetti & Aldrich, 1999). Hypersomnia, and rarely insomnia, may occur from thalamic lesions that may occur during or after stroke (Guilleminault, Quera-Salva, & Goldberg, 1993). The depression that some stroke patients experience can also hinder sleep.

Cardiac disease increases the risk of central apnea, because it can impair respiratory control (Longobardo, Gothe, Goldman, & Cherniak, 1982). As might be expected, individuals with cardiac disease frequently report insomnia (Schwartz et al., 1999). Congestive heart failure can disrupt breathing during sleep and lead to frequent arousals and poor sleep quality (Javaheri, 1999).

Chronic obstructive pulmonary disease (COPD) also confers increased risk of sleep-disordered breathing. Profound changes in respiratory control occur during sleep, including marked reductions in hypoxic and hypercapnic respiratory drive (Douglas, 2000). Most persons with COPD report disturbed sleep, including frequent arousals, increased stage 1 sleep, and decreased total sleep time (Sandek, Andersson, Bratel, Hellstrom, & Lagerstrand, 1999).

Osteoarthritis, the most common cause of chronic pain among the elderly (Cooley et al., 1998), and *rheumatoid arthritis* (Mahowald & Mahowald, 2000) can both give rise to insomnia. Interestingly, pain and sleep disturbance can influence each other bidirectionally. Moldofsky (1989) reported that increased daytime osteoarthritis pain can either precede or follow a night of poor sleep.

Effects of Exercise on Sleep

Popular culture holds that physical activity enhances sleep, with exercise routinely touted in the press as a sleep aid. Descriptions of good sleep hygiene typically include exercise performed 4 to 6 h before bedtime. In a review of the evidence that exercise has a beneficial effect on sleep, Youngstedt (2000) pointed out that the notion that exercise influences sleep has intuitive appeal because exercise is the antithesis of sleeping pills, it offers a simple and low-cost alternative to other treatments, and many people find it relaxing. However, researchers studying the effects of exercise on sleep have reached varying conclusions. Some find that exercise facilitates sleep, others that it harms sleep, and others that it has no effect (Driver & Taylor, 2000). Many of these studies suffer from methodological constraints that make comparisons difficult. These include sample size; the method by which sleep was measured; type, duration, and timing of exercise; subject characteristics, such as fitness; whether the exercise was acute or chronic; whether the exercise was indoors or outdoors (light exposure); and whether a control group was included. Most studies of the effects of exercise on sleep are conducted with men who are either young, good sleepers, or both. These factors limit generalizability of the results and also leave little room for change because of ceiling or floor effects (Youngstedt, 2003).

Sleep Models That Predict Exercise Effects

Thermogenic hypothesis. Circadian sleep rhythms relate closely to body temperature (McGinty & Szymusiak, 1990), and research implicates the anterior hypothalamus in both heat loss and sleep mechanisms. As mentioned earlier, falling body temperature precedes the onset of sleep, and researchers hypothesize that increasing body temperature before bedtime can activate both heat loss and the associated sleep mechanisms (Horne & Staff, 1983; Van Someren, 2000). For example, in two studies Dorsey and colleagues demonstrated that passive body heating, achieved via a hot bath 1.5 to 2 h before bedtime, improved sleep quality in older female insomniacs (Dorsey et al., 1996, 1999). Exercise raises body temperature more effectively than any other stimulus. The purported influence of temperature regulation on sleep gains further support from findings that older adults, depressed people, and insomniacs have an impairment in nocturnal temperature down-regulation (Glotzbach & Heller, 1994), all of whom report sleep problems.

Energy conservation hypothesis. Based on the principle that the body has a certain amount of energy available, the energy conservation hypothesis proposes that if more energy is used during the day, more must be conserved at night during sleep (Adam & Oswald, 1983). Driver and Taylor (2000) reviewed the available evidence and concluded that sleep has some role in energy regulation, but the details of this relationship remain unclear.

Body restoration or compensatory hypothesis. This model predicts that sleep should allow the body to recuperate from daily wear and tear. Exercise, therefore, should serve as a stressor on the body and thereby facilitate sleep. Some evidence favors this theory, but again the details and extent of the relationship require further elucidation (Driver & Taylor, 2000). In their meta-analysis, Kubitz, Landers, Petruzzello, and Han (1996) reported that the exercise and sleep effects they found generally supported the compensatory theory.

Other Mechanisms for Exercise Effects on Sleep

Circadian phase-shifting effects. Light exposure strongly influences the circadian system, and bright light therapy has been used to treat poor sleepers with disrupted circadian rhythms (Chesson et al., 1999). Many older persons experience little light stimulation (Campbell, Kripke, Gillin, & Hrubovcak, 1988). This lack of exposure to light may reduce the environmental cues that the circadian system needs to function well, thus contributing to circadian desynchronization (Youngstedt, Kripke, & Elliott, 2001). Many studies of exercise and sleep have suffered methodologically from the possible confounding effects of daylight, because the exercise was performed outside.

Antidepressant effects. Bright light also counters depression. When depressed individuals exercise outside, the increased light exposure mitigates the depression that contributes to poor sleep. Exercise itself can also alleviate depression among both younger and older adults (Brosse, Sheets, Lett, & Blumenthal, 2002; Singh, Clements, & Fiatarone, 1997).

Anxiolytic effects. Evidence shows that in addition to its antidepressant effects, exercise reduces anxiety, another common contributor to disturbed sleep (Petruzzello, Landers, Hatfield, Kubitz, & Salazar, 1991). Anxiety contributes to insomnia (Edinger, Stout, & Hoelscher, 1988), and it has been suggested that sleep improvements following exercise in normal sleepers may be restricted to days in which individuals are experiencing significant anxiety (Youngstedt, O'Connor, & Dishman, 1997).

Adenosine effects. Exercise stimulates adenosine release through the depletion of central glycogen stores. Recent research identifies adenosine as a sleep regulator (Porkka-Heiskanen et al., 1997). In support of this role, one study found that more positive sleep changes occurred after exercise in subjects with normal adenosine neurotransmission, compared with subjects in whom adenosine neurotransmission was blocked (Youngstedt, Kripke, & Elliott, 1999).

Epidemiological Studies

In his review, Youngstedt (2000) reported that epidemiological studies have provided the majority of the evidence supporting the beneficial effects of exercise on sleep. For example, Sherrill, Kotchou, and Quan (1998) reported on the Tucson Epidemiological Study of Obstructive Airways Disease, which included 722 middle-aged to elderly men and women. The researchers concluded that regular exercise correlated with a reduction in the prevalence and risk of symptoms of disturbed sleep. In another study, of a random sample of 1,600 young to middle-aged Finnish adults, 33% of men and 30% of women reported that exercise promoted sleep and was the single most important variable affecting sleep (Vuroi, Urponen, Hasan, & Partinen, 1988). Although the data from these surveys and others suggest a strong beneficial effect of exercise on sleep, methodological issues limit the conclusions that may be drawn. These studies rely on subjective self-reports rather than polysomnography, the gold standard in sleep measurement. Although self-reported sleep data provide valuable insight into subjects' perceptions, persons with insomnia tend to overestimate the amount of time they are awake. In addition, people often forget nighttime awakenings or the exact time when they fell asleep. Furthermore, some self-report questionnaires lack reliability and validity. Finally, these survey results are retrospective and therefore especially subject to influence by subjects' biases.

Acute Exercise and Sleep

Most investigators of the relationship between exercise and sleep have studied the effects of acute exercise on young, healthy men who sleep normally. Youngstedt and his colleagues (1997) recently conducted a meta-analysis of 38 studies, each of which included a polysomnographic assessment of sleep and a within-subjects design. The authors concluded that acute exercise had almost no effect on the time it took to fall asleep or that there were very small increases in total sleep time (median = 10 min) and slow-wave sleep (median = 1.44 min). REM sleep also decreased by a significant but small amount of time (median = 6 min), and REM latency increased after sleep onset (median = 11.6 min). Such small changes would have very little clinical effect.

The discrepancy between subjective and objective reports on the effects of exercise effects on sleep may relate to the feelings of fatigue that subjects experience following exercise. Subjects often confuse tiredness with sleepiness, but they are two different states (Lichstein, Means, Noe, & Aguillard, 1997). Rather than increasing sleepiness, acute exercise results in greater alertness that relates to the intensity of the exercise and is most pronounced when the exercise is performed in the middle of the night (Driver & Taylor, 2000).

Factors Affecting Acute Exercise and Sleep

Fitness. Youngstedt and colleagues (1997) in their meta-analysis on the effects of acute exercise on sleep concluded that fitness generally did not moderate the influence of exercise on sleep. Equivalent sleep changes followed acute exercise in fit and sedentary individuals.

Duration and intensity. The same meta-analysis found that duration of exercise more consistently moderated sleep quality than did fitness or intensity of exercise (Youngstedt et al., 1997). The most reliable effects arose from exercise lasting more than 1 h, possibly because experimental protocols more clearly described this variable than other conditions such as fitness. Driver and Taylor (2000), reviewing five relevant studies, reported that the data on intensity of exercise varied and that no conclusions could be drawn.

Time of day. Although most sleep hygiene recommendations include the caveat that exercise should not be performed late in the evening, Youngstedt and colleagues (1999) found that vigorous late-night exercise did not disturb sleep. However, exercise may have the ability to influence the circadian system by inducing significant phase shifting (Van Reeth et al., 1994).

Gender. Comparatively few studies on exercise and sleep include women as research subjects, particularly premenopausal women. Those that have included women often have not controlled for menstrual cycle phase, oral contraceptive use, or menopausal status (Driver & Taylor, 2000). One meta-analysis (Kubitz et al., 1996) reported a larger effect of exercise on the sleep of women compared with men. In other studies, gender differences in the response of sleep to exercise were not consistent.

Age. Because sleep quality decreases with age, treatments of older subjects may produce greater relative and absolute improvements than the same treatments applied to younger subjects. Kubitz and colleagues (1996) found that older adults were more likely to experience a larger effect of exercise on sleep compared with younger adults.

Chronic Exercise and Sleep

Researchers examining the effects of chronic exercise on sleep have found more beneficial results than those studying acute exercise, particularly with regard to older adults. For example, in one randomized controlled study of normal sleepers, 30 men and women, mean age 66, were randomly assigned to 6 months of aerobic training or to a stretching and flexibility control group (Vitiello, Prinz, & Schwartz, 1994). After the 6-month training period, only participants in the aerobic training condition significantly increased their stage 3 and 4 sleep time. Neither group improved on other sleep variables. Notably, an objective measure of sleep quality was used in this study.

In another study of older adults, 43 subjects with moderate sleep complaints, aged 50 to 76 years, were randomly assigned to 16 weeks of moderate-intensity aerobic exercise or to a wait-list control group (King, Oman, Brassington, Bliwise, & Haskell, 1997). The exercise consisted of brisk walking or low-impact aerobics. Subjects who exercised reported significantly greater improvements in self-reported sleep quality. In a similar randomized controlled trial, King, Baumann, O'Sullivan, Wilcox, and Castro (2002) examined the effects of moderate-intensity exercise on 100 female family caregivers aged 49 to 82 years. Each concurrently cared for a relative with dementia. Participants were randomized to 12 months of home-based, telephone-supervised, moderate-intensity exercise training or to an attention-control nutrition education group. Compared with the control participants, the exercise group experienced a significant improvement in self-rated sleep quality. Both groups reported reductions in psychological distress. A confounding factor in both of these studies is that subjects who exercised probably received more bright light. For most participants, their exercise consisted of outdoor walking. Therefore, the improvement noted may have arisen from longer periods of light exposure rather than, or in addition to, the effects of exercise.

Singh and colleagues (1997) conducted another controlled randomized study of older adults. A total of 32 depressed or dysthymic older adults, mean age 71, were assigned to a supervised weight-training program or an attention control group. Most participants reported poor sleep at baseline. Results indicated that exercise significantly improved all subjective sleep quality and depression measures. The study did not determine whether exercise exerted its effect on sleep via depression reduction or more directly.

Although the four previous studies included older adults as subjects, another study on chronic exercise and sleep included subjects with a mean age of 44 years (Guilleminault et al., 1995). This study provides evidence that chronic exposure to bright light can enhance sleep and also strengthens the evidence on the effects of exercise on sleep. Because of the lack of a control group, however, these results must be interpreted with caution. Thirty subjects with psychophysiological insomnia were randomly assigned to one of three treatments, each of which lasted 4 weeks: sleep hygiene education, sleep hygiene combined with late afternoon exercise (daily walking), or sleep hygiene plus morning bright light (1 h of exposure daily at 3,000 lux). Pre- and posttreatment measures were self-report sleep logs and actigraphy, an objective measure. All subjects tended to improve, but only the sleep hygiene plus bright light group significantly improved. Their total sleep time increased by an impressive 54 min. The total sleep time for the sleep hygiene with exercise group increased by 17 min, and sleep hygiene training alone resulted in a 3 min increase.

These studies suggest that chronic exercise does enhance sleep, particularly in older adults and people with poor sleep. The factors most subject to change were total sleep time, increased stage 3 and 4 sleep, and decreased sleep onset latency. Methodological issues that reduce the generalizability of some of these results include (1) lack of objective sleep quality measures in addition to self-report measures, (2) the confounding effect of light exposure with exercise, (3) the confounding effect of the mood-altering function of exercise with other exercise effects, and (4) expectancy or other effects attributable to the lack of an attention control or wait-list control group.

A.C. King (personal communication, April 22, 2003) and her colleagues are currently in the last year of a 4-year study that has been designed to avoid the methodological pitfalls listed previously. The study design is a 1-year randomized trial. The objectives of the study are (1) to determine the 6-month and 12-month effectiveness of a physical activity program in promoting improvements in subjectively and objectively measured sleep quality in older adults with moderate sleep complaints, (2) to evaluate the efficacy of the physical activity regimen for promoting initial and long-term changes in a broad array of quality-of-life variables, and (3) to investigate a selected set of potential mediators of the physical activity and sleep relationship. Subjects for this project are 120 sedentary, healthy, community-dwelling older men and women who are being randomized to one of two conditions. The exercise group will perform moderate-intensity physical activity, such as walking, swimming, or cycling, twice a week in groups and three times a week at home. Subjects in the attention control group will participate in successful aging classes once a week and additional activities based on class content. Data will be collected at baseline and at 6 and 12 months using self-rated and objective sleep quality measures collected in the natural environment, along with a wide array of other psychological and physical functioning measures. The researchers expect that about 30 subjects will complete each arm of the study, which means that this will be the largest study of its kind once the results are published.

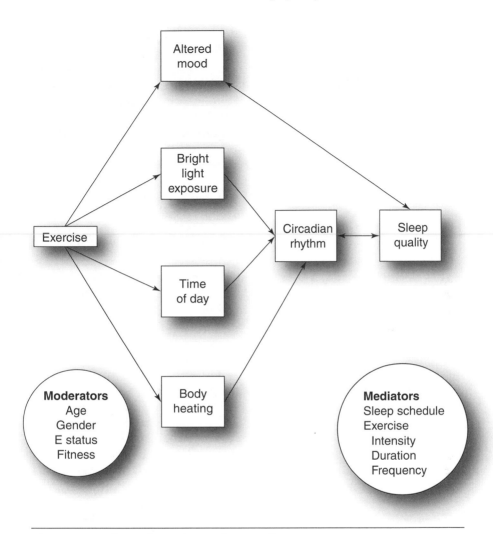

Figure 9.2 Effects of exercise on sleep quality.

A summary of these putative exercise effects on mediators of sleep quality is shown in figure 9.2. This model includes mediators of sleep, the role of circadian rhythm, and the effect of moderators on sleep quality.

Future Research

Although acute exercise confers no clinically significant sleep benefit, chronic exercise shows much more promise (Driver & Taylor, 2000; Youngstedt, 2000). A number of important questions remain to be answered.

Several areas of research exploring the mechanisms of the relationship between exercise and sleep merit further attention. Perhaps the most important are light exposure and the circadian rhythm. The findings of Guilleminault and colleagues (1995) emphasize the potential importance of bright light exposure. Particularly for older adults, light exposure may contribute significantly to the clinical enhancement of sleep. Many older adults are exposed to little natural light compared with younger adults. In addition, some groups of older adults face significant obstacles to chronic exercise, such as those who use wheelchairs, those who are cognitively impaired, and those in nursing homes. The incidence of circadian rhythm abnormalities increases in older adults (Youngstedt et al., 2001), and some evidence suggests that exercise promotes phase shifting (Van Reeth et al., 1994). Thus, for those who can exercise, chronic exercise in brightly lit conditions may be the optimal approach (Driver & Taylor, 2000).

Other researchers are focusing on the mood-altering role of exercise and its effects on sleep. Although clinical major depression and anxiety occur more frequently in younger adults, older adults have higher levels of depressive symptomology. These subclinical negative mood states may worsen sleep, but they appear to respond to chronic exercise (Brosse et al., 2002; Singh et al., 1997).

Another potential mechanism by which exercise influences sleep, the thermogenic hypothesis, deserves future attention. The intriguing evidence that older adults with impaired sleep also down-regulate nocturnal temperature abnormally (Glotzbach & Heller, 1994) calls for continued study of the relationship between the body-heating effects of exercise and sleep quality. The sleep-enhancing properties of passive body heating and exercise should be compared in older adults, given that some elderly cannot exercise for a variety of reasons. Youngstedt and colleagues (1997) suggested that future research in this area should replicate previous work and move forward with innovative experimental designs.

Improvements in experimental design and methodology would facilitate the exploration of many issues. Ideally, designs should be longitudinal and have adequate follow-up, include more subjects, and control for light exposure. Women should serve as subjects more frequently, given their relative neglect in the past, and their estrogen status should be controlled (Driver & Taylor, 2000). Subjects with disturbed sleep should be included, to avoid ceiling or floor effects (Youngstedt, 2003). Especially with older adults, attention control groups are important. Older adults may be lonelier than younger adults, particularly if they are socially isolated for any reason, such as retirement or disability. In addition, both subjective and objective measures of sleep quality should be included. These measures may inform on different and equally valuable aspects of sleep (King et al., 2002).

Investigators using exercise interventions generally have failed to use recent technological advances such as ambulatory activity monitors,

Internet-based programs, and personal data assistant devices (Brosse et al., 2002). These strategies could improve monitoring of exercise adherence and treatment response. In addition, technology now enables the best objective sleep measure, polysomnography, to be conducted in subjects' homes, thus facilitating their participation and increasing generalizability of results. Advances in structural and functional neuroimaging techniques may also improve the identification of neuroanatomic correlates of exercise and sleep mediators.

More information about gender differences and the effect of the menopausal transition on the exercise–sleep relationship is needed in studies of middle-aged and older women. Along the same lines, the effects of age should be explored further, including mediators of the exercise–sleep relationship in older adults with various chronic illnesses. The importance of age, gender, and estrogen status as moderator variables was highlighted by a meta-analysis of studies examining the effects of fitness on the cognitive functioning of older adults (Colcombe & Kramer, 2003). In summary, sleep quality is very difficult to quantify, and the factors that affect it are complex. Investigators should well understand all of the known research design problems and take every precaution to control them.

EDITORS' DISCUSSION SUMMARY

Discussion Highlights

Epidemiological studies support the existence of a relationship between physical activity and sleep quality. Older adults often report disturbances in sleep quality and quantity that are of sufficient magnitude to decrease their quality of life. Evidence is accumulating that poor sleep quality is associated with impaired daytime cognitive performance and motor function. Two aspects of the activity of exercise and four potential mechanisms were discussed as possible ways that exercise might benefit cognition by enhancing sleep.

A number of mechanisms have been proposed to explain the hypothesized link between physical activity and improved sleep. Among the more common mechanisms are exercise-induced increases in body temperature, the need to restore energy used in exercise, antidepressant and anxiolytic effects of exercise, improvements in sleep attributable to exercise-induced adenosine release, and increased light exposure in outdoor activity, which regularizes the circadian rhythm. Bright light exposure also has antidepressant and anxiolytic effects.

Methodological Research Problems

Several confounds are present in the research literature on this topic. First, although epidemiological studies support the existence of a relationship between physical activity and improved sleep, well-controlled studies using polysomnographic assessment of sleep are needed before definitive conclusions can be drawn about the effect of both acute and long-term exercise participation and sleep quality and quantity. Second, studies of women are not prevalent in this literature, and those that are published have infrequently controlled for estrogen levels. Third, the light exposure that occurs in outdoor activities is a confounding variable. Sleep improvements that are attributed to exercise may really be caused by increased light exposure. Fourth, researchers have primarily used subjective self-report techniques, which are known to be especially flawed when used to report sleep experiences. The quality of sleep data is better when measures such as polysomnography are used. Fifth, exercise can alter mood as well as produce physiological changes that are beneficial for sleep. Mood changes should be assessed and controlled in sleep studies.

Future Directions for Research

Randomized controlled trials for both male and female older adults, especially the oldest-old, should be conducted. In addition, an effective way to understand exercise effects on sleep and cognition might be to study them together in special groups: for example, groups with normal and disturbed sleep patterns, or groups with different chronic medical or psychiatric conditions.

CHAPTER 10

Exercise, Sleep, and Cognition: Interactions in Aging

Michael V. Vitiello, PhD

University of Washington

EDITORS' OVERVIEW

Dr. Vitiello investigates the relationships among exercise, sleep, and cognition and explores the neuroendocrine regulation of sleep. The somatotrophic axis and the hypothalamic–pituitary–adrenal (HPA) axis contribute to the regulation of sleep. In early sleep, the somatotrophic axis dominates, as the pituitary gland delivers pulses of growth hormone (GH) to the body. As sleep progresses, GH levels eventually diminish, while levels of cortisol, epinephrine, and norepinephrine rise because of the activities of the hypothalamus and the adrenal

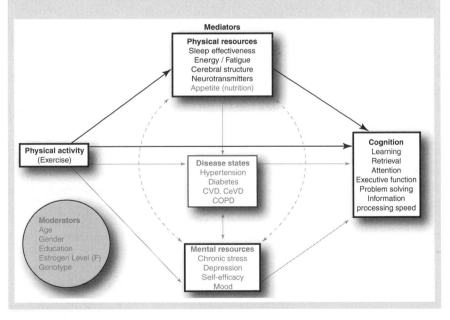

Acknowledgments: I thank the editors for providing me the opportunity to put my thoughts on these important interrelationships into the literature. I also acknowledge the many colleagues who either directly or indirectly helped me formulate the thoughts I have expressed here, in particular, Drs. Beth Kerr, Lawrence H. Larson, Guiliana Mazzoni, George R. Merriam, Karen E. Moe, and Robert S. Schwartz. This work was supported by Public Health Service grants RO1-MH45186, RO1-MH53575, and KO2-MH01158 to Michael V. Vitiello.

medulla. Exercise most likely influences sleep quality via its neuroendocrine effects. Exercise can increase the activity of the somatotrophic axis and decrease the activity of the HPA axis. These neuroendocrine changes in turn improve sleep quality, because the somatotrophic and HPA axes help to regulate the staging and quality of sleep.

Exercise most likely influences cognition via its effects on sleep. However, the effect of exercise on cognition via sleep is confounded by multiple causal pathways, but some effects can be separated. For example, Dr. Vitiello found that cognitive ability remained unaltered in the older adults in a study of endurance exercise, despite longer periods of slow-wave sleep. This finding undermines the proposed directional arrow from exercise to improved cognition via improvements in sleep. Conversely, in another study Dr. Vitiello found that cognition improved in the absence of any improvement in sleep quality. Such contradictory studies reveal the complexity of the interactions among sleep, exercise, cognition, and the neuroendocrine factors believed to mediate the beneficial effects of exercise on sleep.

The evidence in support of the beneficial effect of regular exercise, here meaning both endurance (aerobic) and resistance (weight) training, on health and quality of life in older individuals is considerable (e.g., Drewnowski & Evans, 2001; Karani, McLaughlin, & Cassel, 2001).

Regular exercise is linked to a number of beneficial physiological and health outcomes such as increased aerobic capacity, increased strength, improved body composition (increased lean and decreased fat mass), improved balance and decreased risk of falls, decreased depressive symptoms, increased functional capacity, and improved sense of energy and general well-being.

Regular exercise may also be associated with improved immune function, although the data in support of this relationship are essentially cross-sectional. Furthermore, regular exercise, likely at least in part through body weight and body composition effects, has been demonstrated to lower the risk for a number of diseases including hypertension, stroke, coronary artery disease (CAD), hyperinsulinemia, insulin resistance, and non-insulin-dependent diabetes mellitus (NIDDM) and to decrease related mortality.

That regular exercise improves general somatic function is clear. What are less clear are the benefits of exercise on cerebral functions such as sleep quality and cognitive function. Although there is considerable myth and anecdotal evidence in support of such relationships, and even reasonable support in the epidemiological literature, particularly for exercise and sleep, the experimental literature in support of these conceptualizations is, in reality, quite sparse. Here we shall examine the interrelationships of exercise, sleep, and cognitive function in the context of aging.

Sleep, Sleep Disorders, and Cognition Relationships

Here I review the evidence in support of sleep–cognition relationships and evidence demonstrating the affect of disturbed sleep and sleep disorders on cognitive function.

Sleep and Cognition

Considerable evidence from the animal literature shows that sleep plays a significant role in cognitive function, in particular in memory; see Ambrosini and Giuditta (2001) for a comprehensive review of this area. Similarly, in the human literature there is evidence supporting the impact of sleep quality on memory. Smith (2001) reviewed the human literature attempting to relate sleep states to memory processes. Experimental studies in this area typically present learning material to participants and then examine their ability to recall this material after posttraining sleep or sleep deprivation. Results strongly suggest that rapid eye movement (REM) sleep is involved with the efficient memory processing of cognitive procedural material but not declarative material. Although there are some data to suggest that non-REM (NREM) sleep is necessary for declarative memory consolidation, NREM may in fact simply occur at the same time as another factor that is actually involved in the memory processing (Smith, 2001).

Limited recent results further suggest that the length of the NREM–REM sleep cycle may be important for declarative memory, a possibility also supported by the animal literature (Ambrosini & Giuditta, 2001). Such limited data also suggest that NREM, particularly stage 2 sleep, may be involved with the memory for motor procedural but not cognitive procedural tasks. Smith (2001) as well as Strickgold (2001), in his editorial introducing the reviews discussed here, both caution that sleep researchers would do well to capitalize on the latest advancements in memory research by choosing tasks that represent special memory systems and examining their relationships to specific sleep states.

Jones and Harrison (2001), in their review focusing on sleep and frontal lobe relationships, noted that experimental studies involving total sleep loss, sleep reduction, and clinically related sleep fragmentation report impaired performance on tasks of frontal lobe or executive function, including measures of verbal fluency, creativity, and planning skills. This constellation of impairment has also been observed in sleep-related breathing disorder (SRBD) patients, and the deficit at least partially persists in the face of successful treatment, although the executive impairment appears to be more closely related to nighttime hypoxemic events rather than daytime sleepiness.

Studies of electroencephalographic (EEG) changes throughout the course of sleep and following sleep deprivation, as well as those involving functional neuroimaging and psychophysiological changes (event-related potentials) following sleep deprivation, provide further indication of the relative importance of the frontal regions of the brain to sleep.

However, neurocognitive studies present many inconsistencies, task classification is often ambiguous, and, in the absence of any unifying explanation at the level of cognitive mechanisms, the overall picture is one of a disparate range of impairment following sleep loss and sleep fragmentation (Jones & Harrison, 2001). In addition, these same authors note that poorly defined concepts of frontal lobe function, executive function, memory, and attention, using tasks largely developed with more severe deficit levels in mind, create further difficulties in interpreting the literature in this area.

Sleep Disorders and Cognition

In their comprehensive review of cognitive dysfunction in individuals with sleep disorders, Fulda and Shulz (2001) reviewed 56 studies that explored cognitive dysfunctions in people with SRBDs (24 studies), insomnia (18 studies), or narcolepsy (14 studies). Fulda and Shulz (2001) grouped individual study outcomes according to neuropsychological functions and reviewed the available evidence separately for SRBD, insomnia, and narcolepsy.

The authors noted that consistent evidence was found for impaired driving simulation performance in SRBD patients (92.9% of comparisons with control subjects). Other neuropsychological functions with less pronounced impairments included (a) attention span, divided attention, and sustained attention for SRBD patients; (b) attention span, verbal immediate memory, and vigilance for insomniac patients; and (c) sustained attention, vigilance, and driving simulation performance for narcoleptic patients. Reduced performance in tasks measuring attention was found to be higher for SRBD and narcoleptic patients than for insomniacs (35.9%, 44.2%, and 22.8% of all comparisons, respectively). Impairment of memory performance in comparison with control subjects was less pronounced for all three groups, with 20.0% for insomnia, 17.1% for SRBDs, and 15.6% for narcolepsy. In other areas of cognitive functioning, the data did not allow definite conclusions for any of the three patient groups examined (Fulda & Shulz, 2001).

Narrowing their focus on sleep disorders and cognition to the relationship between sleep apnea and cognitive function in children, Blunden, Lushington, and Kennedy (2001) noted that SRBDs are common in children, and although the sequelae of cardiopulmonary and growth and developmental impairment have been well documented, neurocognitive deficits have been less well studied. Nevertheless, there is an emerging body of evidence that children with SRBDs show reduced neurocognitive functioning, especially in the interrelated areas of attentional capacity and memory. In addition, these children show increased problematic behavior and reduced school performance. Early reports suggest that some of these deficits may be reversible with treatment. The genesis of these defects is unclear but may include hypoxemia and the subtle changes in sleep architecture induced by the periodic arousals that typically terminate an apneic event (Blunden et al., 2001).

Exercise and Cognition

Numerous studies have examined the impact of regular exercise on cognitive function in the context of aging. Although some epidemiological and cross-sectional studies (e.g., Clarkson-Smith and Hartley, 1989; Laurin, Verreault, Lindsay, MacPherson, & Rockwood, 2001; Richards, Hardy, & Wadsworth, 2003) have supported such a relationship, some (Fabre, Chamari, Mucci, Masse-Biron, & Prefaut, 2002; Kramer et al., 1999; Rikli & Edwards, 1991) but far from all (Blumenthal & Madden, 1988; Blumenthal et al., 1989; Hill, Storant, & Malley, 1993; Kerr, Scott, & Vitiello, 1993; Madden, Blumenthal, Allen, & Emery, 1989) randomized controlled studies have found any positive effect of exercise training on the cognitive function of the elderly.

We took advantage of our randomized controlled trial examining the impact of 6 months of endurance training on the subjective and objective sleep quality of the healthy sedentary older men and women, described subsequently (Vitiello, Prinz, & Schwartz, 1994a, 1994b), to examine the impact of such training on cognitive function in this same sample (Kerr et al., 1993). A total of 39 subjects (22 men and 17 women) with an average age of 67 were randomly assigned to either endurance training (ET) or a stretching–flexibility (SF) control group. After 6 months, $\dot{V}O_2$max increased 15% ($p < .002$) in the ET group and was unchanged in the SF group. As is more completely described subsequently, for a somewhat larger group of subjects, the ET group also showed a significant posttraining improvement in sleep quality, whereas the SF group did not. However, across all cognitive and motor function tests (Verbal Recall, Letter Sets, Verbal Fluency, Trails A, Force Maintenance With and Without Visual Feedback), there was no indication that any improvement in either cognition or motor function could be attributed to ET, because any improvements that did occur were present for both groups, most likely indicating practice effects.

Colcombe and Kramer (2003) used meta-analysis to review studies they deemed to be experimentally sound that examined the impact of physical activity and exercise on the cognitive function of older adults. Their analysis included 18 studies that used subject randomization and appropriate control conditions. Colombe and Kramer concluded that interventions that led to increased levels of physical activity resulted in improvements in cognitive function, particularly for those cognitive tasks that involved executive processes.

Despite our own negative findings, review of the literature indicates that there is considerable support from the epidemiological and cross-sectional literature for the beneficial effect of regular exercise on the cognitive function of older adults. Furthermore, the previously mentioned meta-analysis (Colcombe & Kramer, 2003) indicated that there is a positive effect of physical activity on cognitive performance, although the ultimate robustness of this relationship remains to be fully delineated.

Exercise and Sleep Quality

Here I examine the complicated relationship between exercise and sleep quality. Particular attention is paid to randomized, controlled trials of various types of fitness training on a variety of elderly population samples and the implications of these findings for exercise–sleep relationships in the general elderly population.

Effects of Exercise on Sleep

The putative causal relationships between acute and chronic exercise on sleep quality were comprehensively reviewed by Driver and Taylor (2000). They pointed out that considerable epidemiological evidence suggests that regular exercise is associated with good self-reported sleep quality as well as general well-being in elderly populations. However, these authors also noted that the experimental data in support of exercise's beneficial impact on sleep quality is less clear-cut, attributing this lack of clarity in the literature to "differences in the exercise protocols studied (e.g., aerobic or anaerobic, intensity, duration) and interactions between individual characteristics (e.g., fitness, age, and gender) (p. 387). Driver and Taylor also noted that "the tendency to study changes in small groups of good sleepers may also underestimate the efficacy of exercise for promoting sleep" (p. 387).

Although the ultimate functions of sleep continue to be elucidated, both the restorative and energy conservation theories of sleep propose that sleep is in large part a compensatory mechanism following catabolic processes of daytime activity. Age-related declines in activity present one of the theoretical mechanisms by which regular exercise may improve sleep quality. Others include exercise or fitness-based changes in thermoregulation, circadian rhythms, metabolism, hormonal secretion (e.g., growth hormone–releasing hormone), and immune function (e.g., cytokines).

What exactly are the data supporting the beneficial impact of regular exercise on sleep quality in general and on older individuals in particular? Let us examine the evidence, first in studies that have used subjective (questionnaire-based) measures of sleep quality and then in studies that have measured sleep objectively.

Subjective Sleep

Driver and Taylor reviewed the epidemiological literature on this topic and, although recognizing interpretive limitations such as directionality and third variable explanations, concluded, "These studies consistently support the view that acute and chronic exercise promotes sleep" (p. 391). A large (N = 1,190) Finnish study (Vuori, Urponen, Hasan, & Partinen, 1988) provides an excellent example of such epidemiological findings. In response to open-ended questions, both men and women reported exercise as the most important sleep-promoting factor, and respondents who reported getting regular exercise had less daytime sleepiness compared with those who were more sedentary. Most impressive, 43% of those who reported increased amounts of exercise during the previous 3 months (n = 81) reported improved subjective sleep compared with only 1% whose self-reported sleep deteriorated. Conversely, 30% of those subjects who reported decreased exercise in the previous 3 months (n = 73) reported deterioration in their sleep, compared with the 4% who reported improved sleep quality.

As for experimental data, a comprehensive search of the literature reveals that only three randomized, controlled studies of the impact of fitness training on the sleep of sedentary older adults have been reported. The first was our own randomized control trial of 6 months of endurance training (ET) versus a stretching–flexibility (SF) control on the subjective and objective sleep of healthy older adults not complaining of sleep problems (Vitiello et al., 1994a, 1994b).

Since then, two other randomized controlled trials of exercise training effects on the subjective sleep of community-dwelling elderly volunteers with moderate sleep impairment have been published (King, Oman, Brassington, Bliwise, & Haskell, 1997; Singh, Clements, & Fiatarone, 1997). One examined the impact of 16 weeks of ET on a group of elderly volunteers complaining of significant sleep disturbance (King et al., 1997) versus a wait-list control. The other study examined the effect of 10 weeks of resistance training (RT) versus an attention control in a group of clinically depressed older volunteers (Singh et al., 1997).

Finally, a fourth randomized study (Tworoger et al., 2003) examined the impact of either ET or SF on the subjective sleep quality of a large group of community-dwelling, inactive, overweight women (not on estrogen replacement therapy) who may or may not have had sleep complaints.

Overall, these four studies suggest that, despite some methodological limitations, both RT and ET, and likely SF, improve subjective sleep quality in community-dwelling, elderly volunteers who may or may not be sleep impaired or complaining.

Objective Sleep

The impact of exercise on polysomnographic sleep is an area of much controversy, with little consensus (Driver & Taylor, 2000). As discussed previously, it is clear that because of inadequate study design and inappropriate targeting of populations, no firm conclusion can be drawn regarding these changes. The bulk of fitness training studies that have targeted sleep quality as an outcome measure have been performed on small samples of optimally sleeping younger men and women or athletes. The limited cross-sectional data available suggest that fit older subjects have shorter sleep latencies, higher sleep efficiencies, and more slow-wave sleep than sedentary subjects. The elderly, the most likely group to benefit from such an intervention, are virtually unstudied.

Nevertheless, a recent meta-analysis of the effects of chronic exercise on sleep quality (Kubitz, Landers, Petruzzello, & Han, 1996) reported the following effect sizes in respect to exercise effects on sleep measures: increased total sleep time (0.94), increased slow-wave sleep (0.43), decreased sleep latency (0.45), decreased REM sleep (0.57), and decreased nighttime wakefulness (0.40). However, this meta-analysis of 12 studies mixed cross-sectional and prospective studies, and protocols were confounded by exercise sometimes preceding sleep assessments and sometimes not. Finally, these effect sizes, on average, represent relatively small absolute changes in the sleep variables measured.

The only randomized controlled trial of the impact of ET on the objective sleep quality of healthy sedentary elderly persons is from our laboratory (Vitiello et al., 1994a, 1994b), which at this time is published only in abstract form. Our subjects were carefully screened to exclude those with sleep complaints. We found that 6 months of ET resulted in an increase (~33%) in stage 3 to 4 sleep, or slow-wave sleep (SWS), in both elderly men and women. No improvements in any other sleep measure (e.g., measures of fragmentation) were noted for the ET group, nor were changes in any objective sleep measure noted for the control group (an SF attention control). These findings were confirmed when an additional baseline and posttraining night during which periodic blood sampling occurred were examined. As mentioned previously, nonspecific, subjectively reported, retrospective improvements in sleep quality were noted for both ET and SF groups (Vitiello et al., 1994b). Again it must be emphasized that the subjects participating in this study were healthy older men and women who did not complain of sleep disturbances and who were carefully screened to exclude sleep disorders.

Implications

Epidemiological data clearly support the hypothesis that regular exercise is associated with improved sleep quality. However, the experimental literature in support of this relationship is mixed, likely because of methodological differences and issues of subject sample size and sample characteristics. The four randomized studies of exercise effects on subjective sleep quality of the elderly currently published or completed indicate that regular exercise, whether endurance, resistance, or stretching–flexibility, is likely to improve sleep quality.

There are no published randomized controlled trials examining the influence of exercise on the objectively measured sleep either of older individuals complaining of sleep disturbance or of older insomniacs, and there are no randomized controlled trials of the impact of exercise on the subjective sleep of insomniacs. Clearly, such studies will be required before the beneficial impact of regular exercise on sleep quality in older individuals, and the downstream impact of such improved sleep on health, longevity, and quality of life, can clearly be delineated.

Fortunately, one such randomized trial is currently under way and another is currently submitted for funding. A study titled Promoting Exercise, Sleep, and Well-Being in Older Adults, 1 R01 MH58853, A. King, Principal Investigator, is examining the subjective and objective sleep quality of 120 sedentary men and women (ϵ55 years) with moderate sleep complaints before and after randomization to 1 year of moderate endurance training or an attention control. Subjective and objective sleep quality is being assessed at baseline and 6 and 12 months. Although this prospective study is yet to be completed, preliminary baseline data from this study sample support a positive relationship between physical fitness and sleep quality (Woo et al., 2003).

Only after additional well-designed and controlled, randomized trials examining the impact of regular exercise on sleep quality in the elderly are carried out will we have a definitive answer to whether exercise has beneficial effects on sleep quality in various components of the elderly population. Clearly, additional appropriate efficacy studies examining the three kinds of exercise (ET, RT, and SF) need to be conducted in various segments of the elderly population (e.g., healthy noncomplainers; those complaining of significant sleep disturbance; those with an insomnia diagnosis; and both persons in the community and those who are institutionalized) before the true nature of exercise–sleep relationships in the elderly population will be clearly delineated. Then a comparable series of effectiveness studies will be necessary to determine if the beneficial impact of exercise on sleep can be brought to the elderly generally.

Beyond that, the direct impact of improved sleep quality on health, longevity, and quality of life in the elderly also remains to be illuminated.

However, we can, with fair certainty given the clear direct impact of regular exercise on health, longevity, and quality of life, continue to prescribe such exercise with the appropriate caveats to the elderly population in general as a fundamental component of a healthy lifestyle and of good sleep hygiene practice as well.

Neuroendocrinology of Sleep and Its Impact on Cognition

Steiger (2003) offered a comprehensive review of some major components of the neuroendocrine control of sleep. In his review, Steiger (2003) commented on the bidirectional interaction that exists between sleep electroencephalograms (EEG) and endocrine activity in various species including humans. Although many neuroendocrine hormones affect sleep, a key role has been shown for the reciprocal interaction between sleep-promoting growth hormone–releasing hormone (GHRH) and sleep-impairing corticotrophin-releasing hormone (CRH). Changes in the GHRH:CRH ratio result in changes of sleep–endocrine activity. GHRH and its peer growth hormone secretagogues ghrelin and galanin promote SWS, whereas somatostatin, which suppresses GH secretion, is another sleep-impairing factor. Furthermore, there is good evidence that the change of this ratio in favor of CRH contributes to some of the aberrances of sleep seen in aging and depression, such as decreased SWS and increased sleep fragmentation.

HPA Axis: Sleep and Cognition

There is a growing body of literature suggesting that the disturbed objective sleep of primary insomniacs, and possibly their perceived disturbed sleep (Edinger et al., 2000; Morin, 2000; Rosa & Bonnet, 2000), may be at least in part the result of "hyperarousal" or disproportionate activation of the HPA axis (Bonnet & Arand, 1997; Vgontzas et al., 1998; Vgontzas, Bixler, Lin, et al., 2001; Vgontzas, Bixler, Wittman, et al., 2001).

HPA Axis and Sleep

Previously we proposed that a similar overactivation of the sympathetic nervous system (SNS) was a potential explanatory mechanism for at least part of the age-related increase in fragmentation that is observed even in healthy older adults who do not complain of disturbed sleep (Vitiello, Veith, Ralph, Frommlet, & Prinz, 1989; Vitiello, Prinz, & Halter, 1983; Vitiello, Ralph, Veith, & Prinz, 1990; Vitiello, Veith, Ralph, & Prinz, 1992). This SNS hypothesis was further developed by Richardson and colleagues (Richardson, Poe, Seymour, & Roth, 2001) as a possible explanatory mechanism for primary insomnia.

Several lines of evidence support this conceptualization. We demonstrated that elevating sympathetic tone, via a physiological manipulation, will fragment the sleep of healthy young men (Vitiello et al., 1983; Vitiello et al., 1989; Vitiello et al., 1990; Vitiello et al., 1992). Richardson recently replicated this observation and proposed that it serve as an experimental model for primary insomnia (Richardson et al., 2001). Vgontzas and colleagues (Vgontzas et al., 1998; Vgontzas, Bixler, Lin, et al., 2001; Vgontzas, Bixler, Wittman, et al., 2001) have demonstrated that insomniacs have elevated 24-hr adrenocorticotropic hormone and cortisol levels compared with matched controls. Bonnet and Arand (1998) demonstrated that two other measures reflective of sympathetic tone, nighttime heart rate period and variability, are disturbed in insomniacs relative to controls. Similarly, in a related line of evidence, Perlis, Smith, Andrews, Orff, and Giles (2001) and others have shown increased NREM beta/gamma activity in the sleep EEG of insomniacs compared with controls.

Assuming that hyperarousal may explain at least some of the symptoms of primary insomnia, both endurance training and resistance training are likely to provide benefits by mitigating such hyperarousal: for instance, through lower heart rate and blood pressure (Charlton & Crawford, 1997; Goldsmith, Bloomfield, & Rosenwinkel, 2000; O'Sullivan & Bell, 2000; Seals, Taylor, Ng, & Esler, 1994) and by either lowering cortisol (Wang, Tsai, Chen, & Wang, 2001) or moderating its reactivity (de Diego Acosta et al., 2001).

HPA Axis and Cognition

Comparable to this hyperarousal hypothesis of insomnia, there is growing evidence that increased HPA axis activity, in particular elevated cortisol levels, may have adverse effects on cognitive function. This hypothesis was originally proposed by Sapolsky based on work in primates demonstrating that elevated levels of cortisol were associated with hippocampal neuronal death (Sapolsky, 1989; Uno, Tarara, Else, Suleman, & Sapolsky, 1989); later the work was extended to humans (Lee, Ogle, & Sapolsky, 2002; Sapolsky, 2002).

Much of the work of Sapolsky (Sapolsky et al., 2002) and others has focused on the response of the HPA axis to stress and on the role of the HPA axis in posttraumatic stress disorder and major depressive illness (e.g., Elzinga & Bremner, 2002; Hoschl & Hajek, 2001; Lupien et al., 1999). However, there is a growing appreciation of the potential role of HPA activity within the aging process and the generalized cognitive decline that accompanies it.

Admittedly, it is difficult to attribute the increased HPA activity that is seen with advancing age to aging per se as opposed to accumulated environmental insults or the various comorbidities of aging such as cardiovascular disease or type 2 diabetes mellitus (Bjorntorp, 2002). Nevertheless, in a review of the possible relationship between lifetime glucocorticoid (cortisol) exposure and hippocampal impairment, Hibberd and colleagues concluded, "There is now strong evidence which associates hypercortisolemia in aged men with later cognitive dysfunction and this complements a wealth of rodent and other human data" (Hibberd, Yau, & Seckl, 2000, p. 560).

Given this relationship, behaviors that can moderate HPA activity over time should have potentially similar benefits in ameliorating hippocampal death and related cognitive decline. Clearly, regular exercise is one such behavior that is likely to benefit the HPA axis both directly and indirectly through its sleep-enhancing effects as described previously.

Somatotrophic Axis: Sleep and Cognition

Pulsatile pituitary GH secretion, regulated by the hypothalamic releasing factors GHRH and grehlin, the hypothalamic inhibiting factor somatostatin, and their various negative feedback loops, continues with aging but with diminished GH pulse amplitude (Prinz, Weitzman, Cunningham, & Karacan, 1983). In particular, nighttime GH secretion declines so that often there is no longer a clear night–day GH rhythm. SWS also declines with aging, although it is unclear whether the GH decline is attributable to the reduction in SWS, whether SWS deteriorates because of the decline in GH, or whether both are decreased because of a common reduction at a higher level of regulation (e.g., GHRH).

Somatotrophic Axis and Sleep

It has been demonstrated that sleep is influenced by clinical extremes of GH status (Aström & Lindholm, 1990; Aström & Trojaborg, 1992) and that sleep can be improved in response to acute GH administration (Drucker-Colin, Spanis, Hunyadi, Sassin, & McGaugh, 1975) or stimulation of the GH–insulin-like growth factor-I (IGF-I) axis using GHRH (e.g., Obal et al., 1988, 1996). Acute GHRH administration increases SWS, and acute decreases in GH levels following administration of a GHRH antagonist decrease slow-wave amplitude and slow-wave sleep duration in animals (Obal et al., 1996; Obal, Payne, Kapas, Opp, & Kreuger, 1991).

Among hormones, GHRH displays the best-documented sleep-promoting activity and is clearly implicated in the regulation of sleep, specifically NREM sleep. GHRH hypothalamic neurons projecting to the basal forebrain, specifically the medial preoptic area, likely act directly to increase NREM and SWS (Krueger, Obal, & Fang, 1999; Obal & Krueger, 2001).

Three independent laboratories have reported that GHRH promotes sleep in healthy young subjects (Kerkhofs et al., 1993; Marshall et al., 1996; Marshall, Boes, Strasburger, Born, & Fehm, 1997; Shier, Guldner, Colla, Holsboer, & Steiger, 1997; Steiger et al., 1992), although two older studies reported no such effect (Garry et al., 1985; Kupfer, Jarrett, & Ehlers, 1991), and some limited evidence suggests that the effect of GHRH on the sleep of the elderly may be weaker (Guldner et al., 1997; Murck, Frieboes, Schier, & Steiger, 1997).

Effects of Somatotrophic Axis Activity on the Brain

It has been suggested that the declines in GH and IGF-I observed with advancing age may contribute to the impaired cognitive function associated with aging and possibly even to that seen in neurodegenerative diseases such as Alzheimer's disease (Aleman et al., 1999; Connor & Dragunow, 1998; Connor et al., 1997; Rollero et al., 1998; Van Dam et al., 2000). GH and IGF-I bind to specific receptors in CNS structures relevant to learning and memory, such as the hippocampus, and both are present in plasma and cerebrospinal fluid (Adem et al., 1989; Johansson et al., 1995; Nyberg & Burman, 1996). Aging is associated with significant reductions in the density of GH binding sites, particularly in the pituitary, hypothalamus, and hippocampus (Lai et al., 1993; Nyberg, 1997).

Sonntag recently reviewed the interactions of GH, IGF-I, and brain aging (Sonntag et al., 2000; Sonntag, Brunso-Bechtold, & Riddle, 2001). He noted that work in aged rodents has demonstrated that administration of GH, IGF-I, or GHRH results in (1) increased cortical glucose metabolism (Lynch, Lyons, Khan, Bennett, & Sonntag, 2001), (2) increased cortical microvascular density and inferred cerebral blood flow (Sonntag, Lynch, Cooney, & Hutchins, 1997), (3) reversal of age-related declines of spatial and reference memory (Lichtenwalner et al., 2001), and (4) amelioration of age-related declines in hippocampal neurogenesis (Thorton, Ingram, & Sonntag, 2000; Thornton, Ng, & Sonntag, 1999).

At this time it is unclear whether some of these effects are the result of increased microvascularity and related changes in cerebral blood flow per se, the direct paracrine actions of IGF-I (e.g., via up-regulation of *N*-methyl-d-aspartate receptors), or both (Sonntag et al., 2000; Sonntag et al., 2001). However, given the density of IGF-I receptors in cortical areas supporting abilities such as declarative memory, it is conceivable that IGF-I supplementation via GHRH administration will have a facilitatory effect.

Manipulation of the Somatotrophic Axis and Cognitive Function in Humans

GH-deficient children have significant cognitive deficits, which may be moderated by GH treatment (Sartorio et al., 1996; van der Reijden-Lakeman, de

Sonneville, Swaab-Barneveld, Slijper, & Verhulst, 1997). Cognitive deficits are also seen in GH-deficient adults (Deijen, de Boer, Blok, & van der Veen, 1996; Sartorio et al., 1996) and can be normalized by GH therapy (Deijen, de Boer, & van der Veen, 1998). We and others have reported positive correlations between IGF-I and cognition in the healthy elderly (Aleman et al., 1999; Papadakis, Grady, Tierney, Black, Wells, & Grunfeld, 1995; Vitiello et al., 1999), particularly with respect to processing speed.

Previous to our own recent work described subsequently, there had been no direct examination of the effect of GHRH treatment on cognitive function. However, the effect of somatotrophic axis supplementation by GH treatment has been explored. Three placebo-controlled trials (Deijen et al., 1998; Papadakis et al., 1996; Soares et al., 1999) of GH treatment for 6 to 24 months in GHD adults reported improved cognitive function, although a fourth, similar, placebo-controlled study (Baum et al., 1998) observed no such improvement after 18 months of GH treatment.

We have recently concluded a 5-month, double-blind, placebo-controlled trial of GHRH treatment on a number of outcomes, including cognitive function, in a large group ($N = 89$) of healthy older men and women (Vitiello et al., 2000; Vitiello et al., 2002; Vitiello et al., 2006). Our results indicate that long-term GHRH treatment results in significant improvement in certain cognitive functions in healthy older adults, particularly those cognitive abilities that involve working memory and psychomotor processing speed.

Impact of Exercise and Fitness on the HPA and Somatotrophic Axes and Its Implications for Sleep and Cognition

Let us summarize the various areas of research reviewed briefly here. In doing so, we will speak generally and not concern ourselves with the exact reasons for, or mechanisms by which, an endocrine axis either increases or decreases its activity with advancing age. That is, it is relatively unimportant to our thesis whether the changes in hormonal levels are the result of aging per se, of other age-related processes such as comorbid illnesses, or of some combination of both. What is important is that as a general rule, HPA axis activity increases with advancing age and somatotrophic axis activity decreases.

HPA axis activity increases with advancing age, resulting in increased levels of circulating cortisol. Such increased levels of cortisol have been associated with poor sleep quality and impaired cognitive function. Somatotrophic axis activity declines with advancing age, resulting in lower levels of circulating GHRH, GH, and IGF-I. Such decreased levels of somatotrophic hormones have been associated with poor sleep quality and impaired cognitive function.

Let us now consider the impact of regular exercise and improved physical fitness on these relationships. Fitness training clearly lowers levels of physiological arousal, causing decreases in sympathetic tone, blood pressure, and heart rate (Charlton & Crawford, 1997; Goldsmith et al., 2000; O'Sullivan & Bell, 2000; Seals et al., 1994). As for the impact of fitness training on levels of cortisol, some studies report that fitness training results in lower cortisol levels (e.g., Wang et al., 2001), whereas others do not (e.g., Hakkinen, Pakarinen, Kraemer, Hakkinen, Valkeinen, & Alen, 2001). However, even if fitness training does not lower cortisol, it appears to blunt the reactivity of the HPA axis to physical challenge, resulting in lower increases in cortisol in fit compared with unfit subjects (de Diego Acosta et al., 2001). This fitness training–induced blunting of HPA activity and reactivity could well have beneficial effects directly on both sleep and cognition as well as indirectly on cognition via improved sleep.

Conversely, fitness training stimulates somatotrophic axis activity, resulting in increased levels of GH and IGF-I (Poehlman & Copeland, 1990), although fitness training must be maintained or circulating IGF-I returns to pretraining levels within days following cessation of training (Vitiello et al., 1997). Again, this fitness training–induced augmentation of somatotrophic activity is likely to have beneficial effects on both sleep quality and cognitive function, although it is unclear whether these beneficial exercise and fitness effects on cognitive function are direct, indirect via improved sleep, or both. Limited work in the area of somatotrophic activity suggests that both pathways are likely, because preliminary work has uncoupled improvements in sleep from those in cognition. Specifically, following successful endurance training in a group of healthy elderly men and women, sleep quality improved (Vitiello et al., 1994a, 1994b) but cognitive function did not (Kerr et al., 1993). Conversely, augmenting somatotrophic activity by chronic GHRH treatment in healthy older men and women resulted in improvements in cognitive function (Vitiello et al., 2000; Vitiello et al., 2002) but no improvement in sleep quality (Vitiello, Moe, Larsen, Merriam, & Schwartz, 2003).

It is quite possible that methodological limitations precluded finding beneficial effects on both sleep and cognitive function in these studies. The cognitive battery used in the fitness training study lacked sufficient tasks sensitive to the executive functions (Kerr et al., 1993) that more recent work has shown to be most responsive to fitness training (Colcombe & Kramer, 2003). In the GHRH treatment study, the timing of administration and pharmacokinetics of the GHRH preparation may have confounded the observation of any beneficial effect on sleep, which is sensitive to the timing of somatotrophic activity, without obscuring a beneficial impact on cognitive function, which may be responsive to overall levels or somatotrophic activity but not to its timing (Vitiello et al., 2001).

Fitting Together What We Know:
A View to the Future

Here, then, is what we know about how exercise, sleep, and cognitive function interrelate in the context of aging:

1. Sleep quality has a clear effect on cognition:
   - appropriate amounts and timing of sleep appear to be requirements for optimal cognitive function;
   - poor sleep quality results in poor cognitive function;
   - sleep disorders, including sleep-related breathing disorder, are associated with compromised cognitive function; and
   - effective treatment of sleep disorders is commonly associated with improved cognitive function.

2. Physical activity appears to have a beneficial effect on cognition:
   - epidemiological and cross-sectional studies consistently show that regular physical activity or fitness training is associated with higher levels of cognitive functioning, and
   - meta-analysis of the experimental data indicates that fitness training results in improved cognitive function, particularly for tasks tapping executive functions.

3. Physical activity appears to have a beneficial effect on sleep quality:
   - epidemiological and cross-sectional studies consistently show that regular physical activity or fitness training is associated with better quality sleep, and
   - meta-analysis of the experimental data indicates that fitness training results in improved sleep quality.

4. Sleep is at least partially regulated by two neuroendocrine systems that also affect cognitive function:
   - age-related increases in HPA axis activity, operationalized by high cortisol levels, result in more fragmented sleep and poorer cognitive function; and
   - age-related decreases in somatotrophic axis activity, operationalized by low GHRH, GH, and IGF-I levels, result in more fragmented sleep and poorer cognitive function.

5. Regular physical activity or fitness training tends to ameliorate the age-related changes in these two neuroendocrine systems, likely facilitating improved sleep quality and cognitive function.

From these observations we can make the following conjectures concerning the interrelationships among exercise, sleep, and cognition in the context of aging:

1. Sleep is likely a mediator of the impact of exercise on cognitive function.

2. Regular physical activity or exercise likely facilitates good sleep quality directly via
   - its role as a circadian rhythm zeitgaber, or "time-giver";
   - its thermogenic effect;
   - exercise-related changes in body composition and metabolism; and
   - amelioration of age-related changes in activity of the HPA and somatotrophic axes.

3. Regular physical activity or exercise may affect cognition directly, but clearly it affects cognition indirectly through the impact of improved sleep quality, per se, on cognition and through exercise-generated changes in the sleep-related activities of the HPA and somatotrophic axes.

4. Conversely, a lack of exercise likely results in poor sleep quality and may affect cognition adversely, both directly and also indirectly via resulting poor sleep quality and the unmodified age-related changes in somatotrophic and HPA activity.

Although the first five observations detailed here are fairly well supported in the literature, their robustness and the exact mechanisms underlying them still remain to be fully elucidated. For example, the putative causal relationships between exercise and sleep and exercise and cognitive function, although supported by meta-analyses, would be better served with more definitive experimental support. It is hoped that future fitness training studies include both sleep and cognitive function as outcomes and monitor HPA and somatotrophic activities, which would allow for testing of the more conjectural relations detailed here. It is encouraging to know that some such studies are currently under way, and their results are eagerly anticipated.

Regardless of whether these conjectures stand the test of time and experimentation, it is crucial to remember that regular exercise has been clearly demonstrated to address many of the comorbidities that accompany aging, such as cardiac failure, hypertension, falls, depression, pain, and functional decline. Regular exercise by the elderly also has been associated with improved overall subjective quality of life, has no serious adverse consequences, and is relatively inexpensive.

Given the current state of the scientific literature, the evidence that all people should make regular fitness training a part of their lives is overwhelming. What is most encouraging is that the literature also clearly shows that all of these benefits can be derived, albeit in some cases to a lesser degree, even if one begins fitness training in the later years.

All of this being said, if to all of the well-known benefits of regular exercise training can also be added improved sleep quality and cognitive function, this will indeed be very tasty icing on an already substantial and compelling cake, addressing two of the very important declines in function that tend to accompany advancing age. It is hoped such icing will further entice larger portions of the population, both elderly and younger, to incorporate regular and lifelong fitness training into their lives.

EDITORS' DISCUSSION SUMMARY

Discussion Highlights

A lively discussion ensued following Dr. Vitiello's proposal that despite popular belief and some anecdotal evidence, the experimental evidence in support of beneficial relationships among exercise, sleep, and cognitive function in old age is sparse. The discussion focused on the relationship of sleep to cognition, the relationship of exercise to sleep, types of exercise that might be beneficial, and mechanisms by which exercise might modify sleep or cognition.

Strong evidence is available from both animal and human studies that sleep plays a significant role in cognitive function, in particular memory. Experimental studies in humans suggest that increased REM sleep is associated with improvements in procedural memory and that increased NREM sleep may be more important for declarative memory consolidation. Studies of individuals with sleep disorders reveal that these individuals are consistently more susceptible to decrements in attention, verbal memory, vigilance, and driving simulation performance.

Considerable epidemiological evidence suggests that regular exercise is associated with good self-reported sleep quality as well as general well-being in elderly populations. However, experimental data in support of exercise's beneficial impact on sleep quality are less clear-cut. Future studies will likely improve confidence that exercise improves sleep quality. Exercise and sleep may also interact reciprocally with one another, and the effect of sleep on exercise may have either a negative or a positive impact, such that improvements in sleep quality may improve one's ability to exercise, whereas poor sleep may impair performance of exercise.

Both resistance training and endurance training have been associated with modest improvements in subjective sleep quality in community-dwelling older adults. However, few researchers have examined the effect of exercise on objectively measured polysomnographic sleep in older adults, and few definitive conclusions can be drawn. A recent meta-analysis of the effects of chronic exercise on sleep quality suggested that exercise is associated with increased total sleep time, increased slow-wave sleep, decreased sleep latency, decreased REM sleep, and decreased nighttime wakefulness.

Several mechanisms have been proposed for the purported relationships among exercise, sleep, and cognition in aging. Disturbed sleep may be, at least in part, the result of hyperarousal, or disproportionate activation of the HPA axis. In turn, increased HPA axis activity, in particular elevated cortisol levels, may have adverse effects on cognitive function. Interestingly, regular exercise has been, at least in a few studies, associated with decreased reactivity of the HPA axis to physical challenge. Fitness training could blunt HPA activity and reactivity, and this may be one mechanism that links exercise, sleep, and cognition.

Methodological Research Problems

A major measurement problem in this area is the absence of a highly valid, standardized, noninvasive way to quantify sleep quality. Current laboratory techniques of using EEG and polysomnographic recordings are highly invasive and inconvenient. A questionnaire for determining sleep quality is badly needed, but much work is being done on this problem to improve the correlations between objective sleep data and self-reports.

Future Directions

Before definitive conclusions can be drawn about the nature and strength of the relationships among exercise, sleep, and cognitive performance, additional randomized controlled exercise training studies are needed in which both sleep and cognitive function are measured objectively in conjunction with the assessment of HPA activity.

PART IV

Exercise, Chronic Disease, and Cognition

CHAPTER 11

Exercise, Hypertension, and Cognition

Hiro Tanaka, PhD

Miriam Cortez-Cooper, PhD
The University of Texas at Austin

EDITORS' OVERVIEW

Dr. Tanaka and Dr. Cortez-Cooper review what is known about the relationships among aging, hypertension, exercise, and cognition. In this chapter, they review what we know about hypertension and aging, hypertension and cognition, hypertension and habitual exercise, and finally, hypertension, cognition, and exercise. Hypertension is one of the most important risk factors for cerebrovascular disease such as stroke, which often results in cognitive impairment and dementia. Hypertension also contributes to cognitive impairment even in stroke-free individuals. Regular aerobic exercise has been shown to be a clinically efficacious therapeutic intervention to lower blood pressure in hypertensive adults. Evidence from cross-sectional and longitudinal studies suggests that higher physical activity or greater aerobic capacity may also prevent or attenuate age-related reductions in cognitive function. Age-related stiffening of

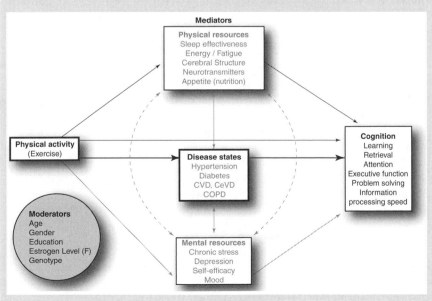

large elastic arteries (or a loss of arterial compliance) contributes to the increase in systolic blood pressure and pulse pressure that occurs with age. The results from long-term longitudinal studies appear to support a relationship between hypertension and cognition.

With advancing age, cognitive function decreases and the prevalence of cognitive impairment increases. Poor cognitive function has been associated with a number of adverse outcomes, including personal discomfort, loss of autonomy and independence, increased societal costs, increased risk of dementia, and even death (Bassuk, Wypij, & Berkman, 2000). In light of these important health and societal implications associated with cognitive function, factors or states that modulate cognitive impairment with age are of considerable interest. In this regard, accumulating evidence indicates that hypertension is a potent risk factor for cognitive impairment in elderly people. It is well established that hypertension is one of the most important risk factors for cerebrovascular disease such as stroke (Collins et al., 1990; Kannel, D'Agostino, & Silbershatz, 1997), which is known to often result in cognitive impairment and dementia (PROGRESS Collaborative Group, 2003). Hypertension also appears to contribute significantly to cognitive impairment even in stroke-free individuals (Elias, Wolf, D'Agostino, Cobb, & White, 1993; Launer, Masaki, Petrovitch, Foley, & Havlik, 1995).

The results of recent clinical trials demonstrate that lowering blood pressure in older adults with essential hypertension reduces the risk of future cardiovascular-disease related mortality and morbidity (Collins et al., 1990; MacMahon & Rodgers, 1993) as well as new-onset cognitive dysfunction and dementia (Forette et al., 1998). In this regard, regular aerobic exercise has been shown to be a clinically efficacious therapeutic intervention for lowering blood pressure in hypertensive adults (Tanaka, DeSouza, & Seals, 1999; Tanaka, Reiling, & Seals, 1998). Moreover, evidence from cross-sectional and longitudinal studies has suggested that higher physical activity or greater aerobic capacity may also prevent or attenuate age-related reductions in cognitive function (Barnes, Yaffe, Satariano, & Tager, 2003; Laurin, Verreault, Lindsay, MacPherson, & Rockwood, 2001; Spirduso & Clifford, 1978). As such, it is possible to hypothesize that regular exercise may prevent cognitive dysfunction through its effect on high blood pressure. Accordingly, the primary aim of this brief review is to examine the relationships among regular exercise, hypertension, and cognition.

Hypertension and Aging

Arterial blood pressure increases with advancing age in most industrialized societies, resulting in a high prevalence of essential hypertension (blood pressure >140/90 mmHg) among older adults (Kannel et al., 1997). Among

Americans aged 65 years or more, more than 50% of Caucasians and more than 70% of African Americans have high blood pressure (American Heart Association, 2003). These elevations in blood pressure are the largest contributor to cardiovascular mortality and morbidity among older adults (Taylor et al., 1991). The cost of hypertensive disease in the United States in 2003, including health expenditure and lost productivity, was estimated at $50 billion (American Heart Association, 2003). The age-related increase in blood pressure is absent in undeveloped societies and, as such, is not an inevitable consequence of biological aging (Pavan et al., 1999).

Until fairly recently, it was thought that elevated diastolic blood pressure posed a greater risk than high systolic blood pressure in the development of cardiovascular disease. As such, diastolic blood pressure was primarily targeted for detection, evaluation, and treatment of hypertension (Kannel, 1999). In recent years, the target has markedly changed to those patients whose systolic blood pressure is greater than 140 mmHg (Kannel, 1999). The need to shift the paradigm to systolic blood pressure is clear based on the available evidence. Cardiovascular and total mortality are far greater for elevated systolic than for diastolic blood pressure, especially in the older population (Sharrett et al., 1999). Moreover, increased pulse pressure, the measure of blood pressure most strongly related to cardiovascular risk, is primarily attributable to increased systolic blood pressure (Safar & London, 2000). In fact, systolic blood pressure increases markedly with advancing age, whereas the age-related increase in diastolic blood pressure is rather modest and tends to even decrease after the age of 60 years (Kannel et al., 1997).

Emerging evidence indicates that age-related stiffening of large elastic arteries (or a loss of arterial compliance) contributes to the increase in systolic blood pressure and pulse pressure that occurs with age (O'Rourke, 1990; Safar & London, 2000). The compliance of central arteries buffers pulsatile ventricular output ejected with each heartbeat through mechanical distention during systole, and the elastic recoil continues to propel blood into the arterial tree during diastole. This compliance function effectively converts the pulsatile flow at the level of the aorta to continuous flow in the capillaries (Nichols & O'Rourke, 1998). This is clinically important because loss of smooth, continuous capillary flow may result in end organ damage. Additionally, reductions in this buffering action, as seen in sedentary aging and hypertension, exert a number of adverse effects on systemic cardio-vascular function and disease risk, including elevations in systolic blood pressure and pulse pressure, increased aortic impedance and left ventricular wall tension, and a reduction in arterial baroreflex gain (Monahan, Dinenno et al., 2001; O'Rourke, 1990; Tanaka, Dinenno et al., 1998).

Arterial stiffness is an important determinant of the magnitude of mechanical deformation and strain caused by the changes in arterial blood pressure and, hence, the sensitivity of baroreceptors (Monahan, Dinenno et al., 2001; Monahan, Tanaka, Dinenno, & Seals, 2001). The arterial baroreflex is the principal mechanism for short-term (i.e., beat-to-beat) blood pressure homeostasis in humans. The age- and hypertension-related reduction in baroreflex sensitivity is thought to restrict the ability to increase heart rate in response to hypotensive stress and, therefore, is thought to contribute to the increased prevalence of orthostatic hypotension with advancing age as well as hypertension (Lipsitz, 1989). Orthostatic hypotension is known to cause generalized cerebral hypoperfusion, resulting in dizziness, nausea, syncope, and falls, and is also associated with the prevalent comorbid conditions of angina pectoris, myocardial infarction, and transient ischemia (Lipsitz, 1989). As described subsequently, such neurocardiovascular instability is very common and is highly prevalent in individuals with cognitive impairment and dementia (Kenny, Kalaria, & Ballard, 2002).

Hypertension and Cognition

With advancing age, cognitive function decreases and the prevalence of cognitive impairment leading to dementia increases. Some older adults do not experience increases in blood pressure with advancing age (Pavan et al., 1999; Seals, Stevenson, Jones, DeSouza, & Tanaka, 1999), and overt cognitive impairment is absent in some elderly as well. However, the reduction in some aspects of cognitive function is known to occur in every species that has been examined (Erickson & Barnes, 2003), suggesting that cognitive impairment may have some biological or physiological basis. Among the various factors proposed to affect cognitive impairment, hypertension has become increasingly discernable as a mediator variable (Alves de Moraes, Szklo, Knopman, & Sato, 2002; Elias et al., 1993; Kilander, Nyman, Boberg, Hansson, & Lithell, 1998; Launer et al., 1995).

Given the close association between high blood pressure and cerebrovascular disease including stroke (Kannel et al., 1997), it is reasonable to hypothesize that hypertension increases the risk for cognitive impairment. However, when considering non-stroke-related cognitive impairment, the observational cross-sectional studies have produced mixed results. This is clearly illustrated by Seux and Forette, who reviewed a number of studies conducted on older normotensive and hypertensive adults (Seux & Forette, 1999). High blood pressure was associated with higher cognitive function (Guo, Fratiglioni, Winblad, & Viitanen, 1997), lower cognitive function (Seux et al., 1998), or no difference in cognitive function (Farmer et al., 1987). Thus, a relationship between hypertension and cognition appears highly contradictory when the findings from observational cross-sectional studies are considered. Such controversial results are likely attributable to methodological problems (Starr, 1999) that are inherent in observational studies, including the differences in population studied, neuropsychological methods used, and blood pressure variables selected (systolic vs. diastolic blood pressure).

The results from long-term longitudinal studies are more consistent and appear to support the relationship between hypertension and cognition. As in many other areas of cardiovascular risks, the Framingham Study has made an important contribution in this area. In this large longitudinal study, elevated blood pressure at baseline was a significant predictor of reduced cognitive function during the follow-up period of 12 to 15 years (Elias et al., 1993). One major strength of this study is that most hypertensive patients enrolled in this study did not receive treatments, thereby eliminating or substantially reducing the potentially confounding influence of antihypertensive therapy. These findings are consistent with the results of the Honolulu–Asia Aging Study (Launer et al., 1995). This 25-year longitudinal study demonstrated that increased midlife systolic, but not diastolic, blood pressure was significantly associated with cognitive impairment in late life. These findings have been confirmed with several other longitudinal studies (Alves de Moraes et al., 2002; Kilander et al., 1998). Collectively, the results of large, well-conducted longitudinal studies indicate that high blood pressure is associated with cognitive impairment in later life. Among various measures of cognitive function, hypertension appears to influence attentional, perceptual–motor, and short-term memory processes (Shapiro, Miller, King, Ginchereau, & Fitzgibbon, 1982). It should be noted, however, that the relationship between cognition and hypertension may not be causal. For example, it is possible that the relationship may be mediated by other factors that are collinearly related to both cognition and hypertension, including psychosocial stress and socioeconomic status.

The mechanisms by which high blood pressure may influence cognitive decline are complex and are not fully understood. One potential mechanism is through the impairment of dynamic vascular autoregulation. Vascular autoregulation in cerebral arteries refers to the ability of the small cerebral arteries to maintain a constant blood flow despite the large oscillations in blood pressure (Panerai, Carey, & Potter, 2003). As systemic blood pressure increases, the cerebral arteries constrict, thereby limiting the increase in cerebral blood flow to prevent swelling of the brain beyond which can be accommodated by the bony cranium. Conversely, when blood pressure falls, the cerebral arteries vasodilate to prevent blood flow from declining to the point of cerebral ischemia. Because of this function, the cerebral vasculature has an ability to adapt to chronically elevated blood pressure but at the expense of changes that increase the risk for cerebrovascular disease. Structural changes, including arteriolar narrowing and wall thickening, would shift the operating pressure levels controlled by autoregulation to higher values and would reduce the tolerance to episodes of hypotension, rendering the brain vulnerable to hypotension-induced ischemia (Phillips & Whisnant, 1992). This is supported by the observation that the vasodilator capacity of the small cerebral arteries is reduced in hypertensive humans and spontaneously hypertensive rats (Jennings, 2003).

Another possibility is that arterial stiffness, a primary mechanism underlying the age-related increase in blood pressure, also acts on the brain to induce cognitive dysfunction. An increase in arterial stiffness, which would result in a loss of arterial wall buffering function, has been shown to lead to the more prominent vessel wall oscillations in cerebral arteries (Keunen, Vliegen, Stam, & Tavy, 1996). The inability to convert the pulsatile flow to continuous flow could damage capillaries in cerebral circulation and could lead to hypertension-induced lesions if it persists. In fact, the arterial structural changes that occur in response to chronically elevated blood pressure are associated with diffuse white matter disease or leukoariosis, the prevalence of which is significantly higher in individuals with moderate or severe hypertension (Johansson, 1994). Whether these increased white matter hyperintensities seen in magnetic resonance imaging are causally related to declines in cognitive function is still a matter of debate. Nevertheless, there is experimental support for the concept linking arterial stiffness to cognitive decline. First, higher pulse pressure, a rough surrogate marker of arterial stiffness, is associated with increased risk of dementia and Alzheimer's disease in older adults (Qiu, Winblad, Viitanen, & Fratiglioni, 2003). Second, neurocardiovascular instability, commonly manifested as orthostatic and postprandial hypotension, is highly prevalent in those with cognitive impairment and dementia (Kenny et al., 2002). In this regard, neurocardiovascular instability is closely associated with arterial stiffness via arterial baroreflex sensitivity (Kenny et al., 2002). Indeed, we have recently demonstrated that arterial stiffness plays an important role in the age-related reduction in arterial baroreflex sensitivity (Monahan, Dinenno et al., 2001; Monahan et al., 2000). These results are consistent with the hypothesis that arterial stiffness may be a putative mechanism underlying cognitive dysfunction. Other possibilities include the reduction in endothelial function, which would result in cerebral hypoperfusion (Lavi, Egbarya, Lavi, & Jacob, 2003). In fact, the alteration in blood flow to the brain changes behavioral performance on a variety of mental tasks (Patterson, 2001).

Hypertension and Habitual Exercise

Current guidelines recommend that for patients with stage 1 and 2 hypertension, lifestyle modifications, including regular aerobic exercise, be used for an initial period of 3 to 6 months, followed by pharmacological interventions, if necessary, to achieve normalization of blood pressure (Joint

National Committee on Prevention, 1997). These recommendations were based on epidemiological and interventional studies that have examined the relationship between regular exercise and blood pressure (Paffenbarger, Wing, Hyde, & Jung, 1983; Seals et al., 1999; Tanaka et al., 1999). In one of the most notable epidemiological studies to date, Paffenbarger and colleagues reported that among Harvard college alumni, vigorous physical activity was associated with the lower incidence of hypertension in later life (Paffenbarger et al., 1983). Recently, we demonstrated that the elevations in blood pressure with age that are usually observed in sedentary adults are absent in those who regularly perform endurance exercise (see figure 11.1) (Seals et al., 1999).

The results of intervention studies are consistent with cross-sectional studies. In young adults with elevated arterial blood pressure at baseline, regular aerobic exercise lowers casually determined systolic and diastolic blood pressure at rest (Fagard & Amery, 1995; Tanaka et al., 1997). We and others have reported that middle-aged and older adults demonstrate similar reductions in response to exercise therapy (Hagberg, Montain, Martin, & Ehsani, 1989; Tanaka et al., 1999; Tanaka, Reiling et al., 1998). However, the magnitude of reduction in blood pressure with exercise appears to be smaller in older compared with the young adults (Ishikawa, Ohta, Zhang, Hashimoto, & Tanaka, 1999), and both men and women may experience similar benefits from regular exercise (Ishikawa et al., 1999). Interestingly, regular exercise at mild intensities may lower blood pressure at rest more than would exercise at higher intensities in older adults (Fagard & Amery, 1995). A factor that is most consistently related to the magnitude of decline in blood pressure with exercise is baseline (preintervention) blood pressure (Fagard & Amery, 1995). That is, the higher the baseline blood pressure, the greater reduction in blood pressure that would be expected with regular exercise. Reductions in arterial blood pressure with exercise therapy have been observed independent of a number of potential influences, including reductions in body mass and body fat, changes in dietary intake, and increases in maximal aerobic capacity (Seals, Silverman, Reiling, & Davy, 1997; Tanaka et al., 1997; Tanaka et al., 1999). These results indicate that hypotensive effects can be attributed to the effect of regular exercise per se. Thus, the available evidence indicates that regular aerobic exercise appears to be a clinically efficacious therapeutic intervention for reducing arterial blood pressure in middle-aged and older adults.

Information concerning the physiological mechanisms by which regular exercise lowers blood pressure is limited. The available data indicate that arterial stiffness may play a role in hypotensive effects of regular exercise (Seals et al., 1999; Seals et al., 2001; Tanaka et al., 2000). As described previously, the stiffness of central arteries is thought to contribute to age-associated increases in systolic blood pressure and pulse pressure (O'Rourke,

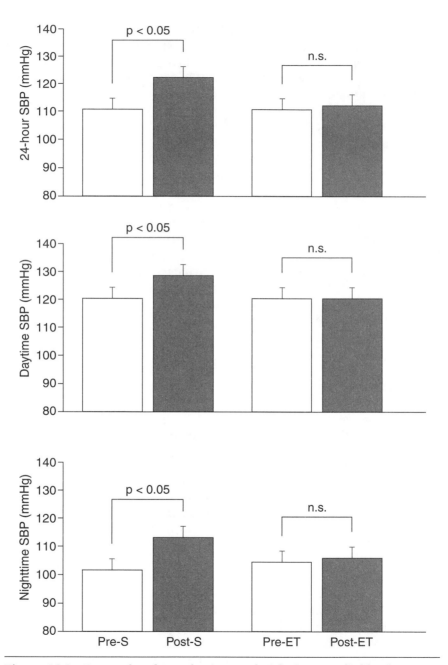

Figure 11.1 Twenty-four-hour, daytime, and nighttime systolic blood pressure (SBP) in premenopausal sedentary (S) and endurance-trained (ET) women.

Reprinted from D.R. Seals et al., 1999, "Lack of age-associated elevations in 24-h systolic and pulse pressures in women who exercise regularly," *American Journal of Physiology: Heart and Circulatory Physiology* 277(3): H947-H955. Used with permission.

1990). We previously reported that the increase in arterial stiffness observed in sedentary adults was absent in adults who habitually engaged in physical activity (figure 11.2) (Tanaka, DeSouza, & Seals, 1998) and that their favorable levels of arterial stiffness were significantly related to the absence of any obvious elevation in blood pressure with age in endurance-trained adults (Seals et al., 1999). Additionally, we recently reported that in older women with elevated baseline blood pressure levels, the reductions in blood pressure induced by lifestyle modifications may be mediated by a decrease in the stiffness of the large elastic arteries (Seals et al., 2001).

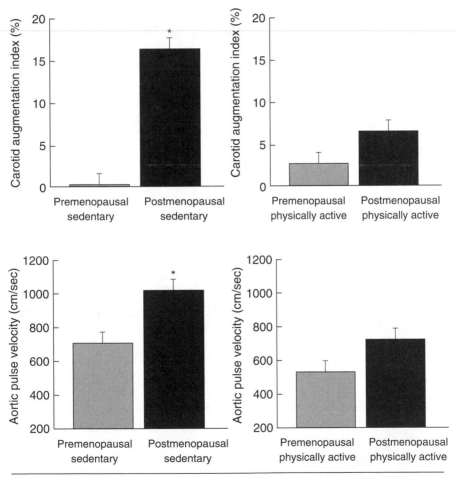

Figure 11.2 Arterial stiffness, as assessed by pulse wave velocity and carotid augmentation index, of sedentary and endurance-trained women.

From H. Tanaka, C.A. DeSouza and D.R. Seals, 1998, "Absence of age-related increase in central arterial stiffness in physically active women," *Arteriosclerosis, Thrombosis, and Vascular Biology* 18(1): 127-132.

These findings provide support for the postulate that reductions in arterial stiffness may play a mechanistic role in the blood pressure–lowering effects of exercise.

Hypertension, Cognition, and Habitual Exercise

From a theoretical point of view, control or prevention of risk factors for cognitive impairment, including hypertension, should contribute to a reduction in the incidence of cognitive impairment. Indeed, because of the close association between hypertension and stroke (Kannel, 1999), habitual exercise should reduce the risk of cognitive impairment by preventing cerebrovascular disease, which is known often to result in cognitive impairment and dementia (PROGRESS Collaborative Group, 2001, 2003). An important question that has not been examined is whether the hypotensive effects of exercise training could reverse the adverse influence of hypertension on cognitive function. To the best of our knowledge, only one study has investigated the effects of aerobic exercise on cognitive function in patients with hypertension (Pierce, Madden, Siegel, & Blumenthal, 1993). Those authors found that a 16-week aerobic training program was not associated with improvements in cognitive and psychosocial functions. However, interpretation of these data is difficult because the authors failed to demonstrate the hypotensive effect of aerobic exercise training. Another unanswered question is whether well-established benefits of regular exercise on cardiovascular disease risks in hypertensive populations are mediated by its influence on the clinical expression of neurodegenerative processes.

Some clues to answer these questions may come from pharmacological studies. The results from recent intervention studies support the idea that hypotensive effects induced by drugs may prevent and improve cognitive dysfunction, although the evidence is far from uniform (Applegate & Little, 1994). The Systolic Hypertension in Europe (Syst-Eur) trial involved a group of 2,418 nondemented subjects with isolated systolic hypertension aged 60 years and older (Forette et al., 1998). Subjects were randomized to either placebo or active treatment with a calcium-channel blocker alone or in association with angiotensin-converting enzyme inhibitor. Mean follow-up was limited to 2 years because the trial was terminated early because of a significant reduction in stroke, which was the primary outcome measure of the study. Nevertheless, the reduction in blood pressure was associated with reduced incidence of cognitive dysfunction and dementia by 50% (Forette et al., 1998). These earlier observations were confirmed by the extended observation of patients who were offered active trial medication for a further period and experienced greater reductions in the incidence of dementia (Forette et al., 2002). More recently, the results of the PROG-RESS study, designed to determine the effects of antihypertensive drugs in hypertensive subjects with a history of stroke or transient ischemic attack, also demonstrated a significant reduction in cognitive impairment and dementia (PROGRESS Collaborative Group, 2001, 2003). Taken together, these results suggest that a blood pressure–lowering regimen may play a role in the prevention of cognitive impairment and dementia in a hypertensive population.

Many putative mechanisms have been proposed to explain the effects of regular exercise in preventing and enhancing cognitive dysfunction. They include maintenance of and increase in cerebral blood flow (which would enhance the supply of oxygen and nutrients to the brain) (Rogers, Meyer, & Mortel, 1990); reduction in brain tissue loss (Colcombe et al., 2003); and growth of new capillaries from the existing blood vessels, termed *angiogenesis* (Lavi et al., 2003). It is also possible that beneficial effects of regular exercise on arterial stiffness may account, at least in part, for the influence of regular exercise on cognitive function. Another possibility is that increase in endothelial function with exercise training (DeSouza et al., 2000) may maintain cerebral blood flow, attenuating or preventing adverse effects of hypertension on brain function (Rao, 2002). It is likely that some of these mechanisms may be applied to postulated benefits of exercise on cognitive function in hypertensive patients. However, this issue has not been investigated in hypertensive patients.

EDITORS' DISCUSSION SUMMARY

Discussion Highlights

For many decades, cerebrovascular health and brain circulation have been proposed as mechanisms that influence cognition. The discussion on this topic was focused on the relationships among exercise, hypertension, and cognitive functioning in old age and how these relationships might reduce blood profusion in the brain. Strong evidence exists that hypertension is a potent risk factor for cognitive impairment in the elderly. Similarly, research evidence from both cross-sectional and longitudinal studies suggests that higher physical activity or greater aerobic capacity can prevent or attenuate age-related reductions in cognitive function. One mechanism by which regular exercise may prevent cognitive dysfunction is through its effect on high blood pressure. Indeed, midlife hypertension poses a greater cognitive risk than old-age hypertension. Midlife hypertension predicts old-age dementia and cognitive impairment better than does old-age hypertension. Therefore, preventive treatment of hypertension should begin during midlife in order to protect cognitive function most effectively.

Hypertension induces small but significant decreases in cerebral blood flow, contributing to regional hypoperfusion of the brain. Other conditions that may reduce perfusion include decreased blood volume during surgery, surgically induced decreases in blood pressure, and decreased heart rate. Increases in neuronal activity can reduce perfusion to inactive areas as perfusion increases in areas recruited for a task. Areas of the brain subject to the greatest damage from transient hypoperfusion include the basal ganglia and the subcortical elements of the frontal control systems, which are normally hypoperfused. In addition, arterial thickening in response to hypertension increases the risk of brain ischemia attributable to a loss of ability of arteries to dilate.

The brain increases regional blood flow in areas that perform any given task. In theory, the increase in local blood flow reflects an increase in the level of functioning of the brain in those areas. The aging brain also demonstrates plasticity to recruit alternative areas for a given task than those normally recruited. When those areas are recruited, regional cerebral blood flow is increased in those areas. However, hypertension may reduce perfusion in areas normally recruited for a given task. The brain may lose some of its ability to redirect local blood flow with age. Evidence for the loss of local control of brain blood flow comes from observations that endothelial function declines with age, flow-mediated dilation declines with age, and acetylcholine-mediated dilation declines with age. All of these effects of aging diminish the capacity for local control of perfusion in the brain. Loss of local control of perfusion may underlie impaired recruitment of alternative brain areas for a given task.

One factor that leads to hypertension is a decrease in baroreceptor sensitivity with age. This decrease is attributable in part to increases in arterial stiffness with age. In addition, hypertension accelerates arterial stiffening, and hence aging and hypertension reduce baroreceptor regulation of blood pressure, because arteries must be compliant for baroreceptors to regulate blood pressure. When arteries stiffen, the brain may increase its role in regulation of blood pressure to compensate for the decline in baroreceptor sensitivity.

It is noteworthy that the brain plays major roles in regulation of heart rate and blood pressure, but it plays a minor role in regulation of baroreceptors. Researchers have shown that primates can regulate their heart rates to avoid electric shock, and electrodes in various brain areas can assist or impede control of heart rate by the brain. Meanwhile, declines in blood pressure predict cognitive decline, whereas low blood pressure is associated with advancing dementia. Hence, neurodegeneration might cause changes in blood pressure. In the healthy adult population, increases or decreases in cognition might either increase or decrease blood pressure. If cognition does affect blood pressure, it is not clear whether it affects ambulatory blood pressure (monitored over 24 h) or only casual blood pressure (a single isolated measurement).

Methodological Research Problems

Two methodological problems that make interpretation of research in this area difficult are the interpretation of regional brain perfusion and the differential results obtained from casual and ambulatory measures of blood pressure. Regional brain perfusion may not reflect function accurately. Measurements of brain function rely heavily on perfusion measurements rather than on direct measurements of function. Direct measurement techniques need to be developed to improve understanding of brain function.

Most researchers use a measure of casual blood pressure, which means that they obtain a single isolated measurement. Ambulatory blood pressure predicts cognitive function better than casual blood pressure. Similarly, ambulatory blood pressure is more sensitive to exercise effects. In a long-term study comparing the effects of walking at 70% of maximal heart rate five times per week on blood pressure values measured by either method, Seals and Reiling (1991) found that endurance exercise decreased casual blood pressure within 6 months but did not alter ambulatory blood pressure in the same period. Within 12 months, however, ambulatory blood pressure declined significantly in response to exercise, whereas casual blood pressure declined only slightly more between 6 and 12 months of exercise. Studies of acute exercise show that a single bout of aerobic exercise lowers ambulatory blood pressure for 10 to 12 hours in mildly to moderately hypertensive patients. Researchers studying aging, blood pressure, and cognition have generally not obtained ambulatory blood pressures.

Future Directions in Research

Studies need to be conducted to discover (a) the effects of regular exercise on cognitive function in patients with hypertension, (b) the hypotensive effects of exercise associated with a corresponding improvement in cognitive function, (c) the ways that arterial stiffness is related to cognitive function, and (d) the underlying physiological mechanisms by which the hypotensive effects of exercise might influence cognitive function in older adults.

CHAPTER 12

Diabetes, Executive Control, Functional Status, and Physical Activity

Donald R. Royall, MD
The University of Texas Health Sciences Center

EDITORS' OVERVIEW

This chapter begins with an introduction of the effects of exercise and physical activity on diabetes and their role as mediators of functional status and executive control function (ECF). ECF has, within the past 6 to 10 years, attracted a substantial amount of attention as a type of cognitive function that is crucial to normal physical and social functioning but that is negatively affected by aging independently of other types of cognition. In this model, physical activity positively affects diabetic symptoms, which benefits mental function, which in turn facilitates ECF.

Because so few studies of diabetes, ECF, functional status, and physical activity exist, the introduction is followed by a completed longitudinal research paper

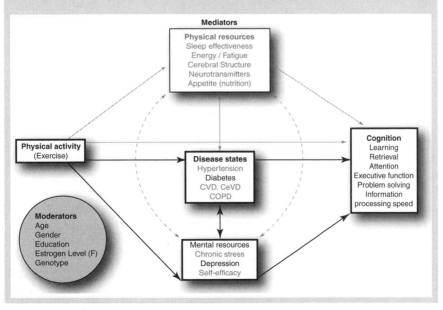

This study was supported by a grant from the National Institute of Aging (AG10939).

written by Dr. Royall and a team of collaborators. In this paper they show that (a) diabetes generally impairs ECF in older adults, (b) physical function mediates part of the relationship between diabetes and ECF, but (c) physical activity's effects are not specific to ECF. Instead, the researchers found that the physical activity levels of diabetics were related to visuospatial cognitive abilities. They suggest that two mechanisms that are known to have detrimental effects on cognition, psychological depression and ischemic vascular disease, have also been shown to be influenced by exercise.

Cognition, particularly executive control function (ECF), has been shown to be significantly associated with exercise in old age (Barnes, Yaffe, Satariano, & Tager, 2003; Binder, Storandt, & Birge, 1999; Blumenthal et al., 1989). Executive functions organize complex goal directed activities and are necessary to the initiation, sequencing, and monitoring of higher behavioral sets (Royall et al., 2002). Thus, ECF may be particularly relevant to the successful completion of functional activities, such as instrumental activities of daily living (IADLs), as well as to the capacity to initiate and sustain an effective exercise program.

Not all cognitive functions may be as relevant to physical activity as ECF is. Moreover, not all dimensions of executive control may be relevant. Binder and colleagues (1999) studied the relationship between performance on psychometric measures, a modified Physical Performance Test (modified PPT), and self-reported activities of daily living, in 125 men and women aged ≥75 years. Two factors, an executive attentional control factor and a memory factor, accounted for 55% of the variance in cognitive test performance. Hierarchical multiple regression analyses demonstrated that age, number of medications, and attentional control were independent predictors of the total modified PPT score.

Executive function is thought to be mediated by specific frontal systems that include various regions within the frontal cortex, the basal ganglia, the thalamus, and their associated white matter connections (Royall et al., 2002). Aerobic fitness appears to protect individuals from age-related frontal atrophy (Colcombe et al., 2003). Thus, it is conceivable that an exercise program might have positive benefits on ECF.

The significance of this is that ECF has a robust association with functional status and level of care (Royall, 1999). Nonetheless, it is unclear whether cognition mediates the effect of exercise on functional status. Wilson and colleagues (2002) reported a significant association between self-reported mental and physical activity and incident Alzheimer's disease (AD) risk in a sample of 1,249 community-dwelling older persons aged ≥65 years. In logistic regression models adjusted for age, education, sex, race, and certain genetic risks, increased cognitive activity was associated with a 64% reduction in the risk of incident AD (odds ratio [OR] 0.36, 95%

confidence interval [CI] 0.20-0.65). In contrast, weekly hours of physical activity were not related to disease risk (OR 1.04, 95% CI 0.98-1.10).

Wilson and colleagues' failure to demonstrate a significant association between physical activity and incident dementia might have been an artifact of the specific physical activities they chose to model. Some physical tasks may be more closely associated with cognition than others. Fried, Ettinger, Lind, Newman, and Gardin (1994) demonstrated that at least four dimensions of physical function can be derived from factor analyses of self-reported physical impairment in the Cardiovascular Health Study. These include activities primarily dependent on mobility and exercise tolerance, complex activities heavily dependent on cognition and sensory input, selected basic self-care activities, and upper-extremity activities. Groups 2 and 3 are similar, but not identical, to IADLs and activities of daily living (ADLs), respectively. In multiple logistic regression analyses, the associations between common chronic diseases, such as diabetes mellitus, and physical performance were strongest for tasks in groups 2 and 3. Thus, although chronic disease can be associated with select physical outcomes, this effect is limited to the more cognitive aspects of physical performance, not its more motor–cardiovascular aspects, supporting the findings of Wilson and colleagues. In a similar study, Bootsma-van der Wiel and colleagues (2002) found that general cognition and depressive symptoms had effects on walking ability that were greater than, and independent of, specific chronic medical conditions, including diabetes mellitus.

Literature Review

There is little other relevant literature from which to assess the associations among exercise, cognition, and functional status in diabetes mellitus. We recently used MEDLINE to search the English-language medical literature between 1966 and June 2003. Of 62,002 articles containing the search terms *cognition, frontal lobe, executive,* or *neuropsychological tests,* only 198 also contained the terms *diabetes* or *diabetes mellitus.* Of these, only four also contained references to *muscle–skeletal, respiration, exertion, exercise test,* or *exercise.*

Only two of those articles were relevant to the current inquiry. As one might guess, a sedentary lifestyle and diabetes mellitus both are modifiable and potentially reversible risks for cognitive impairment in old age (Fillit et al., 2002). However, although it can be shown that exercise and cognition interact to reduce the rate of functional decline in older adults, this effect appears to be independent of diabetes (Wang, van Belle, Kukull, & Larson, 2002).

Nonetheless, previous researchers have shown that diabetes is associated with frontal system dysfunction and executive deficits. Diabetic patients show impairment on tests that are thought to be sensitive to executive control. These include the digit–symbol subtest of the Weschler Adult Intelligence Scale (Keymeulen et al., 1995; Perlmuter, Tun, Sizer, McGlinchey, & Nathan, 1987; Tun, Perlmuter, Russo, & Nathan, 1987), verbal fluency (Perlmuter et al., 1987), abstract reasoning (Desmond, Tatemichi, Paik, & Stern, 1993; Reaven, Thompson, Nahum, & Haskins, 1990), and cognitive flexibility (Van Boxtel et al., 1998), as well as Grooved Pegboard, Trail Making, Stroop Word Naming, and Picture Arrangement (Meneilly, Cheung, Tessier, Yakura, & Tuokko, 1993).

Possible Mechanisms

At least three plausible mechanisms by which diabetes and cognition may relate are stroke, major depression, and hypoglycemia. Subcortical vascular disease and white matter lesions (WMLs), for example, disproportionately affect frontal systems (Ishii, Nishihara, & Imamura, 1986) and are specifically associated with poor performance on tests of executive function (Steingart et al., 1987). Diabetes is an independent risk factor for stroke and WMLs (Awad, Spetzler, Hodak, Awad, & Carey, 1986; Fazekas et al., 1988; Schmidt, 1992).

Frontal systems stroke is also strongly associated with poststroke depressive syndromes (Robinson, Kubos, Starr, Rao, & Price, 1984; Starkstein, Robinson, & Price, 1988). Depression is associated with frontal cerebral blood flow (rCBF) reductions in both unipolar and bipolar presentations (Baxter et al., 1989). Frank major depression may follow subcortical lesions to the globus pallidus, whereas subcortical lesions lead to apathetic states that resemble depression (Lauterbach et al., 1997). The risk of depressive symptoms is increased in diabetes mellitus (Gavard, Lustman, & Clouse, 1993).

However, the association between depression and diabetes mellitus may partially reflect selection biases related to the specific screening measure used. Leedom, Meehan, Procci, and Zeidler (1991) reported that the cognitive items on the Beck Depression Inventory (BDI; Beck, Steer, & Brown, 1996; Steer, Ball, Ranieri, & Beck, 1999) may account for most of the depressive symptoms reported by type 2 diabetic patients. Thus, the BDI may be vicariously sensitive to the frontal system impairments of elderly diabetic patients. The Geriatric Depression Scale (GDS; Sheikh & Yesavage, 1996) offers a less biased alternative for depression screening in diabetic subjects. It was developed specifically for use in older, medically ill patients and has been weighted in favor of the psychological symptoms of depression, rather than its so-called vegetative symptoms (Brink, 1987; Royall, 1997).

Finally, some psychiatric symptoms in diabetic patients may be attributable to insulin itself (Lustman, Griffith, Clouse, & Cryer, 1986). Keymeulen and colleagues (1995) documented regionally specific *frontotemporal* hypoperfusion by single photon emission tomography (SPECT) in long-term type 1 (insulin-dependent) diabetics but not in either recent-onset cases or age-matched controls. Frontal function can also be examined through functional measures such as cortical electroencephalography (EEG) and the P300 event-related potential. Tribl and colleagues (1996) reported frontal EEG slowing in response to insulin-induced hypoglycemia in patients with insulin-dependent diabetes mellitus (IDDM). Blackman and colleagues (1992) reported increased P300 latency in IDDM patients during insulin-induced hypoglycemia but not enforced euglycemia. The hypoglycemic effects on P300 latency persist despite restoration of serum glucose by intravenous glucose or a meal.

Exercise might modify any of these risk factors. However, although exercise is associated with ECF, it is not clear that this relationship is causal in direction. ECF could conceivably affect motivation, perseverance, and the capacity to engage in an effective exercise program. This issue can only be addressed in prospective studies.

New Data

We have developed information on exercise and executive function as part of the Hispanic Established Population for Epidemiological Studies in the Elderly (HEPESE) cohort. HEPESE is a longitudinal study of a representative sample of Mexican Americans, aged ≥65 years, residing in the southwestern United States. The sample was drawn using area probability sampling procedures to represent Mexican American elderly in five southwestern states, Texas, New Mexico, Colorado, Arizona, and California.

HEPESE contains information on cognition (i.e., the MMSE; Folstein, Folstein, & McHugh, 1975) and CLOX: An Executive Clock Drawing Task (Royall, Cordes, & Polk, 1998). CLOX is divided into two parts. CLOX1 is an unprompted task that is sensitive to executive control. CLOX2 is a copied version that is less dependent on executive skills.

CLOX offers two significant advantages over other cognitive assessments. First, CLOX1 is more sensitive to ECF than either the MMSE or other clock drawing tasks (CDTs; Royall, Mulroy, Chiodo, & Polk, 1999). Thus, it can supply information on a domain of cognitive function that has not been well addressed by the epidemiological literature. Second, CLOX provides the capacity to develop two-dimensional assessments of cognition. The pattern of CLOX1 versus CLOX2 performance may have diagnostic significance not conveyed by either measure alone. Finally, it appears that CDTs appear to be less vulnerable to linguistic, cultural, or educational bias than traditional dementia screening instruments (La Rue, Romero, Ortiz, Liang, & Lindeman, 1999). A Spanish-language translation has been developed specifically for use in HEPESE (Royall et al., 2003).

Method

Data were collected in three waves from fall 1993 to spring 1994. They included demographic data, depression scores, cognitive measures, and self-reported and performance indicators of physical function and physical activity.

Subjects

HEPESE subjects were interviewed in their own homes. The baseline response rate for eligible respondents was 83%. The total number of subjects surveyed at baseline (fall 1993 to spring 1994) was 3,050. Of these, 1,713 (56.2%) were still available at wave three (fall 1998 to spring 1999), when the CLOX was introduced. A valid CLOX (either CLOX1 or CLOX2) was obtained in 1,202 subjects (70.2%). Of these, 1,165 had a valid CLOX1, and 1,202 had a valid CLOX2. A sizable fraction of the HEPESE sample (n = 829, 72.5%) was administered the CLOX in Spanish translation.

Demographic data were abstracted from the Older Americans Resources Scale (OARS; Fillenbaum, 1985). The OARS contains self-reported information on general health, health services utilization, exercise, current medication use, and a number of chronic medical conditions, including diabetes mellitus. Self-reported general health was scored on a 4-point metric, ranging from 0 = *poor* to 3 = *excellent*.

Depressive symptoms were measured by the Center for Epidemiological Study–Depression (CES–D) scale (Radloff, 1977). The CES–D is a well-validated self-report depression scale for use in the general adult population. It contains 20 items rating the frequency of depressive symptoms on a 4-point scale ranging from *rarely or none* to *most all of the time*. CES–D scores are distributed across four factors: depressed affect, positive affect, somatic or vegetative symptoms, and interpersonal distress.

Cognitive Measures

CLOX: An Executive Clock Drawing Task (Royall et al., 1998): The CLOX is a brief ECF measure based on a CDT. CLOX1, but not CLOX2, makes a significant independent contribution to the number of categories achieved on the Wisconsin Card Sorting Task (Royall, Chiodo, & Polk, 2001). Each CLOX subtest is scored on a 15-point scale. Lower CLOX scores are impaired. Cutpoints of 10/15 (CLOX1) and 12/15 (CLOX2) represent the 5th percentiles for young adult controls (Royall et al., 1998).

Subjects in this study were divided on the basis of their wave 3 CLOX scores into three groups—no dementia, type 1 dementia, and type 2 dementia—using the nomenclature of Royall and Polk (1998). Type 1 dementia arises from conditions that, like AD, have clinical features that can be specifically attributed to pathology in cortical regions outside the frontal lobes. Type 2 dementias lack such features. Most type 2 disorders exhibit pathology that is limited to the frontal systems that provide executive control over complex behavior. Because executive control depends on systems that include both cortical and subcortical structures, the pathology associated with type 2 presentations may be frontocortical, subcortical, or both, depending on the disorder involved. The pattern of CLOX performance can significantly discriminate AD from both nondemented elderly controls and cases of vascular dementia (74.5% correct by resubstitution, Wilks' lambda = 0.41, $F_{6, 182}$ = 17.2, $p < .001$) (Royall, 2002). Although diabetes mellitus has been associated with dementia, it remains unclear whether a type 1 or a type 2 pattern is involved (Ott et al., 1999).

Those who passed both CLOX subtests were designated not demented (ND). Those who failed both CLOX subtests were designated type 1 dementia (type 1). Because CLOX2 failure suggests a frank constructional dyspraxia, type 1 patients exhibit cortical-type clinical features and may be specifically predisposed to AD and its variants (Royall & Polk, 1998). Subjects who passed CLOX2 but failed CLOX1 were designated type 2 dementia (type 2). This group is probably clinically heterogeneous but can be expected to disproportionately represent non-AD dementias, although both early AD and left hemisphere AD variants without constructional dyspraxia might also be classified as type 2 cases on the basis of their lack of CLOX2 failure in the presence of ECF impairment detected by CLOX1.

A small number of subjects ($n = 59$; MMSE = 21.8 ± 4.8) failed CLOX2 at 12/15 despite passing CLOX1 at 10/15. This pattern of CLOX performance is conceptually uninterpretable. These CLOX records were individually reinspected. They often had borderline CLOX1 scores that might easily have been reclassified as impaired had they done slightly worse. In contrast, their CLOX2 scores were clearly impaired. They were recoded into the type 1 group. This classification is consistent with their impaired wave 3 MMSE scores.

The Mini-Mental State Examination (MMSE) (Folstein et al., 1975): The MMSE is a well-known and widely used test for screening cognitive impairment (Tombaugh & McIntyre, 1992). Scores range from 0 to 30. Scores <24/30 reflect cognitive impairment, but scores as low as 18/30 are considered normal in those with less than 8 years of education. MMSE has no items that specifically address ECF and may underestimate cognitive impairment in the absence of posterior cortical pathology. MMSE scores in this sample were considered impaired if they were <18/30.

Functional Status and Physical Performance

Functional status was defined by self-reported IADL scores using the modified OARS scale. This is a well-validated, self-report IADL scale that also has predictive validity when assessed against mortality (Fillenbaum, 1985).

Change in IADL was modeled as the difference between IADL assessments in wave 3 to wave 1.

Physical activity was measured using the Physical Activity Scale for the Elderly (PASE; New England Research Institute, 1991). The PASE is a brief, easily administered and scored instrument designed specifically to assess physical activity in the elderly (Washburn & Ficker, 1999). The PASE asks 12 questions concerning daily activities, ranging from simple walking activities and routine housework to strenuous sports and recreational activities, including weightlifting. Each question inquires about how many hours per day each activity is performed, ranging from less than 1 h to greater than 4 h. Each question then asks about how many days in a week the subject performs each activity.

The PASE uses a summed weighted score rounded to the nearest integer (New England Research Institute, 1991) with the higher scores correlating with higher levels of physical activity. The validity of the PASE has been well established (Martin et al., 1999; Schuit, Schouten, Westerterp, & Saris, 1997; Washburn, McAuley, Katula, Mihalko, & Boileau, 1999). HEPESE collected PASE data only at baseline. Of the original 2,439 participants recruited, 273 refused to answer the PASE questions, leaving 2,166 to be analyzed. Of these, 1,190 had valid CLOX1 scores at wave 3.

Analysis

Subjects were classified as diabetic if they endorsed diabetes mellitus as a self-reported medical condition at wave 3. Cross-group differences between diabetic and nondiabetic subjects were tested in a series of univariate analyses of variance and multivariate analyses of covariance (ANCOVAs), adjusted for baseline age. Multivariate regression was used to model the specific associations between baseline PASE scores and wave 3 cognitive measures, adjusted for age and wave 3 IADLs.

Results

Table 12.1 presents demographic and clinical characteristics of diabetic versus nondiabetic HEPESE subjects. Diabetic subjects were significantly older than nondiabetic subjects. Although poorly educated (5.2 ± 3.9 years) and likely to prefer Spanish for their interviews (69.6%), diabetic subjects could not be distinguished from nondiabetic subjects by these characteristics.

Diabetic subjects reported significantly increased rate of heart disease, rate of stroke, and use of hypoglycemic medications compared with nondiabetic subjects. Diabetic subjects were observed to have significantly higher systolic blood pressures than nondiabetic subjects. Diabetic subjects were also rated significantly higher on the CES–D than nondiabetic subjects.

Table 12.1   Demographics and Clinical Characteristics

	Nondiabetic (n =878)	Diabetic (n = 312)	Total (N = 1,190)	F^a	p
Age	**71.7 (5.4)**	**70.5 (4.7)**	**71.4 (5.3)**	**10.70**	**.001**
Education	5.3 (3.9)	5.2 (3.9)	5.2 (3.9)	0.18	NS
% Female	40.9	39.1	40.4	0.30	NS
% English	25.8	30.4	27.0	2.29	NS
W3 MMSE	23.5 (5.0)	23.4 (5.0)	23.5 (5.0)	0.01	NS
W3 CLOX1	8.4 (3.3)	8.3 (3.1)	8.4 (3.2)	0.03	NS
W3 CLOX2	12.4 (2.4)	12.1 (2.4)	12.3 (2.4)	3.40	NS
W3 % type 1 dementia	30.5	33.2	31.2	0.75	NS
W3 % type 2 dementia	33.2	32.8	33.2	0.02	NS
W3 health	2.5 (0.8)	2.8 (0.9)	2.6 (0.9)	28.97	<.001
W3 systolic BP	135.4 (16.6)	138.2 (18.0)	136.2 (17.0)	6.43	.01
W3 diastolic BP	76.1 (10.8)	75.8 (11.1)	76.0 (10.8)	0.27	NS
W3 CAD	5.5	10.7	6.9	7.80	.005
W3 stroke	2.1	5.2	3.0	7.26	.007
W3 CES–D	7.4 (8.3)	8.6 (9.5)	7.7 (8.6)	5.02	.03
W3 AODM Meds	2.0 (0.1)	1.3 (0.5)	1.8 (0.4)	756.09	<.001

AODM = adult-onset diabetes mellitus; BP = blood pressure; CAD = coronary artery disease; CES–D = Centers for Epidemiological Studies–Depression screening test; CLOX = CLOX: An Executive Clock Drawing Task; Meds = medications; MMSE = Mini-Mental State Examination; NS = not significant; W3 = wave 3.

^{a}Analysis of variance, $df = 1, 1188$.

Nonetheless, diabetic subjects reported slightly better general health at wave 3 than nondiabetic subjects.

In contrast, there were no significant differences in cognition at wave 3 between diabetic and nondiabetic subjects. Diabetic subjects scored in the normal ranges for CLOX2 and (education-adjusted) MMSE. Nonetheless, they showed ECF impairment on CLOX1, which is not strongly biased by education, acculturation, socioeconomic status, or language in this sample (Royall et al., 2003). We found that 32.8% of diabetic subjects displayed combined CLOX-rated ECF impairment and constructional dyspraxia (e.g., type 1 dementia) at wave 3. An additional 33.2% displayed isolated ECF impairment (i.e., type 2 dementia) at wave 3.

Table 12.2 examines the physical function of diabetic versus nondiabetic HEPESE subjects. Diabetic subjects displayed significantly increased disability relative to nondiabetics, with regard to both self-reported IADL and PASE assessments. Diabetics had significantly increased IADL impairment at baseline and at wave 3 and a greater rate of deterioration in IADL impairment over time.

Multivariate Models: After adjustment for age and education, the presence of diabetes mellitus at wave 3 had a significant effect on CLOX2 scores (by ANCOVA: $F_{1, 1149} = 5.03$, $p = .03$) but neither CLOX1 nor wave 3 MMSE scores. The effect on CLOX2 was not attenuated by the addition of wave 1 IADLs as a covariate (by ANCOVA: $F_{1, 1146} = 5.47$, $p = .05$) or by the addition of PASE performance as a covariate (by ANCOVA: $F_{1, 1068} = 5.45$, $p = .03$). Diabetes mellitus had no significant effects on CLOX-defined dementia type after adjustment for age.

Similarly, in a forward stepwise multivariate regression model, PASE scores among diabetic subjects were not significantly associated with wave 3 CLOX scores (table 12.3). In contrast, PASE scores at baseline were significantly associated with wave 3 IADL and MMSE scores ($F_{3, 254} = 12.4$, $p < .001$, $R^2 = .13$). Age entered the model, but did not contribute significantly, independently of the other variables.

Table 12.2   Physical Performance

	Nondiabetic (n = 878)	Diabetic (n = 312)	Total (N = 1,190)	F^a	p
Baseline IADL	**1.03 (1.84)**	**1.29 (1.92)**	**1.10 (1.87)**	**4.46**	**.04**
W3 IADLs	1.35 (2.36)	2.05 (2.67)	1.53 (2.46)	18.79	<.001
DIADLs	0.12 (0.33)	0.18 (0.39)	0.14 (0.35)	8.36	.004
Baseline PASE	102.29 (56.25)	92.78 (59.50)	99.78 (57.26)	5.89	.02

IADLs = Instrumental Activities of Daily Living; DIADLs = Differences in IADLs between wave 1 (W1) and wave 3 (W3); PASE = Physical Activity Scale for the Elderly; W3 = wave 3.
[a]Analysis of variance, $df = 1, 1188$.

Table 12.3   Forward Stepwise Regression Model of Physical Activity Scale for the Elderly (PASE) Scores in Diabetic Subjects[a]

	Step	Multiple R^2	R^2 Change	F	p
W3 IADLs	1	.10	.102	29.00	<.001
W3 MMSE	2	.12	.019	5.56	.02
Age	3	.13	.007	1.92	NS

IADLs = Instrumental Activities of Daily Living; MMSE = Mini-Mental State Examination; NS = not significant; W3 = wave 3.

[a]$F_{3, 254} = 12.4, p < .001, R = .13$.

Discussion

We have demonstrated a modest but significant cross-sectional association between diabetes and cognition and a longitudinal association between PASE performance and future cognitive function in diabetics. However, in contrast to recent reports of the benefits of exercise in older adults, neither association could be considered strong in its intensity, nor did physical activity have significant effects on ECF (i.e., CLOX1) as distinct from general cognition (i.e., CLOX2 and MMSE).

The failure to detect a significant effect of diabetes mellitus on CLOX1 reflects the high prevalence of ECF impairment in community-dwelling elderly persons, particularly Mexican Americans (Royall, Espino, Polk, Palmer, & Markides, 2004). Sixty-six percent of diabetic HEPESE subjects failed CLOX1, but so did 63.7% of nondiabetic subjects. The high prevalence of ECF impairment in this sample is consistent with previous studies. Thirty-three percent of 1,298 community-dwelling elderly persons *over the age of 60* (our sample frame is older) were found to have ECF impairment in the recent San Luis Valley Health and Aging Study (Grigsby et al., 2002); 45.4% of ($n = 746$) elderly *Hispanics* were impaired. As in the HEPESE, ECF was a significant independent predictor of IADLs, in age- and MMSE-adjusted models (Royall, Espino, et al., 2004).

The significant age- and education-adjusted association between diabetes mellitus and CLOX2 is consistent with earlier findings that fitness is most closely associated with measures of visuospatial function (Shay & Roth, 1992). We also note the strong visuospatial demands of the putative executive measures (e.g., Trail Making and digit-symbol substitution) that have been significantly associated with cardiorespiratory fitness in older persons (Barnes et al., 2003; Kramer et al., 1999). However, in this study, baseline physical activity and IADLs did not appear to mediate the significant association between diabetes and nonexecutive cognition.

Several possibilities need to be considered in light of this negative finding. First, previous studies have examined the effects of exercise in relatively "younger" elderly populations. However, ECF deteriorates linearly with age and is strongly associated with the rate of change in IADLs (Royall, Palmer, Chiodo, & Polk, 2000, 2005, in press), especially among the oldest old (Palmer, Royall, Chiodo, & Polk, 2000). This may reflect structural brain changes that are less amenable to lifestyle interventions.

Second, ECF appears to be a multidimensional construct (Royall et al., 2002). Although CLOX is an independent predictor of both IADLs and level of care in elderly samples (Royall, Chiodo, & Polk, 2000), it may yet not tap a dimension of ECF that is amenable to change with exercise.

Third, the physical activities elicited by the PASE and IADL measures may not be congruent to the highly structured exercises prescribed in previous studies. Nonetheless, the failure of a more naturalistic measure, such as the PASE, to explain variance in an ECF measure among diabetics merely emphasizes the possibility that only specific and highly regimented exercise routines may be associated with clinically significant gains in (perhaps selected) ECF measures. This increases the possibility that previous findings may have reflected assessment biases inherent to the ECF required to adhere to and benefit from such rigorous exercise routines. Moreover, even the methods by which cardiorespiratory fitness is determined may require a certain level of executive control and therefore artificially accentuate the association between poor fitness and ECF impairment (Hollenberg et al., 1998). Future studies should assess the baseline ECF of participants and use this variable as a covariate when examining the effects of exercise on frontal functions.

Fourth, we note that both PASE and IADLs rely on subject self-report. Interestingly, we have previously noted a double dissociation between CLOX2 and self-reported functional status versus CLOX1 and objective functional outcomes (Royall et al., 2000). Researchers who use self-reported outcomes in populations at risk for ECF impairment need to be wary of the possibility that accurate self-report itself depends on frontal system substrates, particularly in the right hemisphere. Impairments of insight may undermine the validity of self-reported physical and functional status measures in such samples (Fan, Royall, Chiodo, Polk, & Mouton, 2003). In this regard, it is interesting that diabetic subjects report significantly better health than nondiabetic subjects, despite increased rates of self-reported medical problems and depressive symptoms. In addition, baseline PASE scores, which may be less subjective, correlated significantly, but weakly, with self-reported IADLs in the HEPESE cohort ($r = -.29$, $p = .05$).

In summary, we have examined the association between physical function and future ECF among a large sample of predominantly Hispanic, community-dwelling elderly diabetic persons. Although baseline physical function had modest significant effects on future general cognition, there was no significant effect on ECF. Previous studies associating exercise and frontal function may not be as widely generalizable as once thought.

EDITORS' DISCUSSION SUMMARY

Discussion Highlights

A growing body of evidence suggests that cognitive tasks that require executive control functioning mediated by frontal systems such as the frontal cortex, basal ganglia, thalamus, and their associated white matter connections may be particularly sensitive to modification by aerobic exercise training. However, most researchers who have examined the relationship between physical activity, cognitive functioning, and old age have examined these associations in relatively healthy individuals. Few have examined these relationships in experimental groups exhibiting a specific chronic condition or disease.

The relationship between exercise and cognition may be especially interesting to examine in patients with diabetes mellitus. Evidence supports the hypothesis that diabetes is associated with frontal system dysfunction and executive control deficits. Furthermore, diabetic patients have been impaired on tests that are thought to be sensitive to executive control. Three plausible mechanisms have been proposed that could account for the cognitive deficits observed in individuals with diabetes: complications associated with stroke, major depression, and hypoglycemia. Because regular exercise has been shown to affect each of these mechanisms, additional research that examines the relationships between exercise, executive control functioning, and aging in individuals with diabetes is a step in the right direction.

Methodological Research Problems

Impairments in executive function that are commonly found in older adults and in diabetics may compromise the measurements that researchers use to determine both health and physical fitness. For example, the ability to cooperate and perform in cardiovascular assessments requires executive function. Allen and colleagues (2003) reported that lung capacity assessments and medication compliance in patients with chronic obstructive pulmonary disease are affected by executive function. Persons with lower executive function cannot follow a command such as "blow into this little tube until I tell you to stop." The sequencing of the many steps of the test requires executive control: The patient has to hold his breath, push it out, then wait, and then draw the air back. Moving through these several stages in the correct order requires executive function. Thus, executively impaired patients' cardiovascular assessments may not reflect their true cardiovascular performance. The correlations that have been published between function and cognition in populations at risk for executive impairment may be spuriously high.

Executive function surely also affects the accuracy of self-reports. Self-reported variables including health, financial decision-making capacity, IADLs, and depression ratings obtained from executively impaired populations such as elderly, depressed, and diabetic persons may be compromised.

Future Directions

First, studies of physical activity and cognition have been of relatively young and healthy older adults. Physical activity effects on older adults, and those with low executive control scores, should be determined. These may not be amenable to lifestyle interventions. The results from previous studies may have been biased by including only those subjects who could adhere to a relatively complex exercise protocol. Second, identifying the dimensions of executive control and developing tests that can predict future disability are a critical next step. Some aspects of executive control may not be amenable to exercise-induced change. Third, it would be useful to know the extent to which executive deficits distort physical measures such as vital capacity and maximum aerobic capacity; similarly, we need to know how executive control affects self-report in areas such as general health and financial decision making. For example, a surprisingly large fraction of people with executive impairment do not accurately report their general health and financial decision making. Finally, in the study of exercise effects on cognitive effects in diabetics, we need to know whether diabetics who have insulin levels controlled have the same executive control deficits as those with uncontrolled insulin levels.

CHAPTER 13

Exercise, Chronic Obstructive Pulmonary Disease, and Cognition

Charles F. Emery, PhD
The Ohio State University

EDITORS' OVERVIEW

In this chapter, Dr. Emery reviews the evidence that many patients with chronic obstructive pulmonary disease (COPD) also have deficits in neuropsychological performance, including impairments in verbal memory, abstract reasoning, information processing, attention, and psychomotor speed. He discusses the hypothesis that exercise has a positive effect on cognitive function among patients with COPD by increasing blood circulation and availability of blood oxygen in the brain. Increased cerebral blood flow associated with exercise may enhance neurotransmitter release in the brain. Dr. Emery points out that because patients with COPD are at risk for cognitive impairment and are usually quite sedentary, they provide an ideal opportunity to examine the relationship between exercise and cognitive function. He has been one of few researchers who have studied exercise and cognitive function among patients with COPD, finding that exer-

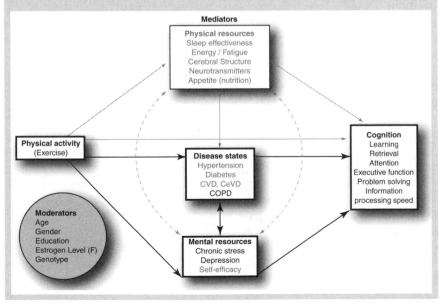

cise is associated with enhanced cognitive performance. Dr. Emery proposes three broad categories of causes for exercise-related improvements in cognition: psychological factors, psychophysiological factors, and physiological factors. All three mechanisms provide plausible explanations for cognitive outcomes of both short-term and long-term exercise interventions.

Dr. Emery provides a working model by which exercise might influence cardiopulmonary and psychosocial functioning and health behaviors and thus benefit brain function. He concludes the chapter by suggesting several research questions about this COPD population that researchers need to solve over the next 10 years and also discusses how the answers to some of these questions may expand our knowledge about the role of exercise and cognition in the older adult population.

Chronic obstructive pulmonary disease (COPD) is the fourth leading cause of death in the United States and a primary cause of disability among older adults (American Lung Association, 2004). COPD is characterized by chronic expiratory air-flow obstruction and encompasses diagnoses of chronic bronchitis, emphysema, and asthma. However, patients with purely asthma symptoms are not diagnosed with COPD because the airway obstruction in asthmatics can be reversed acutely with the administration of bronchodilator medication. Airway obstruction among patients with COPD is, by definition, irreversible. Several of the changes in lung function among patients with COPD, such as loss of elastic recoil, are similar to changes observed in normal aging, but the changes occur at an accelerated rate for COPD patients. Other changes, including airway obstruction and pulmonary blood flow abnormalities, are true pathological changes in the lungs of COPD patients. Morphological changes in the lung (breakdown of alveoli) contribute to reduced lung elasticity. The act of breathing for the patient with COPD is increasingly dependent on accessory muscles in the thoracic cavity because the lung does not passively expel air following inspiration. Cumulative changes in lung functioning eventually result in decreased oxygen uptake in the bloodstream and, ultimately, a state of chronic hypoxia, manifested by a reduced partial pressure of oxygen (PaO_2) and a reduced hemoglobin oxygen saturation (SaO_2). The chronic hypoxia of COPD patients has been associated with physical symptoms such as fatigue and respiratory symptoms such as shortness of breath. Most patients with COPD experience significant reductions in physical activity attributable to pulmonary symptoms. Reduced physical activity, in turn, contributes to loss of muscle mass and diminished ability to engage in physical activity.

Diagnosis of COPD follows from a thorough medical history and physical examination, including lung spirometry. Values derived from spirometry testing include forced expiratory volume in 1 s (FEV_1) and forced vital capacity (FVC). The ratio of these two values (FEV$_1$:FVC) provides an indicator of lung elasticity and a primary diagnostic criterion for COPD. Specifically, during the first second of a forced exhalation, the patient with COPD expels less than 70% of the air in the lung (FEV$_1$:FVC <.70). In addition, FEV$_1$ itself provides a marker of lung elasticity, and normative reference group data are available for FEV$_1$ values according to age, sex, height, and ethnicity. Normal lung functioning is characterized as percent of predicted FEV$_1$ ≥80%. Mild COPD is characterized as FEV$_1$ 65% to 79% of predicted values, moderate is 50% to 64%, and severe is <50% predicted.

The clinical course of COPD is marked by a progressive decrease in physical endurance, increased shortness of breath, and substantial impairments in quality of life (Cugell, 1988). Patients with COPD may experience difficulty conducting activities of daily living such as dressing, showering, and housework (McSweeny, Grant, Heaton, Adams, & Timms, 1982). In addition, social roles often are compromised for patients because they experience reduced ability to engage in social activities as well as increased dependence on spouses or other family members (McSweeny et al., 1982). Patients with COPD also may experience mood changes, especially depression and anxiety, and impaired cognitive and neuropsychological performance (Agle & Baum, 1977; Emery, Leatherman, Burker, & MacIntyre, 1991).

Cognitive Factors Associated With COPD

Ample evidence has documented deficits in neuropsychological performance among patients with COPD, including impairments in verbal memory, abstract reasoning, information processing, attention, and psychomotor speed (Incalzi et al., 1997; Prigatano, Parsons, Wright, Levin, & Hawryluk, 1983). Verbal intelligence does not seem to be affected, but the impairment among COPD patients appears to be rather diffuse and has a significant impact on verbal functions including verbal memory (Incalzi et al., 1997). On the other hand, studies contrasting performance of patients with COPD to that of patients with Alzheimer's disease indicate that the impairment associated with COPD is relatively mild and that patients with COPD perform significantly better on most indicators than do patients with dementia (Incalzi et al., 1997; Kozora, Filley, Julian, & Cullum, 1999).

Disease-Related Factors
Associated With Cognitive Function

Although population-based studies have revealed an association of pulmonary function (e.g., FEV$_1$) with cognitive function among community-residing older adults (Albert et al., 1995; Emery, Huppert, & Schein, 1997;

Emery, Pedersen, Svartengren, & McClearn, 1998), studies of patients with COPD suggest negligible associations of FEV_1 with cognitive function (Grant, Heaton, McSweeny, Adams, & Timms, 1982; Prigatano et al., 1983). One group of researchers found additional markers of pulmonary function (e.g., FVC) associated with cognitive performance (Etnier et al., 1999), but the overall effects were less than would be expected by chance. The absence of an association between pulmonary function and cognitive function among patients with COPD is likely attributable, in part, to the restricted range of pulmonary function indicators for these patients. Among community-residing older adults, decreases in pulmonary function and diminished cognitive capabilities both may reflect a terminal decline phenomenon (Albert et al., 1995; Emery, Pedersen, et al., 1998). In contrast, patients with COPD may survive for a relatively prolonged period of time with a reduced lung capacity (low FEV_1) that is unrelated to change in cognitive function. Thus, although pulmonary function may be a reasonable marker of cognitive capacity in healthy older adults, it is not useful among patients with COPD.

The second primary disease-related factor associated with neuropsychological impairment is blood oxygenation level. Patients with COPD are at risk for chronic reductions in blood oxygenation, and blood oxygenation influences cognitive function, as initially described in reports from the combined Nocturnal Oxygen Therapy Trial and Intermittent Positive Pressure Breathing Trial (Grant et al., 1987). These data indicated that healthy control subjects performed better than mildly hypoxemic patients on tests of cognitive function. In turn, mildly hypoxemic patients (PaO_2 >60 mmHg) performed better than patients who were moderately (PaO_2 = 50-59 mmHg) or severely (PaO_2 <50 mmHg) hypoxemic. Likewise, patients with severe hypoxemia manifested greater neuropsychological impairment than patients with moderate or mild hypoxemia. Differences were observed on a variety of types of cognitive tasks, including measures of immediate verbal and figural memory (Wechsler Memory Scale), psychomotor speed (Digit Symbol from the Weschler Adult Intelligence Scale), motor speed (finger tapping), perceptual organizational skills (Block Design from the Weschler Adult Intelligence Scale), and sequencing (Trail Making Part B). However, data from these studies and others have indicated that neuropsychological functioning is only moderately associated with hypoxemia.

Further evidence supporting the relevance of blood oxygenation for cognitive function is found in studies documenting improved cognitive performance among patients with COPD who receive long-term (>6 months) treatment with oxygen therapy (Heaton, Grant, McSweeny, Adams, & Petty, 1983; Krop, Block, & Cohen, 1973). Cognitive improvement was observed on tests of sequencing and psychomotor speed (Trail Making Part B, finger tapping). It has been suggested that enhanced cognitive performance following oxygen therapy results from improved oxygen delivery to the brain, facilitating neurotransmitter release and other aspects of central nervous system (CNS) metabolic activity.

Extending this line of research, it was hypothesized that exercise would have a positive effect on cognitive function among patients with COPD by increasing blood circulation and availability of blood oxygen in the brain. Among healthy older adults, it has been suggested that increased cerebral blood flow associated with exercise may facilitate enhanced neurotransmitter release in the brain (Dustman et al., 1984). Because patients with COPD are at risk for cognitive impairment and are usually quite sedentary, this population provides an ideal opportunity to examine the relationship between exercise and cognitive function.

Exercise in COPD

Data from numerous experimental evaluations of exercise among patients with COPD consistently indicate positive physical health benefits of exercise activity among patients with COPD, including improvement in upper- and lower-body strength, reductions in shortness of breath, and reduction of health care utilization. As a result of these data, exercise rehabilitation is now the standard of care for patients with COPD (ACCP/AACVPR, 1997). From a practical perspective, it is critical to examine the influence of exercise on cognitive performance among patients with COPD because exercise is commonly recommended for patients with COPD and physical exercise may have a positive affect on cognitive function.

Several different lines of research have been used to examine the influence of exercise on cognitive function among patients with COPD, including cross-sectional studies evaluating the association of exercise performance with cognitive performance, intervention studies evaluating the influence of short-term exercise training interventions on change in cognitive performance, intervention studies documenting effects of longer term (12 months or more) exercise participation on cognitive performance, and effects of acute bouts of exercise on cognitive performance. Primary physiological outcomes that have been examined among patients with COPD include pulmonary function (e.g., FEV_1) and exercise endurance measured by maximal oxygen consumption ($\dot{V}O_2max$) during a stress test or by a timed (e.g., 6 min) walk test. The reliability of exercise outcomes among patients with COPD has been questioned because motivational factors may influence performance during exercise testing. In this population, motivation may be very low and, conversely, fear of exercise-induced dyspnea may be high. In addition, the utility of standard outcomes such as $\dot{V}O_2max$ has been questioned because of the difficulty of achieving maximal exercise performance among patients with COPD who are highly sensitized to exercise-induced shortness of breath. However, most researchers continue to use standard exercise outcome measures in studies of patients with COPD to facilitate comparison with other patient groups and with healthy adults.

Cross-Sectional Studies

Data from cross-sectional studies indicate an association of cognitive performance with exercise capacity, as measured by exercise ergometry (Grant et al., 1982; Grant et al., 1987; Prigatano et al., 1983) and by the 6 min walk test (Etnier et al., 1999). Exercise performance has been most closely associated with indicators of motor speed and strength. However, data also indicate that maximal exercise performance ($\dot{V}O_2$max) may not be associated with cognitive functioning in this population (Etnier et al., 1999). The apparent inconsistency in these data may be related to the reduced reliability in measurement of exercise capacity in this population.

Intervention Studies

Exercise interventions among patients with COPD are usually structured with three exercise sessions per week over the course of 6 to 12 weeks. Each session of exercise rehabilitation may last several hours, allowing patients to take breaks between exercise activities and to participate in educational components of the rehabilitation program. Although daily sessions of rehabilitation may last for several hours, patients generally do not exercise for more than 90 min during each session.

Outcomes of exercise training among patients with COPD include increases in physical endurance, as measured by oxygen consumption ($\dot{V}O_2$max or $\dot{V}O_2$peak) and 6 min walk distance (Emery, Schein, Hauck, & MacIntyre, 1998; Ries, Kaplan, Limberg, & Prewitt, 1995), as well as increased upper-body strength (Lake, Henderson, Briffa, Openshaw, & Musk, 1990). In addition, studies indicate that exercise is associated with reduced shortness of breath (Ries et al., 1995; Sassi-Dambron, Eakin, Ries, & Kaplan, 1995). However, exercise among patients with COPD is not associated with changes in pulmonary function (Emery et al., 1998; Ries et al., 1995).

Exercise also has been associated with psychological outcomes, including reduced depression and anxiety (Emery et al., 1991; Emery et al., 1998; Kozora, Tran, & Make, 2002), enhanced illness-specific quality of life (Goldstein, Gort, Stubbing, Avendano, & Guyatt, 1994), increased positive affect (Emery et al., 1991), and increased self-efficacy expectations (Kaplan, Ries, Prewitt, & Eakin, 1994). However, several investigators have found no significant change in psychological functioning associated with exercise (e.g., Ries et al., 1995). The equivocal nature of the data regarding psychological outcomes is consistent with data from studies of healthy older adults and may reflect variability in the degree to which patients with COPD experience symptoms of distress as well as variation in the measurement of psychological outcomes across studies.

The few studies that have been conducted of exercise and cognitive function among patients with COPD indicate that exercise is associated with enhanced cognitive performance (Emery et al., 1991; Emery et al., 1998; Etnier & Berry, 2001). In particular, there is evidence of an association of exercise with verbal fluency and other cognitive measures reflecting components of fluid intelligence (sequencing, problem solving, abstract reasoning). In one study, no overall improvement in cognitive performance was seen following a 3-week intervention, but the patients who were more impaired at baseline experienced significant improvement in cognitive function (Kozora et al., 2002). Overall, these data are consistent with results of recent studies among healthy older adults indicating a positive effect of exercise on cognitive tasks reflecting executive function (e.g., purposive behavior, self-control, ability to shift attention; Khatri et al., 2001; Kramer et al., 1999). However, the experimental evidence is still limited regarding the influence of exercise interventions on cognitive performance among patients with COPD.

Long-Term Follow-Up of Exercise Effects on Cognitive Performance

In addition to investigating the effects of short-term exercise interventions on cognitive functioning, two relatively recent studies have examined the effect of long-term exercise behavior on cognitive functioning among patients with COPD. In one study, a change in physical fitness was associated with a change in cognitive performance (Culture Fair Intelligence Test, a measure of fluid intelligence) over the course of an 18-month training program of aerobic and strength training exercises (Etnier & Berry, 2001). In a second study (Emery, Shermer, Hauck, Hsiao, & MacIntyre, 2003), exercise nonadherence was associated with a decline in cognitive performance during a 12-month follow-up. This study provided follow-up data from an exercise intervention among patients with COPD in which improvements in verbal fluency had been observed (Emery, Schein, et al., 1998). Although performance on the verbal fluency task was maintained regardless of exercise activity during follow-up, participants who were nonadherent during the follow-up period experienced a significant decline in performance on a task reflecting alertness and psychomotor speed (Digit Symbol subtest from the Weschler Adult Intelligence Scale–Revised). The nonadherent group also experienced significant declines in exercise endurance ($\dot{V}O_2max$), but there was no association between decline in $\dot{V}O_2max$ and decline in cognitive performance. Although Etnier and Berry (2001) found an association of improved exercise capacity with improved cognitive performance, neither of these long-term follow-up studies evaluated additional mechanisms (mediators or moderators) in the relationship between exercise and cognitive performance.

Acute Effects of Exercise on Cognitive Performance

One study evaluated acute effects of exercise on cognitive performance among patients with COPD (Emery, Honn, Diaz, Lebowitz, & Frid, 2001). The authors used an experimental paradigm common in studies of acute exercise effects, with subjects serving as their own controls, exercising during one session and listening to an educational tape about the value of exercise during an alternate session. The study also included a control group of healthy adults matched by age and educational attainment. Results indicated that patients with COPD experienced significant increases in verbal fluency following a 20 min bout of exercise activity. The video-watching condition was not associated with cognitive change. In addition, no change was observed among the healthy control subjects in either condition. Thus, although there may be benefits of acute exercise for cognitive performance, cognitive effects may be more likely among those who are experiencing cognitive impairment or who are at risk for cognitive impairment. Because studies of healthy older adults often select individuals who are relatively high functioning, those individuals may be less likely to benefit from exercise training. The latter observation is consistent with reports from intervention studies among healthy older adults in which no improvement in cognitive function followed exercise (Blumenthal et al., 1989; Emery & Gatz, 1990).

Mechanisms of the Effect of Exercise on Cognitive Performance

To the extent that exercise has positive effects on cognitive performance among adults with COPD, it is important to examine the mechanisms hypothesized to explain the effect. The common explanations can be clustered into three broad categories: psychological factors, psychophysiological factors, and physiological factors. All three mechanisms provide plausible explanations for cognitive outcomes of both short-term and long-term exercise interventions.

Psychological factors are relevant because studies have demonstrated that psychological distress, especially depression and anxiety, may have a negative influence on cognitive functioning. Depression and anxiety are the most commonly reported psychological problems among patients with COPD, and exercise has been found to have a positive effect on symptoms of depression and anxiety. Thus, it has been suggested that reduced psychological distress may mediate the relationship between exercise and cognitive outcomes. However, prior studies in which depression has been statistically controlled indicate that exercise activity has an influence on cognitive outcomes above and beyond the influence of depression (Etnier et al., 1999).

Because hyperarousal of the sympathetic nervous system is associated with impaired cognitive performance, the psychophysiological hypothesis suggests that exercise may contribute to enhanced cognitive function by reducing sympathetic hyperarousal, decreasing sympathetic tone, and contributing to greater oxygen-carrying capacity of the blood. This, in turn, may contribute to enhanced neurotransmitter regulation (Dustman et al., 1990).

Hypothesized physiological mechanisms include neuroendocrine changes associated with exercise (e.g., hormone response in cortisol, growth hormone, insulin-like growth factor, and endorphins) and stimulation of brain structures, such as the reticular activating system.

Future Research

Research in this area will benefit from addressing further the mechanisms by which exercise may contribute to cognitive outcomes. The working model included in figure 13.1 incorporates a number of factors that may influence cognitive function among patients with COPD, including age-related changes in cognitive function (most patients with COPD are older than 55 years); influences of emotion or stress on cognitive performance; disease-related factors (e.g., pulmonary function, blood oxygen level, exercise capacity) that influence exercise and, in turn, cognitive function; and effects of related health behaviors, including smoking, drinking, diet, sleep, and medication adherence. In this model, COPD is a moderator of the relationship between exercise and cognitive function. As severity of COPD increases, disease processes influence cognitive function via health behavior and cardiopulmonary functioning. In the population-based model of exercise and cognitive function, COPD is a mediator. Thus, in the absence of disease, COPD is a mediator of the relationship between exercise and cognitive performance, but in the presence of the disease, severity of COPD is likely to be a moderator.

Three aspects of functioning that are absent from the research to date are nutritional status, sleep patterns, and changes in medical status. Further investigation is needed to evaluate the influence of each of these factors on the relationship between exercise and cognitive performance. Malnutrition is an independent risk factor for mortality among patients with COPD (Chapman & Winter, 1996); thus, nutritional status is especially important in studies of this population. Because of the interactive influence of nutritional status and exercise activity in the presence of chronic

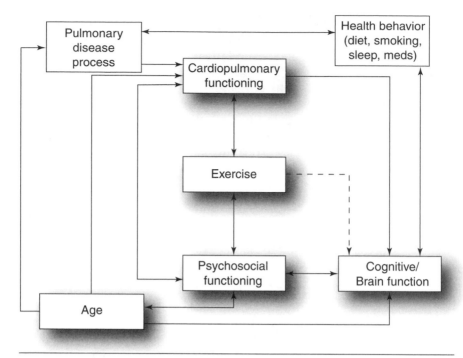

Figure 13.1 Schematic model of the relationships among exercise, cognitive function, and related variables. (Solid lines connect variables for which there is empirical evidence of a relationship; dotted lines connect variables for which the evidence is less strong.)

disease (Blair et al., 1996), models of exercise and cognitive function might be more accurate if nutritional status were included as a moderator of the relationship between exercise and cognitive function.

Many patients with COPD suffer from sleep apnea (Berry & Block, 1988), and there is evidence of the negative effect of sleep apnea on cognitive performance (Decary, Rouleau, & Montplaisir, 2000). Thus, sleep behavior is a critical component of functioning to incorporate in studies of exercise and cognitive function. It is plausible that sleep behavior may mediate the relationship between exercise and cognitive performance, at least for a subset of patients with COPD.

The symptom of fatigue may also be especially important for further study. Fatigue has a negative influence on both physical and cognitive performance. However, studies have not addressed the influence of fatigue on cognitive performance among patients with COPD or the effect of exercise activity on symptoms of fatigue.

Self-care (e.g., medication adherence, symptom management) may have a significant influence on both physical health and cognitive performance among patients with COPD. Adherence to exercise may be associated with adherence to other self-care behaviors. Further investigation is needed into the relationship between cognitive function and behavioral factors such as adherence, especially because exercise adherence itself is likely to be cognitively mediated. Adherence requires planning, organizing, and initiating activity, all of which reflect executive cognitive function, in part.

The overriding need for future studies in this area is to disentangle the various factors associated with pulmonary disease and cognitive function (e.g., interrelationships between cognitive function and depression, anxiety, physical limitations). Large-scale studies will be required, recruiting participants with comorbid diagnoses or using samples that are large enough to justify statistical control of comorbid conditions. One especially important area for further investigation is the interaction of exercise capacity with disease processes and cognitive outcomes. Although it is likely that exercise capacity interacts with disease processes to influence cognitive function, fitness level per se is not associated with cognitive function in this population. Thus, although increased fitness is a likely mechanism by which exercise might influence cognitive function among patients with COPD, it does not explain a substantial portion of the variance in cognitive function.

Imaging studies, as in the work conducted by Kramer and colleagues (Colcombe et al., 2003), will facilitate exploration of brain mechanisms that may be responsible for cognitive change associated with exercise. The technology of functional magnetic resonance imaging may be useful in relating exercise-associated cognitive performance to brain activity among patients with COPD and may help clarify factors contributing to differential effects of an exercise stimulus when comparing groups of patients and healthy controls.

Given the range of types of exercise used among patients with COPD and the variety of cognitive capacities evaluated in prior studies, it also may be useful to evaluate the extent to which various types of exercise (e.g., acute, short-term, long-term, aerobic, strength training) are associated with specific cognitive processes (e.g., attention, concentration, psychomotor speed, verbal processing). Without further documentation of mechanisms associated with cognitive change following exercise, the relevance of type of exercise and intensity of exercise remains unknown.

Grant and colleagues (1987) used factor analysis to derive four cognitive factors (verbal intelligence, perceptual learning and problem solving, alertness and psychomotor speed, and simple motor learning) in their cross-sectional study of cognitive function and hypoxemia among patients with COPD and healthy controls. This factor analytic approach would be appropriate to consider in future intervention studies to minimize the risk of false-positive cognitive results and to work toward establishing conceptually relevant markers of cognitive function.

Summary

The extant data suggest that exercise among patients with COPD is associated with improved performance in verbal fluency and other measures reflecting fluid intelligence and frontal lobe function (e.g., Digit Symbol, Trail Making). Psychomotor speed appears to be an important component of change in cognitive performance associated with exercise. Although there remains a strong rationale for further examination of cognitive outcomes of exercise among patients with COPD, studies in this area have not yet revealed mechanisms by which exercise may influence cognitive performance. Changes in pulmonary function, exercise capacity, and depression do not appear to be related to changes in cognitive function. Further work is needed to evaluate psychophysiological, physiological, and behavioral mechanisms that may help to explain the observed outcomes. Knowledge in this area is limited by the very small number of studies available and reliance on individual neuropsychological outcomes (i.e., focusing on discrete indicators of cognitive functioning) when evaluating cognitive performance. Future research on this topic will be strengthened by extending the evaluation of moderating and mediating variables in addition to focusing on conceptually relevant constructs in the assessment of cognitive functioning.

EDITORS' DISCUSSION SUMMARY

Discussion Highlights

Three themes emerged from the discussion of this topic. First, exercise has beneficial effects on the cognition of patients with COPD, and, second, these benefits may very well accrue from indirect effects on other factors that modify cognition. Third, researchers face a challenge in quantifying these beneficial effects.

Exercise may modify several psychological factors that influence cognition of COPD patients. Beyond the effects of exercise on depression and anxiety, other psychologically based improvements in cognition may come from the effects of sunlight or social contact that frequently occur during exercise. Furthermore, self-efficacy may improve through exercise, because exercisers report improvements in cognition that contradict objective measures but that nonexercisers do not report. Exercise-related mood enhancement may similarly affect cognition.

Another indirect way that exercise may enhance cognition in COPD patients is through decreasing fatigue. In this chapter, the argument is made that fatigue can impair cognition, whereas exercise may improve cognition by alleviating fatigue. Developed further, these concepts can form the basis for a dual model of cognitive performance. The first part of the model would account for transitory states, such as energetics, motivation, or fatigue, that temporarily affect cognition. The second part of the model would describe capacity and long-term mediators of performance of the central nervous system and the brain. For example, HPA axis dysregulation and hyperactivity with age can lead to degeneration of the hippocampus and may otherwise alter brain metabolism. The transitory model would reflect individual fluctuations and the ability to use available capacity. It could help greatly with COPD patients, who fatigue quickly and may be less motivated and hence perform worse. More physically fit people may also be more motivated and hence use more of the available capacity because of their greater stamina.

Although exercise may enhance cognition in many healthy adults, Dr. Emery emphasized that in aged or COPD individuals, exercise may only maintain, rather than improve, cognition. However, maintenance in these cases is a small victory. Researchers have reported a decline in measures of psychomotor function among nonexercisers when compared with persons who maintained exercise activity over a 1-year period.

Research Methodological Problems

Methodological problems in studies of exercise effects among COPD patients, the third theme of the discussion, are extremely challenging. Three types of challenges were discussed: the wide disparity in cognitive assessments used, the difficulty of separating the negative effects on cognition of other COPD-generated symptoms from the positive effects of exercise, and the difficulty of measuring exercise-related change in COPD patients. First, measurements of cognition cannot be compared among studies when researchers measure widely divergent types of brain activity. Cognition can be measured by many different types of tests, such as measurements of psychomotor speed, memory retention, or fluid intelligence. Each type of test measures only a component of cognition.

A second methodological problem is that sleep fragmentation or disruption, rather than hypoxemia alone, may impair cognition in COPD patients. The number of sleep awakenings alone may contribute more to cognitive impairment in COPD patients than does nighttime hypoxemia. When studying the role of any intervention on the cognitive capacity of COPD patients, therefore, researchers should gather more sleep data beyond self-reports from COPD patients and should account for these effects in order to understand fully the effect of the intervention. Almost no reports are available of sleep characteristics in exercise studies. It is also possible that exercise effects on sleep in COPD may be differentially more important to COPD patients than to older adults without COPD.

A final methodological challenge in research of COPD patients is the difficulty of obtaining a valid quantification of their cardiorespiratory capacity. True $\dot{V}O_2$max measurements are often impossible to gather in COPD patients as well as in healthy older individuals. Volitional end points of maximal trials reflect the subject's psychological and physical limits. A solution for this has been to use repeated measures on the same person over time to establish baseline values that can be used as controls. Thus, any improvements in fitness can be determined for each subject, even if true maximal end points are not reached during exercise tests. However, such data based on individual $\dot{V}O_2$ peaks may not be comparable to $\dot{V}O_2$max data from the population at large.

Because of the difficulty of measuring cardiorespiratory capacity in this population, it is difficult to compare the results from the COPD population to the healthy at-large population. The type of exercise test appropriate for most healthy subjects, such as the Rockport 1-mile walk test, is too difficult for a COPD patient. Thus, it is hard to determine whether exercise benefits COPD patients in the same way that it does nondiseased persons.

Future Directions

Discussion of future research in this area, led by Dr. Emery, produced two promising directions. First, mechanisms by which exercise may contribute to maintaining or improving cognition should be investigated in the COPD population. The potential sources of mechanisms include virtually all of the factors shown in the working model of this volume. Functional magnetic resonance imaging is a tool with great promise for understanding factors that may mediate differential effects of exercise on cognition.

Second, information about the influence of nutritional status, sleep patterns, and changes in medical status on cognitive function is largely absent in the COPD literature. This is a wide-open and promising field.

Third, fatigue may be an exceptionally important factor to study as a mediator of cognition in this population. This potential mediator has been neither controlled nor analyzed as a mediating variable in past research.

Fourth, large-scale studies of the effects of comorbidities on cognition should be conducted. Large samples or population studies of persons with comorbidities would provide enough subjects to allow for statistical control of comorbidities.

Finally, we need to know which types of exercise may be more appropriate for COPD patients. It would be useful to know the extent to which different types of exercise (acute, short-term, long-term, aerobic, resistance training, as well as others) are effective.

CHAPTER 14

Conclusions and Future Research Directions

Waneen W. Spirduso, EdD; Leonard W. Poon, PhD; and Wojtek Chodzko-Zajko, PhD

As is clear from the chapters of this book, opinions among experienced researchers are mixed as to how strong the physical activity–cognition relationship is, because the necessary research has not been done. A close look at the epidemiological and cross-sectional evidence for the exercise–cognition relationship is very supportive and compelling, but most of the evidence is based on preselected subgroups (exercisers vs. nonexercisers). The results of exercise intervention studies have been less compelling, although the meta-analysis that was conducted by Colcombe and Kramer (2003) provided evidence that the effects of exercise on cognition were large if only the results from true experimental studies meeting rigorous criteria were considered. What, then, can we say about physical activity and cognition?

Many of the potential links between exercise and mediators, or mediators and cognition, are well established. Such relationships as exercise and stress reactivity; exercise and depression; depression and cognition; exercise and sleep; sleep and cognition; and hypertension, stress reactivity, and cognition are robust. Plausible mechanisms have been described and validated. What are missing are the three-way interactions that link exercise through these mediators to cognition. For example, the link between exercise and some types of depression has been accepted, and the negative effects of depression on cognition are well known. But no one has conducted any type of multivariate modeling to analyze pathways or test causality of a model similar to that proposed in chapter 1, which proposes direct and indirect effects of exercise and depression on cognition. Much more information is needed regarding the potential mechanisms by which these relationships might be mediated.

Several questions also were raised about the mediators of the model (Dr. Etnier, chapter 2). The model contains a number of mediators, but there may be others that should be included and some that prove to be ineffective. Some may prove to be more promising than others to research. We should question whether we have sufficient information about each mediator to include it in the model.

As is clear from the information in chapter 8 (Dr. Joseph), the model also has a missing link, that of the relationships among physical activity, nutrition, and cognition. If not entirely missing, this mediator is at least not well examined. Exercise physiologists, nutritionists, and psychologists have not collaborated to examine the way that the strong links between dietary substrates and exercise-induced changes in blood chemistry interact to affect brain function. The more we learn about relationships between diet and brain substrates such as folic acid, homocysteine, antioxidants, oxidants, and other components of the diet, and the more we learn about exercise-mediated effects on these same factors, suggest that defining exercise and diet as a lifestyle approach to enhancing cognition might be a very forward-thinking strategy.

In addition to having a missing link, the model that we propose as a working model is also directional; that is, it hypothesizes that physical activity influences cognition either directly or indirectly through mediators. The flow of causality is from left (physical activity) to right (cognition). But, as several of our experts pointed out, the relationship between exercise and dysfunction can be modeled in the other direction also, to depict the impact that failing cognition might have on the other components of the model. We know that dementia, for example, has disastrous effects on all the mediators of our model. In this case, the flow of causality would be from right to left in the model.

Pressing Research Problems

Although the participants could not reach consensus on the strength of the physical activity–cognition relationship, we did agree that understanding the relationship is important enough to merit an investment of time by groups of researchers so that in 5 to 10 years we will have answers to some of the more complex research questions. We also reached some consensus about what is needed to ensure that within a reasonable amount of time we will have some answers. We have a clearer picture of what the research questions should be, what we need to know, what our problems are, and what we need to pursue. The problems that we need to resolve and the areas that we need to pursue are shown next and described in more detail in the paragraphs following the list.

1. Defining cognition and quantifying it more effectively
2. Defining physical activity and quantifying it more effectively
3. Determining whether exercise mechanisms influence brain health, functional capacity, and performance state independently or interactively or whether the effects depend on the nature of the physical activity
4. Resolving whether physical activity and cognitive function are related similarly throughout the life span

Defining Cognition and Quantifying It More Effectively

What cognitive constructs are affected by physical activity? Before we can understand the characteristics of physical activity (type, length, duration, intensity) that may be related to cognitive function, we need first to understand what types of cognitive constructs are affected. If we can determine the performance tasks that tap these constructs and encourage researchers to use and analyze them in a standard way, then we could establish continuity among studies. In chapter 7, Dr. Salthouse recommends that cognitive functions be analyzed into higher-order constructs so that potential influences of physical activity on cognition can be studied in terms of which level of a hierarchy of cognitive functions might be affected. The least useful strategy is for each researcher to use a different small set of cognitive tests that may or may not be related to each other. We should know what the shared common variance is and be working at the first-order factor level rather than at the individual variable level. And we should all be using the same or at least similar factors.

Defining Physical Activity and Quantifying It Effectively

What do we mean by physical activity? What is a meaningful way to measure it? Perhaps the strongest consensus came in our growing conviction that we have to develop a better understanding of the appropriate measurements for physical activity. We need to use a measurement approach and identify constructs of physical activity that are pertinent to this research question. We have a good start on understanding cognition from all of the research that Dr. Salthouse has published over the past decade that identifies latent cognitive constructs. He has recommended for years that researchers use these latent cognitive constructs as dependent variables in lieu of observed variables. However, almost none of this work has been done to identify latent physical constructs that represent levels of physical function. We need broad recommendations as to what types of tests are appropriate, and all researchers should be encouraged to use them.

213

Before real progress can be made in understanding how physical activity can influence cognition, physical activity constructs must identified, perhaps in a way similar to that recommended by Dr. Salthouse in his chapter. What outcome from physical activity is important to better mental function in adults? Is it brain stimulation? Brain health? Better glucose or insulin regulation? Increased cerebral circulation? How much and in which region of the brain? If it is any or all of these potential outcomes, how much activity and what type are necessary to change the mechanism in the necessary amount? Our 2-day discussions ended with most of the group questioning the validity of maximum fitness, or $\dot{V}O_2$max, as the gold standard marker of physical activity effects on cognition. This doubt is discussed in Dr. Etnier's chapter, where she showed that (1) changes in $\dot{V}O_2$max in intervention studies do not always correlate with changes in cognitive function, and (2) many researchers have found that moderate exercise, far below that necessary to challenge aerobic capacity, has beneficial effects on many mental functions such as some neuropsychological functions, depression, stress adaptation, and self-efficacy. These observations suggested to us that we need to find other indicators of increased physical activity that represent the quantity and quality of physical activity necessary to produce a wide array of physiological mechanisms that could account for cognitive changes.

We need to know what we should measure, and that will give us the answers for how to do it. Can we measure physical activity with a questionnaire? Can we use a pedometer? Should we be measuring submaximal fitness? The terms *exercise, physical activity,* and *physical fitness* are often used interchangeably throughout the physical activity and cognition literature. Although these constructs are undoubtedly related, they are not identical, and it is imperative that researchers in the field work toward achieving a consensus about how best to define and assess the activity-related variables in future studies. Specialists in physical function and in measurement need to collaborate to make these decisions, and then all researchers need to use them. At the fall 2002 meeting of the National Blueprint advisory committee, the research subgroup determined that this problem should be the highest priority and that the National Blueprint should use whatever means it can to foster a national, standardized test of physical function. In that context, the committee believed that only by this strategy can researchers provide reliable, objective, and consistent data that can support recommendations of the benefits of exercise as public policy. However, it is also likely that only by using this strategy will we be able to identify mechanisms by which exercise enhances cognitive function. A nationally validated physical function test could be used as a standard by which changes in physical activity are quantified. Each of the large population studies funded by the National Institute of Aging has used different combinations of test items.

Determining Whether Exercise Influences Brain Health, Functional Capacity, and Performance State Independently or Interactively

Evidence suggests that exercise has a profound influence on the central nervous system and perhaps how brain neurons develop, but can we distinguish these effects as affecting the health of the organism, the functional capacity, the performance state, or all three? A reciprocal relationship exists between the state of the organism and the health of the organism and what it is experiencing. Changing the state of the organism via exercise, acutely or chronically, may develop the brain in a way that it can be influenced by what it experiences. In other words, exercise may not change an individual's ability to problem solve better, but it would change the state of the brain so that a teacher could be more effective in teaching an individual how to problem solve. Dr. Bartholomew and Dr. Ciccolo discuss this concept in more depth in chapter 3. In animal literature, exercise does not actually change the end point of learning, but it does accelerate the rate of learning. It is almost as though exercise primes the brain, getting it ready in case something occurs that it needs to encode. If something occurs that requires coding, then the brain will do so; but if the system is not pushed, then the effect is not observed. The benefit of accelerated learning is that the animal (or human) can go on to another task or something new.

Brain health is one way to conceptualize the idea that exercise might increase and enhance the brain's resources. A large number of fairly disparate conditions and diseases (e.g., diabetes, CVD, COPD) have negative effects on cognition, but many of the models that researchers in these different fields have developed to explain the effects and improve the symptoms of these conditions come down to very similar underlying physiological mechanisms. The HPA axis status and activation seem to be implicated by almost all researchers. It might be useful to separate the concept of brain health and functional capacity from performance issues, that is, situational effects that affect an individual's ability to execute a task. If we separate these issues, it might help us understand the relationships better.

Resolving Whether Physical Activity Influences Cognitive Function Similarly Throughout the Life Span

We know from the literature that life events and behaviors that happen in our 30s predict some functions in our 70s, yet we focus our research attention on 60-year-olds and use physical activity measures that only reflect the activities of the past week, month, or year. Is that adequate, or do we need physical activity measures that ask for retrospection from our 30s throughout our life history? Even if physical activity is quantified by

215

pedometers for a week, or 3 months, does that indicate how consistent physical activity in a lifestyle might affect cognition in old age?

Aging is a continuous process. It begins at least at age 18 in some variables, and age-related differences between adjacent decades are substantial throughout the life span. In parallel, many physiological measures follow the same aging pattern as that seen for cognitive measures. Sleep and circadian rhythms change, and many neuroendocrine functions follow that similar pattern. Electroencephalographic data from slow-wave sleep and metabolism across age ranges show a similar life span pattern. The decline starts in the 20s. But researchers usually do not quantify variable changes for 18- to 90-year-olds because the necessary tests are intrusive and expensive. Deleterious changes in physiological mechanisms that influence cognition may be happening throughout the life span and perhaps may even be cumulative. But we have a literature that is composed primarily of cross-sectional studies and, basically, of the two end points of the life span.

More research is needed to study the time course of physical activity, cognition, and aging interaction. Particularly, we need to understand how exercise in the middle period of life might change the physical and mental resources of an aging brain. Perhaps the earlier people adopt a healthy lifestyle, the more general protection the brain has and the more resources it has in reserve. If earlier adherence to a healthy lifestyle indeed translates to better cognitive function in old age, it might change the rate of decline. But even if it does not, it would certainly shift the age-related declining curve higher, resulting in a longer period of life in which an individual functions with intact cognition. Quantifying the influence of regular exercise over the course of the life span on cognition, in younger and middle-aged as well as older groups, is essential. At the same time, this information could be very instructive in terms of understanding what mechanisms are operative in influencing cognition.

Longitudinal studies of both physiological and cognitive latent variables are clearly the path we should take, but the obstacles are formidable. However, other designs, such as cross-sequential studies, can be effective. This design uses multiple age groups, in which each has a short-term intervention that is tested as the differences from 20 to 30, 30 to 40, and so forth. This kind of analysis provides some indication of what the age-related effect would be if a study were continued for quite a long time.

Realizing Recommended Research Directions

Several recommendations of potentially fruitful research directions have been made to this point. How might they be realized? Because the recommendations have involved testing a multidimensional model with many variables, mediators, and moderators, they will require many researchers, each with expertise in these model components and interactions, to work together. A good strategy would be to form a cadre of researchers who will develop a program project proposal making the case that lifestyle moderation will be the most exciting, cost-effective, and powerful way to alter brain cognitive functioning and quality of life for older adults. It will require strong collaboration not only among investigators but among universities. The universities would form a consortium, all would adopt a consensus standard for how specific variables would be measured, and each individual member of the consortia would use the same measures of physical activity, physical function, and cognition. Then each researcher would use his or her expertise to measure specific mediators so that multivariate models are built. Establishing a consensus approach to the predictor and the outcome variable will allow comparison of the studies at all of the different sites. The group should develop an action plan for a multisite project that uses many assessments of cognition and physical activity across the life span. With this type of research project and $15 million from a collaboration of government agencies, foundations, and private corporations over a 5-year period, substantial progress could be made in following our recommendations.

Implications for Public Policy

When you think about public policy justifications for promoting physical activity, there is very seldom reference to cognitive outcomes. Right now, exercise–cognition researchers are not contributing to public policy decision making with respect to why people should participate in physical activity. But there may be a subset of people who are at risk for cognitive decline, and it would be very important to study these people if physical activity can be shown to affect that subset of the population. It might be useful to identify those individuals and to see whether physical activity has a more profound effect on that targeted population than on others.

Public policy on this issue might be informed by following the Mayo Clinic's lead in its appeal for policy changes with regard to Alzheimer's disease. Researchers at the Mayo Clinic shifted the paradigm by asking what happens if we delay the progression of Alzheimer's disease by 5 years? They produced economic, caregiver, and other types of relevant data suggesting that the implications at a national level are astounding. This same type of question could be translated to physical activity. What if physical activity delayed the clinical onset of certain dementias or enabled older adults to balance their checkbook and live independently for 2 additional years? There are good data that the Exit Test is a very good predictor of an individual's ability to balance a checkbook at age 75 or 80. But these tests have not been associated with exercise, and longitudinal prospective studies are needed to see if this really happens. At present, those kinds of data are not available.

In recent years there has been a concerted effort to place physical activity and aging issues at the center stage of the national agenda. A major strategic planning document known as the National Blueprint: Increasing Physical Activity Among Adults Age 50 and Older was developed to serve as a guide for multiple organizations, associations, and agencies to inform and support their planning work related to increasing physical activity among America's aging population. More than 50 national organizations and agencies have implemented a wide variety of projects and programs that have been designed to promote physical activity and healthy aging in the age 50 and older population.

A common feature of many of the Blueprint projects has been a concerted effort to translate the outcomes of small, well-controlled clinical trials into practical interventions that can be implemented cost-effectively on a large scale at the local community level. For example, large national U.S. organizations such as AARP and the National Council on the Aging have initiated local community demonstration projects in an attempt to assess the extent to which physical activity interventions housed in locations where seniors regularly gather can be shown to improve health and quality of life. Perhaps most significant, in fall 2004 the Federal Administration on Aging launched a major physical activity and nutrition program known as *You Can! Steps to Healthy Aging*. The goal of the *You Can!* program is to substantively increase the number and scope of physical activity programs throughout the aging network across the United States. From the perspective of this chapter, it is significant to note that the *You Can!* program links both physical activity and healthy nutrition in a single intervention program targeting health and quality of life.

National Blueprint strategies have not focused much attention on cognitive outcomes as a justification for increased attention to physical activity and healthy nutrition at the national level. Instead, attention has been focused on the importance of physical activity and healthy nutrition in the prevention and treatment of chronic conditions, the preservation of independence, and the maintenance and restoration of quality of life. One of the reasons that cognitive benefits have not been emphasized is the virtual absence of studies that have translated outcomes from laboratory-based studies of physical activity and cognitive function into effective and easy-to-implement community programs. For this to occur it will be necessary to solve some of the many theoretical and methodological issues and challenges raised in this book. Although this may seem a daunting task, if, as suggested throughout this book, there is indeed a relationship between physical activity and cognitive decline, the long-term benefits could be substantial.

The evidence is compelling that physical activity has many profoundly positive effects on health outcomes and physical outcomes. However, it remains to be seen how much cognitive improvement might be gained from good health and physical outcomes. Most of us do believe, however, that cognition is such an important component of quality of life that even small gains attributable to exercise would make changes in public policy worthwhile. Our brains, particularly the frontal lobe, are what make us human and what distinguish each of us from everyone else. And these are the very areas that recent research suggests receive the most benefit from exercise.

REFERENCES

Chapter 1

Hockey, G.R.J., Coles, M.G.H., & Gaillard, A.W.K. (1986). Energetical issues in research on human information process. In G.R.J. Hockey, A.W.K. Gaillard, & M.G.H. Coles (Eds.), *Energetics and human information processing* (pp. 3-40). Boston: Martinus Nijhoff.

Jenkins, J.J. (1979). Four points to remember: A tetrahedral model of memory experiments. In L.S. Cermak & F.I.M. Craik (Eds.), *Levels of processing in human memory* (pp. 429-446). Hillsdale, NJ: Erlbaum.

Kahneman, D. (1973). *Attention and effort*. Englewood Cliffs, NJ: Prentice Hall.

Underwood, B.J. (1975). Individual differences as a crucible in theory construction. *American Psychologist, 30*, 128-134.

Chapter 2

Abbott, R.D., White, L.R., Ross, G.W., Masaki, K.H., Curb, J.D., & Petrovitch, H. (2004). Walking and dementia in physically capable elderly men. *Journal of the American Medical Association, 292*(12), 1447-1453.

Albert, M.S., Jones, K., Savage, C.R., Berkman, L., Seeman, T., Blazer, D., et al. (1995). Predictors of cognitive change in older persons: MacArthur studies of successful aging. *Psychology and Aging, 10*(4), 578-589.

Aleman, A., de Haan, E.H., Verhaar, H.H., Samson, M.M., de Vries, W.R., & Koppeschaar, H.P. (2000). Relationship between physical and cognitive function in healthy older men: A role for aerobic power? *Journal of the American Geriatrics Society, 48*(1), 104-105.

American College of Sports Medicine. (2000). *ACSM's guidelines for exercise testing and prescription* (6th ed.). Philadelphia: Lippincott Williams & Wilkins.

Bäckman, L., Small, B.J., & Wahlin, A. (2001). Aging and memory: Cognitive and biological perspectives. In J.E. Birren & K.W. Schaie (Eds.), *Handbook of the psychology of aging* (5th ed., pp. 349-366). San Diego: Academic Press.

Baranowski, T., Anderson, C., & Carmack, C. (1998). Mediating variable framework in physical activity interventions. How are we doing? How might we do better? *American Journal of Preventive Medicine, 15*(4), 266-297.

Baron, R.M., & Kenny, D.A. (1986). The moderator-mediator variable distinction in social psychological research: Conceptual, strategic, and statistical considerations. *Journal of Personality and Social Psychology, 51*(6), 1173-1182.

Barry, A.J., Steinmetz, J.R., Page, H.F., & Rodahl, K. (1966). Effects of physical conditioning on older individuals. 2. Motor performance and cognitive function. *Journal of Gerontology, 21*(2), 192-199.

Baylor, A.M., & Spirduso, W.W. (1988). Systematic aerobic exercise and components of reaction time in older women. *Journal of Gerontology, 43*(5), P121-P126.

Blumenthal, J.A., Emery, C.F., Madden, D.J., Schniebolk, S., Walsh-Riddle, M., George, L.K., et al. (1991). Long-term effects of exercise on psychological functioning in older men and women. *Journal of Gerontology, 46*(6), P352-P361.

Blumenthal, J.A., & Madden, D.J. (1988). Effects of aerobic exercise training, age, and physical fitness on memory-search performance. *Psychology and Aging, 3*(3), 280-285.

Botwinick, J. (1977). Intellectual abilities. In J.E. Birren & K.W. Schaie (Eds.), *Handbook of the psychology of aging* (pp. 580-605). New York: Van Nostrand Reinhold.

Boutcher, S.H. (1993). Conceptualization and quantification of aerobic fitness and physical activity. In P. Seraganian (Ed.), *Exercise psychology: The influence of physical exercise on psychological processes* (pp. 64-79). New York: Wiley.

Caplan, G.A., Ward, J.A., & Lord, S.R. (1993). The benefits of exercise in postmenopausal women. *Australian Journal of Public Health, 17*(1), 23-26.

Cheong, J.W., MacKinnon, D.P., & Khoo, S.T. (2003). Investigation of mediational processes using parallel process latent growth curve modelling. *Structural Equation Modeling, 10*(2), 238-262.

Chodzko-Zajko, W.J., Schuler, P., Solomon, J., Heinl, B., & Ellis, N.R. (1992). The influence of physical fitness on automatic and effortful memory changes in aging. *International Journal of Aging and Human Development, 35*(4), 265-285.

Christensen, H., & Mackinnon, A. (1993). The association between mental, social and physical activity and cognitive performance in young and old subjects. *Age and Ageing, 22*(3), 175-182.

Clarkson-Smith, L., & Hartley, A.A. (1989). Relationships between physical exercise and cognitive abilities in older adults. *Psychology and Aging, 4*(2), 183-189.

Colcombe, S., & Kramer, A.F. (2003). Fitness effects on the cognitive function of older adults: A meta-analytic study. *Psychological Science, 14*(2), 125-130.

Corbin, C., & Pangrazi, B. (1996). What you need to know about The Surgeon General's Report on Physical Activity and Health. *Physical Activity and Fitness Digest, 2*, 1-8.

Crook, T., Bartus, R.T., Ferris, S.H., Whitehouse, P., Cohen, G.D., & Gershon, S. (1986). Age-associated memory impairment: Proposed diagnostic criteria and measures of clinical change—Report of a National Institute of Mental Health Work Group. *Developmental Neuropsychology, 2*(4), 261-276.

Denney, N.W., & Palmer, A.M. (1981). Adult age differences on traditional and practical problem-solving measures. *Journal of Gerontology, 36*(3), 323-328.

References

Denney, N.W., Pearce, K.A., & Palmer, A.M. (1982). A developmental study of adults' performance on traditional and practical problem-solving tasks. *Experimental Aging Research*, *8*(2), 115-118.

Dustman, R.E., Emmerson, R.Y., Ruhling, R.O., Shearer, D.E., Steinhaus, L.A., Johnson, S.C., et al. (1990). Age and fitness effects on EEG, ERPs, visual sensitivity, and cognition. *Neurobiology and Aging*, *11*(3), 193-200.

Dustman, R.E., Emmerson, R., & Shearer, D. (1994). Physical activity, age, and cognitive-neuropsychological function. *Journal of Aging and Physical Activity*, *2*, 143-181.

Dustman, R.E., Ruhling, R.O., Russell, E.M., Shearer, D.E., Bonekat, H.W., Shigeoka, J.W., et al. (1984). Aerobic exercise training and improved neuropsychological function of older individuals. *Neurobiology and Aging*, *5*(1), 35-42.

Elsayed, M., Ismail, A.H., & Young, R.J. (1980). Intellectual differences of adult men related to age and physical fitness before and after an exercise program. *Journal of Gerontology*, *35*(3), 383-387.

Emery, C.F., & Gatz, M. (1990). Psychological and cognitive effects of an exercise program for community-residing older adults. *Gerontologist*, *30*(2), 184-188.

Emery, C.F., Schein, R.L., Hauck, E.R., & MacIntyre, N.R. (1998). Psychological and cognitive outcomes of a randomized trial of exercise among patients with chronic obstructive pulmonary disease. *Health Psychology*, *17*(3), 232-240.

Era, P., Jokela, J., & Heikkinen, E. (1986). Reaction and movement times in men of different ages: A population study. *Perceptual and Motor Skills*, *63*(1), 111-130.

Etnier, J.L., & Berry, M. (2001). Fluid intelligence in an older COPD sample after short- or long-term exercise. *Medicine and Science in Sports and Exercise*, *33*(10), 1620-1628.

Etnier, J.L., & Landers, D.M. (1997). The influence of age and fitness on performance and learning. *Journal of Aging and Physical Activity*, *5*, 175-189.

Etnier, J.L., & Landers, D.M. (1998). Motor performance and motor learning as a function of age and fitness. *Research Quarterly for Exercise and Sport*, *69*(2), 136-146.

Etnier, J.L., Nowell, P.M., Landers, D.M., & Sibley, B.A. (2006). A meta-regression to examine the relationship between aerobic fitness and cognitive performance. *Brain Research Reviews*, *52*, 119-130.

Etnier, J.L., Romero, D.H., & Traustadottir, T. (2001). Acquisition and retention of motor skills as a function of age and aerobic fitness. *Journal of Aging and Physical Activity*, *9*(4), 425-437.

Etnier, J.L., Salazar, W., Landers, D.M., Petruzzello, S.J., Han, M., & Nowell, P. (1997). The influence of physical fitness and exercise upon cognitive functioning: A meta-analysis. *Journal of Sport and Exercise Psychology*, *19*, 249-277.

Fillit, H.M., Butler, R.N., O'Connell, A.W., Albert, M.S., Birren, J.E., Cotman, C.W., et al. (2002). Achieving and maintaining cognitive vitality with aging. *Mayo Clinic Proceedings*, *77*(7), 681-696.

Flicker, C., Ferris, S.H., & Reisberg, B. (1991). Mild cognitive impairment in the elderly: predictors of dementia. *Neurology*, *41*(7), 1006-1009.

References

Hasher, L., & Zacks, R.T. (1979). Automatic and effortful processes in memory. *Journal of Experimental Psychology: General, 108*(3), 356-388.

Hassmen, P., Ceci, R., & Backman, L. (1992). Exercise for older women: A training method and its influences on physical and cognitive performance. *European Journal of Applied Physiology and Occupational Physiology, 64*(5), 460-466.

Hawkins, H.L., Kramer, A.F., & Capaldi, D. (1992). Aging, exercise, and attention. *Psychology and Aging, 7*(4), 643-653.

Hill, R.D., Storandt, M., & Malley, M. (1993). The impact of long-term exercise training on psychological function in older adults. *Journal of Gerontology, 48*(1), P12-P17.

Institute of Medicine. (2002). *Dietary reference intakes for energy, carbohydrate, fiber, fat, fatty acids, cholesterol, protein, and amino acids*. Retrieved December 17, 2002, from http://www.nap.edu/books/0309085373/html/

Izquierdo-Porrera, A.M., & Waldstein, S.R. (2002). Cardiovascular risk factors and cognitive function in African Americans. *Journals of Gerontology. Part B, Psychological Sciences and Social Sciences, 57*(4), P377-P380.

Jacewicz, M.M., & Hartley, A.A. (1987). Age differences in the speed of cognitive operations: resolution of inconsistent findings. *Journal of Gerontology, 42*(1), 86-88.

Khatri, P., Blumenthal, J.A., Babyak, M.A., Craighead, W.E., Herman, S., Bealdewicz, T., et al. (2001). Effects of exercise training on cognitive functioning among depressed older men and women. *Journal of Aging and Physical Activity, 9*(1), 43-57.

Kramer, A.F., Hahn, S., Cohen, N.J., Banich, M.T., McAuley, E., Harrison, C.R., et al. (1999). Ageing, fitness and neurocognitive function. *Nature, 400*(6743), 418-419.

Laurin, D., Verreault, R., Lindsay, J., MacPherson, K., & Rockwood, K. (2001). Physical activity and risk of cognitive impairment and dementia in elderly persons. *Archives of Neurology, 58*(3), 498-504.

Lewis, B.A., Marcus, B.H., Pate, R.R., & Dunn, A.L. (2002). Psychosocial mediators of physical activity behavior among adults and children. *American Journal of Preventive Medicine, 23*(2 Suppl), 26-35.

Lytle, M.E., Vander Bilt, J., Pandav, R.S., Dodge, H.H., & Ganguli, M. (2004). Exercise level and cognitive decline: The MoVIES project. *Alzheimer Disease and Associated Disorders, 18*(2), 57-64.

MacCorquodale, K., & Meehl, P.E. (1948). On a distinction between hypothetical constructs and intervening variables. *Psychological Review, 55*, 95-107.

MacKinnon, D.P. (2001). Mediating variable. In N.J. Smelser & P.B. Baltes (Eds.), *International encyclopedia of the social and behavioral sciences* (pp. 9503-9507). Oxford, UK: Pergamon.

MacKinnon, D.P., Lockwood, C.M., Hoffman, J.M., West, S.G., & Sheets, V. (2002). A comparison of methods to test mediation and other intervening variable effects. *Psychological Methods, 7*(1), 83-104.

References

MacKinnon, D.P., Taborga, M.P., & Morgan-Lopez, A.A. (2002). Mediation designs for tobacco prevention research. *Drug and Alcohol Dependence, 68*(Suppl 1), S69-S83.

Madden, D.J., Blumenthal, J.A., Allen, P.A., & Emery, C.F. (1989). Improving aerobic capacity in healthy older adults does not necessarily lead to improved cognitive performance. *Psychology and Aging, 4*(3), 307-320.

Moul, J.L., Goldman, B., & Warren, B. (1995). Physical-activity and cognitive performance in the older population. *Journal of Aging and Physical Activity, 3*(2), 135-145.

Normand, R., Kerr, R., & Metivier, G. (1987). Exercise, aging and fine motor performance: An assessment. *Journal of Sports Medicine and Physical Fitness, 27*(4), 488-496.

Offenbach, S.I., Chodzko-Zajko, W.J., & Ringel, R.L. (1990). Relationship between physiological status, cognition, and age in adult men. *Bulletin of the Psychonomic Society, 28*, 112-114.

Okumiya, K., Matsubayashi, K., Wada, T., Kimura, S., Doi, Y., & Ozawa, T. (1996). Effects of exercise on neurobehavioral function in community-dwelling older people more than 75 years of age. *Journal of the American Geriatrics Society, 44*(5), 569-572.

Ordovas, J.M. (2003). Cardiovascular disease genetics: A long and winding road. *Current Opinion in Lipidology, 14*, 47-54.

Palleschi, L., Vetta, F., DeGennaro, E., Idone, G., Sottosanti, G., Gianni, W., et al. (1996). Effect of aerobic training on the cognitive performance of elderly patients with senile dementia of Alzheimer type. *Archives of Gerontology and Geriatrics, 5*, 47-50.

Panton, L.B., Graves, J.E., Pollock, M.L., Hagberg, J.M., & Chen, W. (1990). Effect of aerobic and resistance training on fractionated reaction time and speed of movement. *Journal of Gerontology, 45*(1), M26-M31.

Perri, S., & Templer, D.I. (1985). The effects of an aerobic exercise program on psychological variables in older adults. *International Journal of Aging and Human Development, 20*(3), 1984-1985.

Rikli, R., & Busch, S. (1986). Motor performance of women as a function of age and physical activity level. *Journal of Gerontology, 41*(5), 645-649.

Rikli, R.E., & Edwards, D.J. (1991). Effects of a three-year exercise program on motor function and cognitive processing speed in older women. *Research Quarterly for Exercise and Sport, 62*(1), 61-67.

Ritchie, K., Artero, S., & Touchon, J. (2001). Classification criteria for mild cognitive impairment: A population-based validation study. *Neurology, 56*(1), 37-42.

Rowe, J.W., & Kahn, R.L. (2000). Successful aging and disease prevention. *Advances in Renal Replacement Therapy, 7*(1), 70-77.

Salthouse, T.A. (2003). Memory aging from 18 to 80. *Alzheimer Disease and Associated Disorders, 17*(3), 162-167.

Schaie, K.W. (1994). The course of adult intellectual development. *American Psychologist, 49*(4), 304-313.

Science Directorate. (1993). *Vitality for life: Psychological research for productive aging. Human capital initiative document.* Washington, DC: American Psychological Association.

Spirduso, W.W. (1975). Reaction and movement time as a function of age and physical activity level. *Journal of Gerontology, 30*(4), 435-440.

Spirduso, W.W., MacRae, H.H., MacRae, P.G., Prewitt, J., & Osborne, L. (1988). Exercise effects on aged motor function. *Annals of the New York Academy of Sciences, 515,* 363-375.

Stevenson, J.S., & Topp, R. (1990). Effects of moderate and low intensity long-term exercise by older adults. *Research in Nursing Health, 13*(4), 209-218.

Swainson, R., Hodges, J.R., Galton, C.J., Semple, J., Michael, A., Dunn, B.D., et al. (2001). Early detection and differential diagnosis of Alzheimer's disease and depression with neuropsychological tasks. *Dementia and Geriatric Cognitive Disorders, 12*(4), 265-280.

van Boxtel, M.P., Paas, F.G., Houx, P.J., Adam, J.J., Teeken, J.C., & Jolles, J. (1997). Aerobic capacity and cognitive performance in a cross-sectional aging study. *Medicine and Science in Sports and Exercise, 29*(10), 1357-1365.

Weuve, J., Kang, J.H., Manson, J.E., Breteler, M.M., Ware, J.H., & Grodstein, F. (2004). Physical activity, including walking, and cognitive function in older women. *Journal of the American Medical Association, 292*(12), 1454-1461.

Williams, P., & Lord, S.R. (1997). Effects of group exercise on cognitive functioning and mood in older women. *Australian and New Zealand Journal of Public Health, 21*(1), 45-52.

Willis, S.L. (2001). Methodological issues in behavioral intervention research with the elderly. In J.E. Birren & K.W. Schaie (Eds.), *Handbook of the psychology of aging* (5th ed., pp. 78-102). San Diego: Academic Press.

Yaffe, K., Barnes, D., Nevitt, M., Lui, L.Y., & Covinsky, K. (2001). A prospective study of physical activity and cognitive decline in elderly women: Women who walk. *Archives of Internal Medicine, 161*(14), 1703-1708.

Chapter 3

Adler, G., Bramesfeld, A., & Jajcevic, A. (1999). Mild cognitive impairment in old-age depression is associated with increased EEG slow-wave power. *Neuropsychobiology, 40,* 218-222.

Alexopoulos, G.S. (1997, November 6). *Epidemiology, nosology and treatment of geriatric depression.* Paper presented at Exploring Opportunities to Advance Mental Health Care for an Aging Population, meeting sponsored by the John A. Hartford Foundation, Rockville, MD.

Alexopoulos, G.S., Meyers, B.S., Young, R.C., Campbell, S., Silbersweig, D., & Charlson, M. (1997). "Vascular depression" hypothesis. *Archives of General Psychiatry, 54,* 915-922.

References

American Psychiatric Association. (2000). *Diagnostic and statistical manual for mental disorders* (4th ed.). Washington, DC: American Psychiatric Association.

Babyak, M., Blumenthal, J.A., Herman, S., Khatri, P., Doraiswamy, M., Moore, K., et al. (2000). Exercise treatment for major depression: Maintenance of therapeutic benefit at 10 months. *Psychosomatic Medicine, 62,* 633-638.

Bachman, D.L., Wolf, P.A., Linn, R., Knoefel, J.E., Cobb, J., Belanger, A., et al. (1992). Prevalence of dementia and probable senile dementia of the Alzheimer type in the Framingham Study. *Neurology, 42,* 115-119.

Baker, S.C., Frith, C.D., & Dolan, R.J. (1997). The interaction between mood and cognitive function studied with PET. *Psychological Medicine, 27,* 565-578.

Bartholomew, J.B., Ciccolo, J.T., & Morrison, D. (2003). *The effects of an acute bout of exercise on patients with MDD.* Unpublished data.

Bench, C.J., Frackowiak, R.S., & Dolan, R.J. (1995). Changes in regional cerebral blood flow on recovery from depression. *Psychological Medicine, 25,* 247-261.

Benedict, R.H., Dobraski, M., & Goldstein, M.Z. (1999). A preliminary study of the association between changes in mood and cognition in a mixed geriatric psychiatry sample. *Journals of Gerontology. Series B, Psychological Sciences and Social Sciences, 54,* 94-99.

Blazer, D.G. (1996). Epidemiology of psychiatric disorders in late life. In E.W. Busse & D.G. Blazer (Eds.), *The American Psychiatric Press textbook of geriatric psychiatry* (2nd ed., pp. 155-171). Washington, DC: American Psychiatric Press.

Blumenthal, J.A., Babyak, M.A., Moore, K.A., Craighead, W.E., Herman, S., Khatri, P., et al. (1999). Effects of exercise training on older patients with major depression. *Archives of Internal Medicine, 25,* 2349-2356.

Blumenthal, J.A., Williams, R.S., Needles, T.L., & Wallace, A.G. (1982). Psychological changes accompany aerobic exercise in healthy middle-aged adults. *Psychosomatic Medicine, 44,* 529-536.

Branconnier, R.J., DeVitt, D.R., Cole, J.O., & Spera, K.F. (1982). Amitriptyline selectively disrupts verbal recall from secondary memory of the normal aged. *Neurobiology of Aging, 3,* 55-59.

Brody, A.L., Saxena, S., Silverman, D.H., Alborzian, S., Fairbanks, L.A., Phelps, M.E., et al. (1999). Brain metabolic changes in major depressive disorder from pre- to post-treatment with paroxetine. *Psychiatric Research, 11,* 127-139.

Bruce, M.L., & Hoff, R.A. (1994). Social and physical health risk factors for first-onset major depressive disorder in a community sample. *Social Psychiatry and Psychiatric Epidemiology, 29,* 165-171.

Burt, D.B., Zembar, M.J., & Niederehe, G. (1995). Depression and memory impairment: A meta-analysis of the association, its pattern and specificity. *Psychological Bulletin, 117,* 285-305.

Butler, R.N. (1974). Successful aging and the role of the life review. *Journal of the American Geriatrics Society, 22,* 529-535.

Butler, R.N., Lewis, M.I., & Sunderland, T. (1991). *Aging and mental health: Positive psychosocial and biomedical approaches.* Columbus, OH: Merrill.

References

Byrne, D. (1977). Affect and vigilance performance in depressive illness. *Journal of Psychiatry Research, 13*, 185-191.

Caine, E.D., Lyness, J.M., & Conwell, Y. (1996). Diagnosis of late-life depression: Preliminary studies in primary care settings. *American Journal of Geriatric Psychiatry, 4*, S45-S50.

Carmelli, D., Swan, G.E., LaRue, A., & Eslinger, P.J. (1997). Correlates of change in cognitive function in survivors from the Western Collaborative Group Study. *Neuroepidemiology, 16*, 285-295.

Christensen, H., Griffiths, K., Mackinnon, A., & Jacomb, P. (1997). A quantitative review of cognitive deficits in depression and Alzheimer-type dementia. *Journal of the International Neuropsychological Society, 3*, 631-651.

Cotman, C.W., & Engesser-Ceaser, C. (2002). Exercise enhances and protects brain function. *Exercise and Sport Sciences Reviews, 30*, 75-79.

Craft, L.L., & Landers, D.M. (1998). The effects of exercise on clinical depression and depression resulting from mental illness: A meta-regression analysis. *Journal of Sport and Exercise Psychology, 20*, 339-357.

Czeh, B., Michaelis, T., Watanabe, T., Frahm, J., de Biurrun, G., van Kampen, M., et al. (2001). Stress-induced changes in cerebral metabolites, hippocampal volume, and cell proliferation are prevented by antidepressant treatment with tianeptine. *Proceedings of the National Academy of Sciences, 23*, 12320-12322.

Degl'Innocenti, A., Agren, H., & Backman, L. (1998). Executive deficits in major depression. *Acta Psychiatric Scandinavia, 97*, 182-188.

Dimeo, F., Bauer, M., Varahram, I., Proest, G., & Halter, U. (2001). Benefits from aerobic exercise in patients with major depression: A pilot study. *British Journal of Sports Medicine, 35*, 114-117.

Dishman, R.K. (1997). Brain monoamines, exercise, and behavioral stress: Animal models. *Medicine and Science in Sports and Exercise, 29*, 63-74.

Doyne, E.J., Ossip-Klein, D.J., Bowman, E.D., Osborn, K.M., McDougall-Wilson, I.B., & Neimeyer, R.A. (1987). Running versus weight lifting in the treatment of depression. *Journal of Consulting and Clinical Psychology, 55*, 748-754.

Dunn, A.L., Trivedi, M.H., & O'Neal, H.A. (2001). Physical activity dose-response effects on outcomes of depression and anxiety. *Medicine and Science in Sports and Exercise, 33*, S587-S597.

Fossati, P., Amar, G., Raoux, N., Ergis, A.M., & Allilaire, J.F. (1999). Executive functioning and verbal memory in young patients with unipolar depression and schizophrenia. *Psychiatric Research, 89*, 171-187.

Gallo, J.J., & Lebowitz, B.D. (1999). The epidemiology of common late-life mental disorders in the community: Themes for the new century. *Psychiatric Services, 50*, 1158-1166.

Gareri, P., De Fazio, P., & De Sarro, G. (2002). Neuropharmacology of depression in aging and age-related diseases. *Aging Research Reviews, 1*, 113-134.

Gould, E., McEwen, B.S., Tanapat, P., Galea, L.A., & Fuchs, E. (1997). Neurogenesis in the dentate gyrus of the adult tree shrew is regulated by psychosocial stress and NMDA receptor activation. *Journal of Neuroscience, 17*, 2492-2498.

Gurland, B.J., Cross, P.S., & Katz, S. (1996). Epidemiological perspectives on opportunities for treatment of depression. *American Journal of Geriatric Psychiatry, 4,* S7-S13.

Haines, M.E., Norris, M.P., & Kashy, D.A. (1997). The effects of depressed mood on academic performance in college students. *Journal of College Student Development, 37,* 519-526.

Helmes, E., & Duggan, G.M. (2001). Assessment of depression in older adult males by general practitioners. Ageism, physical problems and treatment. *Australian Family Physician, 30,* 291-294.

Hein, S., Bonsignore, M., Barkow, K., Jessen, F., Ptok, U., & Heun, R. (2003). Lifetime depressive and somatic symptoms as preclinical markers of late-onset depression. *European Archives of Psychiatry and Clinical Neuroscience, 253,* 16-21.

Herman, S., Blumenthal, J.A., Babyak, M., Khatri, P., Craighead, W.E., Krishnan, K.R., et al. (2002). Exercise therapy for depression in middle-aged and older adults: Predictors of early dropout and treatment failure. *Health Psychology, 21,* 553-563.

Jacobs, B.L. (1994). Serotonin, motor activity and depression-related disorders. *American Scientist, 82,* 456-463.

Jacobs, B.L. (2002). Adult brain neurogenesis and depression. *Brain, Behavior and Immunity, 16,* 602-609.

Katon, W., Von Korff, M., Lin, E., Bush, T., & Ormel, J. (1992). Adequacy and duration of antidepressant treatment in primary care. *Medical Care, 30,* 67-76.

Katula, J.A., Blissmer, B.J., & McAuley, E. (1999). Exercise intensity and self-efficacy effects on anxiety reduction in healthy, older adults. *Journal of Behavioral Medicine, 22,* 233-247.

Kapur, S., & Mann, J.J. (1992). Role of the dopaminergic system in depression. *Biological Psychiatry, 32,* 1-17.

Landro, N.I., Stiles T.C., & Sletvold, H. (2001). Neuropsychological function in nonpsychotic unipolar major depression. *Neuropsychiatry, Neuropsychological Behavior and Neurology, 14,* 233-240.

Lauer, R.E., Giodrani, B., Boivan, M.J., Halle, N., Glasgow, B., Alessi, N.E., et al. (1994). Effects of depression on memory performance and metamemory in children. *Journal of the American Academy of Child and Adolescent Psychiatry, 33,* 679-685.

Magarinos, A.M., Deslandes, A., & McEwen, B.S. (1999). Effects of antidepressants and benzodiazepine treatments on the dendritic structure of CA3 pyramidal neurons after chronic stress. *European Journal of Pharmacology, 371,* 113-122.

Martinsen, E.W., Medhus, A., & Sandvik, L. (1985). Effects of aerobic exercise on depression: A controlled study. *British Medical Journal, 291,* 109.

McAuley, E., Blissmer, B., Katula, J., Duncan, T.E., & Mihalko, S.L. (2000). Physical activity, self-esteem, and self-efficacy relationships in older adults: A randomized controlled trial. *Annals of Behavioral Medicine, 22,* 131-139.

McAuley, E., Jerome, G.J., Marquez, D.X., Elavsky, S., & Blissmer, B. (2003). Exercise self-efficacy in older adults: Social, affective, and behavioral influences. *Annals of Behavioral Medicine, 25,* 1-7.

McAuley, E., Marquez, D.X., Jerome, G.J., Blissmer, B., & Katula, J. (2002). Physical activity and physique anxiety in older adults: Fitness, and efficacy influences. *Journal of Aging and Mental Health, 6*, 222-230.

McNeil, J.K., LeBlanc, E.M., & Joyner, M. (1991). The effect of exercise on depressive symptoms in the moderately depressed elderly. *Psychology and Aging, 6*, 487-488.

Mendes de Leon, C.F., Kasl, S.V., & Jacobs, S. (1994). A prospective study of widowhood and changes in symptoms of depression in a community sample of the elderly. *Psychological Medicine, 24*, 613-624.

Miller, F.E. (2001). Strategies for the rapid treatment of depression. *Human Psychopharmacology, 16*, 125-132.

North, T.C., McCullagh, P., & Tran, Z.V. (1990). Effect of exercise on depression. *Exercise and Sport Sciences Reviews, 18*, 379-415.

Pennix, B.W.J.H., Rejeski, W.J., Pandya, J., Miller, M.E., Bari, M.D., Applegate, W.B., et al. (2002). Exercise and depressive symptoms: A comparison of aerobic and resistance exercise effects on emotional and physical function in older persons with high and low depressive symptomatology. *Journal of Gerontology: Psychological Sciences, 57*, P124-P132.

Rapaport, M.H., Judd, L.L., Schettler, P.J., Yonkers, K.A., Thase, M.E., Kupfer, D.J., et al. (2002). A descriptive analysis of minor depression. *American Journal of Psychiatry, 159*, 637-643.

Reischies, E.M., & Neu, P. (2000). Comorbidity of mild cognitive disorder and depression—A neuropsychological analysis. *European Archives of Psychiatry and Clinical Neuroscience, 250*, 186-193.

Resnick, B., Orwig, D., Magaziner, J., & Wynne, C. (2002).The effect of social support on exercise behavior in older adults. *Clinical Nursing Research, 11*, 52-70.

Reynolds, C.F., & Kupfer, D.J. (1999). Depression and aging: A look to the future. *Psychiatric Services, 50*, 1167-1172.

Romanoski, A.J., Folstein, M.F., Nestadt, G., Chahal, R., Merchant, A., Brown, C.H., et al. (1992). The epidemiology of psychiatrist-ascertained depression and DSM-III depressive disorders. Results from the Eastern Baltimore Mental Health Survey Clinical Reappraisal. *Psychological Medicine, 22*, 629-655.

Russo-Neustadt, A., Ha, T., Ramirez, H.R., Kesslak, J.P. (2001). Physical activity antidepressant treatment combination: Impact on brain-derived neurotropic factor and nerve growth in rat brain. *Behavioral Brain Research, 726*, 87-95.

Sapolsky, R.M. (1996). Why stress is bad for your brain. *Science, 273*, 749-750.

Sapolsky, R.M. (2001). Depression, antidepressants, and the shrinking hippo-campus. *Proceedings of the National Academy of Sciences, 98*, 12320-12322.

Saunders, P.A., Copeland, J.R., Dewey, M.E., Davidson, I.A., McWilliam, C., Sharma, V., et al. (1991). Heavy drinking as a risk factor for depression and dementia in elderly men. Findings from the Liverpool longitudinal community study. *British Journal of Psychiatry, 159*, 213-216.

Schneider, L.S. (1996). Pharmacological considerations in the treatment of late life depression. *American Journal of Geriatric Psychiatry, 4*, S51-S65.

Serby, M., & Yu, M. (2003). Overview: Depression in the elderly. *Mount Sinai Journal of Medicine, 70*, 38-44.

Sharp, L.K, & Lipsky, M.S. (2002). Screening for depression across the lifespan: A review of measures for use in primary care settings. *American Family Physician, 15*, 1001-1008.

Sheline, Y., Sanghavi, M., Mintun, M., & Gado, M. (1999). Depression duration but not age predicts hippocampal volume loss in medically healthy women with recurrent major depression. *Journal of Neuroscience, 19*, 5034-5041.

Singh, N.A., Clements, K.M., & Fiatarone, M.A. (1997). A randomized controlled trial of progressive resistance training in depressed elders. *Journal of Gerontology, 52*, M27-M35.

Singh, N.A., Clements, K.M., & Singh, M.A. (2001). The efficacy of exercise as a long-term antidepressant in elderly subjects: A randomized, controlled trial. *Journal of Gerontology, 56*, M497-M504.

Siuciak, J.A., Lewis, D.R., Wiegand, S.J., & Lindsay, R.M. (1997). Anti-depressant-like effect of brain-derived neurotropic factor (BDNF). *Pharmacology, Biochemistry and Behavior, 56*, 131-137.

Steinkamp, W., & Kelly, J.R. (1987). Social integration, leisure activity, and life satisfaction in older adults: Activity theory revisited. *International Journal of Aging and Human Development, 25*, 293-307.

Steffens, D.C., & Krishnan, K.R. (1998). Structural neuroimaging and mood disorders: Recent findings, implications for classification, and future directions. *Biological Psychiatry, 43*, 705-712.

Thase, M.E., Nierenberg, A.A., Keller, M.B., & Panagides, J. (2001). Efficacy of mirtazapine for prevention of depressive relapse: A placebo-controlled double-blind trial of recently remitted high-risk patients. *Journal of Clinical Psychiatry, 6*, 782-788.

Tsutsumi, T., Don, B.M., Zaichkowsky, L.D., & Delizonna, L.L. (1997). Physical fitness and psychological benefits of strength training in community dwelling older adults. *Applied Human Science, 16*, 257-266.

Unutzer, J., Katon, W., Callahan, C.M., Williams, J.W., Jr., Hunkeler, E., Harpole, L., et al. (2003). Depression treatment in a sample of 1,801 depressed older adults in primary care. *Journal of the American Geriatrics Society, 51*, 505-514.

U.S. Department of Health and Human Services, Office of the Surgeon General, SAMHSA. (1999). *Mental health: A report of the Surgeon General.* Rockville, MD: U.S. Department of Health and Human Services—Substance Abuse and Mental Health Services Administration, Center for Mental Health Services, National Institutes of Health, National Institute of Mental Health.

Van Broekhoven, F., & Verkes, R.J. (2003). Neurosteroids in depression: A review. *Psychopharmacology, 165*, 97-110.

van der Pompe, G., Bernards, N., Meijman, T.F., & Heijnen, C.J. (1999). The effect of depressive symptomatology on plasma cortisol responses to acute bicycle exercise among post-menopausal women. *Psychiatry Research, 18*, 113-117.

Van Hoomissen, J.D., Chambliss, H.O., Holmes, P.V., & Dishman, R.K. (2003). Effects of chronic exercise and imipramine on mRNA for BDNF after olfactory bulbectomy in rat. *Brain Research, 6*, 228-235.

Veiel, H.O. (1997). A preliminary profile of neuropsychological deficits associated with major depression. *Journal of Clinical Experimental Neuropsychology, 19*, 587-603.

Wells, K.B., Stewart, A., Hays, R.D., Burnam, M.A., Rogers, W., Daniels, M., et al. (1989). The functioning and well-being of depressed patients. Results from the Medical Outcomes Study. *Journal of the American Medical Association, 262*, 914-919.

Whitehead, A. (1973). Verbal learning and memory in elderly depressives. *British Journal of Psychiatry, 123*, 203-208.

Williams, P., & Lord, S.R. (1997). Effects of group exercise on cognitive functioning and mood in older women. *Australian New Zealand Journal of Public Health, 21*, 45-52.

Chapter 4

Adlard, P.A., & Cotman, C.W. (2004). Voluntary exercise protects against stress-induced decreases in brain-derived neurotrophic factor protein expression. *Neuroscience, 124*, 985-992.

Alonso, M., Vianna, M.R., Izquierdo, I., & Medina, J.H. (2002). Signaling mechanisms mediating BDNF modulation of memory formation in vivo in the hippocampus. *Cellular and Molecular Neurobiology, 22*(5-6), 663-674.

Blumenthal, J.A., Babyak, M.A., Moore, K.A., Craighead, W.E., Herman, S., Khatri, P., et al. (1999). Effects of exercise training on older patients with major depression. *Archives of Internal Medicine, 159*(19), 2349-2356.

Blumenthal, J.A., Fredrikson, M., Kuhn, C.M., Ulmer, R.L., Walsh-Riddle, M., & Appelbaum, M. (1990). Aerobic exercise reduces levels of cardiovascular and sympathoadrenal responses to mental stress in subjects without prior evidence of myocardial ischemia. *American Journal of Cardiology, 65*(1), 93-98.

Byrne, A., & Byrne, D.G. (1993). The effect of exercise on depression, anxiety and other mood states: A review. *Journal of Psychosomatic Research, 37*(6), 565-574.

Carrasco, G.A., & Van de Kar, L.D. (2003). Neuroendocrine pharmacology of stress. *European Journal of Pharmacology, 463*(1-3), 235-272.

Chrousos, G.P. (1998). Stressors, stress, and neuroendocrine integration of the adaptive response. The 1997 Hans Selye Memorial Lecture. *Annals of the New York Academy of Sciences, 851*, 311-335.

Colcombe, S.J., Erickson, K.I., Raz, N., Webb, A.G., Cohen N.J., McAuley, E., & Kramer A.F. (2003). Aerobic fitness reduces brain tissue loss in aging humans. *Journals of Gerontology. Series A, Biological Sciences and Medical Sciences, 58*(2), 176-180.

Colcombe, S., & Kramer, A.F. (2003). Fitness effects on the cognitive function of older adults: A meta-analytic study. *Psychological Science, 14*(2), 125-130.

References

Cotman, C.W., & Berchtold, N.C. (2002). Exercise: A behavioral intervention to enhance brain health and plasticity. *Trends in Neuroscience, 25*(6), 292-298.

Cotman, C.W., Berchtold, N.C., & Christie, L.A. (in press). Exercise builds brain health: An interplay of central and peripheral factors. *Trends in Neuroscience.*

Deuster, P.A., Chrousos, G.P., Luger, A., DeBolt, J.E., Bernier, L.L., Trostmann, U.H., et al. (1989). Hormonal and metabolic responses of untrained, moderately trained, and highly trained men to three exercise intensities. *Metabolism, 38*(2), 141-148.

Deuster, P.A., Petrides, J.S., Singh, A., Lucci, E.B., Chrousos, G.P., & Gold, P.W. (1998). High intensity exercise promotes escape of adrenocorticotropin and cortisol from suppression by dexamethasone: Sexually dimorphic responses. *Journal of Clinical Endocrinology and Metabolism, 83*(9), 3332-3338.

DiLorenzo, T.M., Bargman, E.P., Stucky-Ropp, R., Brassington, G.S., Frensch, P.A., & Lafontaine, T. (1999). Long-term effects of aerobic exercise on psychological outcomes. *Preventive Medicine, 28(1),* 75-85.

Ding, Y.H., Young, C.N., Luan, X., Li, J., Rafols, J.A., Clark, J.C., et al. (2005). Exercise preconditioning ameliorates inflammatory injury in ischemic rats during reperfusion. *Acta Neuropathologica (Berl), 109*(3), 237-246.

Duman, R.S., Heninger, G.R., & Nestler, E.J. (1997). A molecular and cellular theory of depression. *Archives of General Psychiatry, 54*(7), 597-606.

Dunn, A.L., Trivedi, M.H., Kampert, J.B., Clark, C.G., & Chambliss, H.O. (2002). The DOSE study: A clinical trial to examine efficacy and dose response of exercise as treatment for depression. *Controlled Clinical Trials, 23*(5), 584-603.

Friedland, R.P., Fritsch, T., Smyth, K.A., Koss, E., Lerner, A.J., Chen, C.H., et al. (2001). Patients with Alzheimer's disease have reduced activities in midlife compared with healthy control-group members. *Proceedings of the National Academy of Sciences of the United States of America, 98*, 3440-3445.

Fujimaki, K., Morinobu, S., & Duman, R.S. (2000). Administration of a cAMP phosphodiesterase 4 inhibitor enhances antidepressant-induction of BDNF mRNA in rat hippocampus. *Neuropsychopharmacology, 22*(1), 42-51.

Garcia, R. (2002). Stress, synaptic plasticity, and psychopathology. *Reviews in the Neurosciences, 13*(3), 195-208.

Gould, E., & Tanapat, P. (1999). Stress and hippocampal neurogenesis. *Biological Psychiatry, 46*(11), 1472-1479.

Greenwood, B.N., Foley, T.E., Burhans, D., Maier, S.F., & Fleshner, M. (2005). The consequences of uncontrollable stress are sensitive to duration of prior wheel running. *Brain Research, 1033*(2), 164-178.

Greenwood, B.N., Foley, T.E., Day, H.E., Campisi, J., Hammack, S.H., Campeau, S., et al. (2003). Freewheel running prevents learned helplessness/behavioral depression: Role of dorsal raphe serotonergic neurons. *Journal of Neuroscience, 23*(7), 2889-2898.

Hassmen, P., Koivula, N., & Uutela, A. (2000). Physical exercise and psychological well-being: A population study in Finland. *Preventive Medicine, 30*(1), 17-25.

Kamarck, T.W., Everson, S.A., Kaplan, G.A., Manuck, S.B., Jennings, J.R., Salonen, R., et al. (1997). Exaggerated blood pressure responses during mental stress are associated with enhanced carotid atherosclerosis in middle-aged Finnish men: Findings from the Kuopio Ischemic Heart Disease Study. *Circulation, 96*(11), 3842-3848.

Kaplan, J.R., Manuck, S.B., Clarkson, T.B., Lusso, F.M., Taub, D.M., & Miller, E.W. (1983). Social stress and atherosclerosis in normocholesterolemic monkeys. *Science, 220*(4598), 733-735.

Kim, J.J., & Yoon, K.S. (1998). Stress: Metaplastic effects in the hippocampus. *Trends in Neuroscience, 21*(12), 505-509.

Kirschbaum, C., Prussner, J.C., Stone, A.A., Federenko, I., Gaab, J., Lintz, D., et al. (1995). Persistent high cortisol responses to repeated psychological stress in a subpopulation of healthy men. *Psychosomatic Medicine, 57*(5), 468-474.

Konsman, J.P., Parnet, P., & Dantzer, R. (2002). Cytokine-induced sickness behaviour: Mechanisms and implications. *Trends in Neuroscience, 25*(3), 154-159.

Lampinen, P., Heikkinen, R.L., & Ruoppila, I. (2000). Changes in intensity of physical exercise as predictors of depressive symptoms among older adults: An eight-year follow-up. *Preventive Medicine, 30*(5), 371-380.

Laurin, D., Verreault, R., Lindsay, J., MacPherson, K., & Rockwood, K. (2001). Physical activity and risk of cognitive impairment and dementia in elderly persons. *Archives of Neurology, 58*(3), 498-504.

Lawlor, D.A., & Hopker, S.W. (2001). The effectiveness of exercise as an intervention in the management of depression: Systematic review and meta-regression analysis of randomised controlled trials. *BMJ, 322*(7289), 763-767.

Lee, J., Duan, W., & Mattson, M.P. (2002). Evidence that brain-derived neurotrophic factor is required for basal neurogenesis and mediates, in part, the enhancement of neurogenesis by dietary restriction in the hippocampus of adult mice. *Journal of Neurochemistry, 82*(6), 1367-1375.

Lee, A.L., Ogle, W.O., & Sapolsky, R.M. (2002). Stress and depression: Possible links to neuron death in the hippocampus. *Bipolar Disorders, 4*(2), 117-128.

Luger, A., Deuster, P.A., Kyle, S.B., Gallucci, W.T., Montgomery, L.C., Gold, P.W., et al. (1987). Acute hypothalamic-pituitary-adrenal responses to the stress of treadmill exercise. Physiologic adaptations to physical training. *New England Journal of Medicine, 316*(21), 1309-1315.

Madden, K.S. (2003). Catecholamines, sympathetic innervation, and immunity. *Brain, Behavior, and Immunity, 17 Suppl 1*, S5-10.

Magarinos, A.M., & McEwen, B.S. (1995). Stress-induced atrophy of apical dendrites of hippocampal CA3c neurons: Involvement of glucocorticoid secretion and excitatory amino acid receptors. *Neuroscience, 69*(1), 89-98.

Maier, S.F., & Seligman, M.E. (1976). Learned helplessness: Theory and evidence. *Journal of Experimental Psychology: General, 105*(1), 3-46.

Manuck, S.B., Kaplan, J.R., & Clarkson, T.B. (1983). Behaviorally induced heart rate reactivity and atherosclerosis in cynomolgus monkeys. *Psychosomatic Medicine, 45*(2), 95-108.

References

McAllister, A.K., Katz, L.C., & Lo, D.C. (1999). Neurotrophins and synaptic plasticity. *Annual Review of Neuroscience, 22*, 295-318.

McEwen, B.S. (1999). Stress and the aging hippocampus. *Frontiers in Neuroendocrinology, 20*(1), 49-70.

McEwen, B.S., & Sapolsky, R.M. (1995). Stress and cognitive function. *Current Opinion in Neurobiology, 5*(2), 205-216.

McEwen, B.S., & Seeman, T. (1999). Protective and damaging effects of mediators of stress. Elaborating and testing the concepts of allostasis and allostatic load. *Annals of the New York Academy of Sciences, 896*, 30-47.

Negrao, A.B., Deuster, P.A., Gold, P.W., Singh, A., & Chrousos, G.P. (2000). Individual reactivity and physiology of the stress response. *Biomedicine and Pharmacotherapy, 54*(3), 122-128.

Nibuya, M., Morinobu, S., & Duman, R.S. (1995). Regulation of BDNF and trkB mRNA in rat brain by chronic electroconvulsive seizure and antidepressant drug treatments. *Journal of Neuroscience, 15*(11), 7539-7547.

Nickerson, M., Elphick, G.F., Campisi, J., Greenwood, B.N., & Fleshner, M. (2005). Physical activity alters the brain Hsp72 and IL-1beta responses to peripheral E. coli challenge. *American Journal of Physiology. Regulatory, Integrative, and Comparative Physiology, 289*(6), R1665-R1674.

Nieman, D.C. (1997). Exercise immunology: Practical applications. *International Journal of Sports Medicine, 18*(Suppl 1):S91-S100.

Pacak, K., & Palkovits, M. (2001). Stressor specificity of central neuroendocrine responses: Implications for stress-related disorders. *Endocrine Reviews, 22*(4), 502-548.

Perry, V.H. (2004). The influence of systemic inflammation on inflammation in the brain: Implications for chronic neurodegenerative disease. *Brain, Behavior, and Immunity, 18*(5), 407-413.

Pollock, K.M. (2001). Exercise in treating depression: Broadening the psychotherapist's role. *Journal of Clinical Psychology, 57*(11), 1289-1300.

Rogers, R.L., Meyer, J.S., & Mortel, K.F. (1990). After reaching retirement age physical activity sustains cerebral perfusion and cognition. *Journal of the American Geriatrics Society, 38*(2), 123-128.

Russo-Neustadt, A., Beard, R.C., & Cotman, C.W. (1999). Exercise, antidepressant medications, and enhanced brain derived neurotrophic factor expression. *Neuropsychopharmacology, 21*(5), 679-682.

Sapolsky, R.M. (2003). Stress and plasticity in the limbic system. *Neurochemical Research, 28*(11), 1735-1742.

Sapolsky, R.M., Romero, L.M., & Munck, A.U. (2000). How do glucocorticoids influence stress responses? Integrating permissive, suppressive, stimulatory, and preparative actions. *Endocrine Reviews, 21*(1), 55-89.

Seligman, M.E. (1972). Learned helplessness. *Annual Review of Medicine, 23*, 407-412.

Sheps, D.S., & Sheffield, D. (2001). Depression, anxiety, and the cardiovascular system: The cardiologist's perspective. *Journal of Clinical Psychiatry, 62*(Suppl. 8), 12-16; discussion 17-18.

Shinkai, S., Konishi, M., & Shephard, R.J. (1997). Aging, exercise, training, and the immune system. *Exercise Immunology Review, 3,* 68-95.

Strawbridge, W.J., Deleger, S., Roberts, R.E., & Kaplan, G.A. (2002). Physical activity reduces the risk of subsequent depression for older adults. *American Journal of Epidemiology, 156*(4), 328-334.

Tong, L., Shen, H., Perreau, V., Balazs, R., & Cotman, C.W. (2001). Effects of exercise on gene-expression profile in the rat hippocampus. *Neurobiology of Disease, 8*(6), 1046-1056.

Tsatsoulis, A., & Fountoulakis, S. (2006). The protective role of exercise on stress system dysregulation and comorbidities. *Annals of the New York Academy of Sciences, 1083,* 196-213.

Venjatraman, J.T., & Fernandes, G. (1997). Exercise, immunity and aging. *Aging (Milano), 9*(1-2), 42-56.

Woods, J.A., Lowder, T.W., & Keylock, K.T. (2002). Can exercise training improve immune function in the aged? *Annals of the New York Academy of Sciences, 959,* 117-127.

Yan, H., Kuroiwa, A., Tanaka, H., Shindo, M., Kiyonaga, A., & Nagayama, A. (2001). Effect of moderate exercise on immune senescence in men. *European Journal of Applied Physiology, 86*(2), 105-111.

Chapter 5

Albert, M.S., Jones, K., Savage, C.R., Berkman, L., Seeman, T., Blazer, D., et al. (1995). Predictors of cognitive change in older persons: MacArthur Studies of Successful Aging. *Psychology and Aging, 10*(4), 578-589.

Avorn, J., & Langer, E. (1982). Induced disability in nursing home patients: A controlled trial. *Journal of the American Geriatrics Society, 30*(6), 397-400.

Bandura, A. (1977). Self-efficacy: Toward a unifying theory of behavioral change. *Psychological Review, 84*(2), 191-215.

Bandura, A. (1986). *Social foundations of thought and action: A social cognitive theory.* Englewood Cliffs, NJ: Prentice Hall.

Bandura, A. (1989). Regulation of cognitive processes through perceived self-efficacy. *Developmental Psychology, 25*(5), 729-735.

Bandura, A. (1997). *Self-efficacy: The exercise of control.* New York: Freeman.

Bandura, A., Reese, L., & Adams, N.E. (1982). Microanalysis of action and fear arousal as a function of differential levels of perceived self-efficacy. *Journal of Personality and Social Psychology, 43*(1), 5-21.

Bandura, A., Taylor, C.B., Williams, S.L., Mefford, I.N., & Barchas, J.D. (1985). Catecholamine secretion as a function of perceived coping self-efficacy. *Journal of Consulting and Clinical Psychology, 53*(3), 406-414.

References

Berry, J. (1999). Memory self-efficacy in its social cognitive context. In T.M. Hess & F. Blanchard-Fields (Eds.), *Social cognition and aging* (pp. 69-96). San Diego, CA: Academic Press.

Berry, J.M., West, R.L., & Dennehy, D.M. (1989). Reliability and validity of the memory self-efficacy questionnaire. *Developmental Psychology, 25*, 701-713.

Cavanaugh, J.C., & Poon, L.W. (1989). Metamemorial predictors of memory performance in young and older adults. *Psychology and Aging, 4*(3), 365-368.

Churchill, J.D., Galvez, R., Colcombe, S., Swain, R.A., Kramer, A.F., & Greenough, W.T. (2002). Exercise, experience and the aging brain. *Neurobiology of Aging, 23*(5), 941-955.

Cioffi, D. (1991). Beyond attentional strategies: Cognitive-perceptual model of somatic interpretation. *Psychology Bulletin, 109*(1), 25-41.

Colcombe, S.J., Erickson, K.I., Raz, N., Webb, A.G., Cohen, N.J., McAuley E., et al. (2003). Aerobic fitness reduces brain tissue loss in aging humans. *Journal of Gerontology. Series A: Biological Sciences and Medical Sciences, 58*(2), 176-180.

Colcombe, S., & Kramer A.F. (2003). Fitness effects on the cognitive function of older adults: A meta-analytic study. *Psychological Sciences, 14*(2), 125-130.

Colcombe, S.J., Kramer, A.F., Erickson, K.I., Scalf, P., McAuley, E., Cohen, N.J., et al. (2004). Cardiovascular fitness, cortical plasticity, and aging. *Proceedings of the National Academy of Sciences of the United States of America, 101*, 3316-3321.

Dixon, R.A., Hultsch, D.F., & Hertzog, C. (1988). The Metamemory in Adulthood (MIA) questionnaire. *Psychopharmacology Bulletin, 24*, 675-688.

Duncan, T.E., & McAuley, E. (1993). Social support and efficacy cognitions in exercise adherence: A latent growth curve analysis. *Journal of Behavioral Medicine, 16*(2), 199-218.

Jerome, G., Marquez, D.X., McAuley, E., Canaklisova, S., Snook, E., & Vickers, M. (2002). Self-efficacy effects on feeling states in women. *International Journal of Behavioral Medicine, 5*(3), 139-154.

Kaplan, R., Reis, A., Prewitt, L., & Eakin, E. (1994). Self-efficacy expectations predict survival for patients with chronic obstructive pulmonary disease. *Health Psychology, 13*(4), 366-368.

Katula, J.A., Blissmer, B.J., & McAuley, E. (1999). Exercise intensity and self efficacy effects on anxiety reduction in healthy, older adults. *Journal of Behavioral Medicine, 22*(3), 233-247.

King, A.C., Haskell, W.L., Young, D.R., Oka, R.K., & Stefanick, M.L. (1995). Long-term effects of varying intensities and formats of physical activity on participation rates, fitness, and lipoproteins in men and women aged 50 to 65 years. *Circulation, 91*, 2596-2604.

Kramer, A.F., Hahn, S., Cohen, N.J., Banich, M.T., McAuley, E., Harrison, C.R., et al. (1999). Aging, fitness and neurocognitive function. *Nature, 400*, 418-419.

Kramer, A.F., Hahn, S., & McAuley, E. (2000). Influence of aerobic fitness on the neurocognitive function of older adults. *Journal of Aging and Physical Activity, 8*, 379-385.

References

Lachman, M.E., Bandura, M., Weaver, S.L., & Elliott, E. (1995). Assessing memory control beliefs: The Memory Controllability Inventory. *Aging and Cognition, 2*(1), 67-84.

Lox, C.L., & Freehill, A.J. (1999). Impact of pulmonary rehabilitation on self-efficacy, quality of life, and exercise tolerance. *Rehabilitation Psychology, 44*(2), 208-221.

Marquez, D.X., Jerome G.J., McAuley, E., Snook, E.M., & Canaklisova, S. (2002). Self-efficacy manipulation and state anxiety responses to exercise in low active women. *Psychology and Health, 17*(6), 783-791.

McAuley, E. (1992). The role of efficacy cognitions in the prediction of exercise behavior in middle-aged adults. *Journal of Behavioral Medicine, 15,* 65-88.

McAuley, E. (1993). Self-efficacy and the maintenance of exercise participation in older adults. *Journal of Behavioral Medicine, 16,* 103-113.

McAuley, E., & Blissmer, B. (2000). Self-efficacy determinants and consequences of physical activity. *Exercise and Sport Sciences Reviews, 28*(2), 85-88.

McAuley, E., Courneya, K.S., Rudolph, D.L., & Lox, C.L. (1994). Enhancing exercise adherence in middle-aged males and females. *Preventive Medicine, 23,* 498-506.

McAuley, E., Jerome, G.J., Elavsky, S., Marquez, D.X., & Ramsey, S.N. (2003). Predicting long-term maintenance of physical activity in older adults. *Preventive Medicine, 37,* 110-118.

McAuley, E., Jerome, G.J., Marquez, D.X., Canaklisova, S., & Blissmer, B. (2003). Exercise self-efficacy in older adults: Social, affective, and behavioral influences. *Annals of Behavioral Medicine, 25,* 1-7.

McAuley, E., & Katula, J. (1998). Physical activity interventions in the elderly: Influence on physical health and psychological function. *Annual Review of Gerontology and Geriatrics, 18,* 111-154.

McAuley, E., Katula, J., Mihalko, S.L., Blissmer, B., Duncan, S.C., Pena, M., et al. (1999). Mode of physical activity and self-efficacy in older adults: A latent growth curve analysis. *Journals of Gerontology: Medical Sciences, 54B,* 283-292.

McAuley, E., Kramer, A.F., & Colcombe, S.J. (2004). Cardiovascular fitness and neurocognitive function in older adults: A brief review. *Brain, Behavior, and Immunity, 18,* 214-220.

McAuley, E., Lox, C., & Duncan, T. (1993). Long-term maintenance of exercise, self-efficacy, and physiological change in older adults. *Journal of Gerontology, 48,* 218-224.

McAuley, E., & Mihalko, S.L. (1998). Measuring exercise-related self-efficacy. In J.L. Duda (Ed.), *Advances in sport and exercise psychology measurement* (pp. 371-392). Morgantown, WV: Fitness Information Technology.

McAuley, E., Mihalko, S.L., & Rosengren, K. (1997). Self-efficacy and balance correlates of fear of falling in the elderly. *Journal of Aging and Physical Activity, 5,* 329-340.

References

McAuley, E., Talbot, H.-M., & Martinez, S. (1999). Manipulating self-efficacy in the exercise environment in women: Influences on affective responses. *Health Psychology*, *18*(3), 288-294.

Mueller, P., & Major, B. (1989). Self-blame, self-efficacy, and adjustment to abortion. *Journal of Personality and Social Psychology*, *57*, 1059-1068.

Oman, R., & King, A. (1998). Predicting the adoption and maintenance of exercise participation using self-efficacy and previous exercise participation rates. *American Journal of Health Promotion*, *12*, 154-161.

Park, D.C., Lautenschlager, G., Hedden, T., Davidson, N., Smith, A.D., & Smith, S.K. (2002). Models of visual, spatial, and verbal memory across the lifespan. *Psychology and Aging*, *17*, 299-320.

Rejeski, W.J., Ettinger, W.H., Martin, K., & Morgan, T. (1998). Treating disability in knee osteoarthritis with exercise therapy: A central role for self-efficacy and pain. *Arthritis Care and Research*, *11*(2), 94-101.

Rodin, J. (1986). Aging and health: Effects of the sense of control. *Science*, *233*, 1271-1276.

Rodin, J., & McAvay, G. (1992). Determinants of change in perceived health in a longitudinal study of older adults. *Journal of Gerontology*, *47*(6), 373-384.

Sallis, J.F., Haskell, W.L., Fortmann, S.P., Vranizan, K.M., Taylor, C.B., & Solomon, D.S. (1986). Predictors of adoption and maintenance of physical activity in a community sample. *Preventive Medicine*, *15*, 331-341.

Sanderson, W.C., Rapee, R.M., & Barlow, D.H. (1989). The influence of an illusion of control on panic attacks induced via inhalation of 5.5% carbon dioxide-enriched air. *Archives of General Psychiatry*, *46*, 157-162.

Satariano, W.A., & McAuley, E. (2003). Promoting physical activity among older adults: From ecology to the individual. *American Journal of Preventive Medicine*, *25*, 184-192.

Schaie, K.W. (2000). The impact of longitudinal studies on understanding development from young adulthood to old age. *International Journal of Behavioral Development*, *24*(3), 257-266.

Seeman, T., McAvay, G., Merrill, S., Albert, M., & Rodin, J. (1996). Self-efficacy beliefs and change in cognitive performance: MacArthur Studies of Successful Aging. *Psychology and Aging*, *11*(3), 538-551.

Seeman, T., Rodin, J., & Albert, M. (1993). Self-efficacy and cognitive performance in high functioning older individuals: McArthur Studies of Successful Aging. *Journal of Aging and Health*, *5*, 455-474.

Skinner, E. (1996). A guide to constructs of control. *Journal of Personality and Social Psychology*, *71*, 549-570.

Tabbarah, M., Crimmins, E.M., & Seeman, T.E. (2002). The relationship between cognitive and physical performance: MacArthur Studies of Successful Aging. *Journals of Gerontology. Series A, Biological Sciences and Medical Sciences*, *57*(4), M228-M235.

Taylor, C.B., Bandura, A., Ewart, C.K., Miller, N.H., & Debusk, R.F. (1985). Exercise testing to enhance wives' confidence in their husbands' cardiac capability soon after acute myocardial infarction. *American Journal of Cardiology*, *55*, 635-638.

Turner, E.E., Rejeski, W.J., & Brawley, L.R. (1997). Psychological benefits of physical activity are influenced by the social environment. *Journal of Sport and Exercise Psychology*, *19*(2), 119-130.

Welch, D., & West, R. (1995). Self-efficacy and mastery: Its application to issues of environmental control, cognition, and aging. *Developmental Review*, *15*, 150-171.

Wiedenfeld, S.A., Bandura, A., Levine, S., O'Leary, A., Brown, S., & Raska, K. (1990). Impact of perceived self-efficacy in coping with stressors on components of the immune system. *Journal of Personality and Social Psychology*, *59*, 1082-1094.

Chapter 6

Anderson, J.R. (1983). *The architecture of cognition*. Cambridge, MA: Harvard University Press.

Atkinson, R., & Shiffrin, R.M. (1971). The control of short-term memory. *Scientific American*, *225*, 82-90.

Baltes, P.B., Staudinger, U., & Lindenberger, U. (1999). Lifespan psychology: Theory and application to intellectual functioning. In J.T. Spence, J.M. Darley, & D.J. Foss (Eds.), *Annual review of psychology* (Vol. 50, pp. 471-507). Palo Alto, CA: Annual Reviews.

Baron, R.M., & Kenny, D.A. (1986). The moderator-mediator variable distinction in social psychological research: Conceptual, strategic, and statistical considerations. *Journal of Personality and Social Psychology*, *51*, 1173-1182.

Birren, J.E. (1960). Behavioral theories of aging. In N.W. Shock (Ed.), *Aging: Some social and biological aspects*. Washington, DC: American Association for the Advancement of Science.

Buckworth, J., & Dishman, R.K. (2002). *Exercise psychology*. Champaign, IL: Human Kinetics.

Churchill, J.D., Galvez, R., Colcombe, S., Swain, R.A., Kramer, A.F., & Greenough, W.T. (2002). Exercise, experience and the aging brain. *Neurobiology of Aging*, *23*(5), 941-955.

Colcombe, S., & Kramer, A.F. (2003). Fitness effects on the cognitive function of older adults: A meta-analytic study. *Psychological Science*, *14*, 125-130.

Crews, D.J., & Landers, D.M. (1987). A meta-analytic review of aerobic fitness and reactivity to psychosocial stressors. *Medicine and Science in Sports and Exercise*, *19*(Suppl. 5), S114-S120.

Davis, J.M. (1995). Carbohydrates, branch-chain amino acids and endurance: The central fatigue hypothesis. *International Journal of Sport Nutrition*, *5*(Suppl), S29-S38.

Dienstbier, R.A. (1989). Arousal and physiological toughness: Implications for mental and physical health. *Psychological Review, 96*, 84-100.

Dienstbier, R.A. (1991). Behavioral correlates of sympathoadrenal reactivity: The toughness model. *Medicine and Science in Sports and Exercise, 23*, 846-852.

Dishman, R.K., & Jackson, E.M. (2000). Exercise, fitness, and stress. *International Journal of Sport Psychology, 31*, 175-203.

English, H.B., & English, A.C. (1958). *A comprehensive dictionary of psychological and psychoanalytical terms.* New York: Longman Green.

Essen-Moller, E. (1956). Individual traits and morbidity in a Swedish rural population. *Acta Psychiatrica Scandinavica Supplementum, 100*, 1-160.

Faulkner, J.A., Brooks, S.V., & Zerba, E. (1990). Skeletal muscle weakness and fatigue in old age: Underlying mechanisms. In V.J. Cristofalo & M.P. Lawton (Eds.), *Annual review of gerontology and geriatrics* (Vol. 10, pp. 147-166). New York: Springer.

Finch, C.E., & Seeman, T.E. (1999). Stress theories of aging. In V.L. Bengtson & K.W. Schaie (Eds.), *Handbook of theories of aging* (pp. 81-97). New York: Springer.

Folkman, S., & Lazarus, R.S. (1985). If it changes it must be a process: Study of emotions and coping during stages of a college examination. *Journal of Personality and Social Psychology, 48*, 150-170.

Gaillard, A.W.K., & Wientjes, C.J.E. (1994). Mental workload and work stress as two types of energy mobilization. *Work and Stress, 8*, 141-152.

Griffiths, A. (1997). Ageing, health and productivity: A challenge for the new millennium. *Work and Stress, 11*, 197-214.

Hammond, E. (1964). Some preliminary findings on physical complaints from a prospective study of 1,064,004 men and women. *American Journal of Public Health, 54*, 11-23.

Hebb, D.O. (1955). Drives and the C.N.S. (conceptual nervous system). *Psychological Review, 62*, 243-254.

Hergenhahn, B.R. (1992). *An introduction to the history of psychology* (2nd ed.). Belmont, CA: Wadsworth.

Hilgard, E.R. (1980). The trilogy of the mind: Cognition, affection, and conation. *Journal of the History of the Behavioral Sciences, 16*, 107-117.

Hockey, G.R., Gaillard, A.W.K., & Coles, M.G.H. (Eds.). (1986). *Energetics and human information processing.* Boston: Martinus Nijhoff.

Hockey, G.R.J., & Hamilton, P. (1983). The cognitive patterning of stress states. In G.R.J. Hockey (Ed.), *Stress and fatigue in human performance* (pp. 331-360). Chichester, UK: Wiley.

Hockey, G.R.J., Payne, R.L., & Terry, R.J. (1996). Intra-individual patterns of hormonal and affective adaptation to work demands: An n = 2 study of junior doctors. *Biological Psychology, 42*(3), 393-411.

Holding, D. (1983). Fatigue. In R. Hockey (Ed.), *Stress and fatigue in human performance* (pp. 145-167). New York: Wiley.

References

Kahneman, D. (1973). *Attention and effort*. Englewood Cliffs, NJ: Prentice Hall.

Koelega, H.S. (1996). Sustained attention. In O. Neumann & A.F. Sanders (Eds.), *Handbook of perception and action* (Vol. 3, pp. 277-331). London: Academic Press.

Kramer, A.F., & Willis, S.L. (2002). Enhancing the cognitive vitality of older adults. *Current Directions in Psychological Science, 11*(5), 173-176.

Kramer, A.F., Hahn, S., Cohen, N.J., Banich, M., McAuley, E., Harrison, C.R., Chason, J., Vakil, E., Bardell, L., Boileau, R.A., & Colcombe, A. (1999). Ageing, fitness and neurocognitive function. *Nature, 400*, 418-419.

Kramer, A.F., et al. (2002). Exercise, aging, and cognition: Healthy body, healthy mind? In W.A. Rogers & A.D. Fisk (Eds.), *Human factors interventions for health care of older adults* (pp. 91-120). Mahwah, NJ: Erlbaum.

Kramer, A.F., & Weber, T. (2000). Applications of psychophysiology to human factors. In G.G. Berntson (Ed.), *Handbook of psychophysiology* (2nd ed., pp. 794-814). Cambridge, MA: Cambridge University Press.

Lazarus, R.S. (1993a). From psychological stress to the emotions: A history of changing outlooks. *Annual Review of Psychology, 44*, 1-24.

Lazarus, R.S. (1993b). Why we should think of stress as a subset of emotion. In L. Goldberg & S. Breznitz (Eds.), *Handbook of stress: Theoretical and clinical aspects* (2nd ed., pp. 21-39). New York: Free Press.

Miller, G.A., Galanter, E., & Pribram, K.H. (1960). *Plans and the structure of behavior*. New York: Holt.

Pandorf, K.B. (1982). Differential ratings of perceived exertion during physical exercise. *Medicine and Science in Sports and Exercise, 14*, 397-405.

Posner, M.I., & Raichle, M.E. (1997). *Images of mind*. New York: Scientific American Library.

Pribram, K.H., & McGuinness, D. (1975). Arousal, activation and effort in the control of attention. *Psychological Review, 82*, 116-149.

Robbins, T.W., & Everitt, B.J. (1995). Arousal systems and attention. In M.S. Gazzaniga (Ed.), *The cognitive neurosciences* (pp. 703-720). Cambridge, MA: MIT Press.

Roth, G.S. (1990). Mechanisms of altered hormone-neurotransmitter action during aging: From receptors to calcium mobilization. In V.J. Cristofalo (Ed.), *Annual Review of gerontology and geriatrics* (Vol. 10, pp. 132-146). New York: Springer.

Rummelhart, D.E., & McClelland, J.L. (Eds.). (1986). *Parallel distributed processing: Explorations in the microstructure of cognition* (Vol. 1). Cambridge, MA: MIT Press.

Sanders, A.F. (1983). Toward a model of stress and human performance. *Acta Psychologica, 53*, 61-97.

Sanders, A.F. (1998). *Elements of human performance*. Mahwah, NJ: Erlbaum.

Selye, H. (1974). *Stress without distress*. Philadelphia: Lippincott.

Shephard, R.J. (1999). Age and physical work capacity. *Experimental Aging Research, 25*, 331-343.

References

Snow, R.E., & Jackson, D.N. (1994). Individual differences in conation: Selected constructs and measures. In H.F. O'Neal, Jr., & M. Drillings (Eds.), *Motivation: Theory and research* (pp. 71-99). Hillsdale, NJ: Erlbaum.

Sothmann, M.S., Buckworth, J., Claytor, R.P., Cox, R.H., White-Welkley, J.E., & Dishman, R.K. (1996). Exercise training and the cross-stressor adaptation hypothesis. *Exercise and Sport Sciences Reviews, 24,* 267-287.

Spirduso, W.W. (1995). *Physical dimensions of aging.* Champaign, IL: Human Kinetics.

Staudinger, U.M., Marsiske, M., & Baltes, P.B. (1993). Resilience and levels of reserve capacity in later adulthood: Perspective from life-span theory. *Development and Psychopathology, 5,* 541-566.

Sternberg, S. (1969). Memory-scanning: Mental processes revealed by reaction time experiments. *American Scientist, 57,* 421-457.

Stones, M.J., & Kozma, A. (1988). Physical activity, age, and cognitive/motor performance. In M.L. Howe and C.J. Brainerd (Eds.), *Cognitive development in adulthood: Progress in cognitive development research* (pp. 273-321). New York: Springer-Verlag.

Tibblin, G., Bengtsson, C., Furunes, B., & Lapidus, L. (1990). Symptoms by age and sex. *Scandinavian Journal of Primary Care, 8*(1), 9-17.

Tomporowski, P.D. (1997). The effects of physical and mental training on the mental abilities of older adults. *Journal of Aging and Physical Activity, 5,* 9-27.

Tomporowski, P.D. (2003a). Effects of acute bouts of exercise on cognition. *Acta Psychologica, 112,* 297-324.

Tomporowski, P.D. (2003b). Performance and perceptions of workload among young and older adults: Effects of practice during cognitively demanding tasks. *Educational Gerontology, 29,* 447-466.

Tomporowski, P.D. (2006). Physical activity, cognition, and aging: A review of reviews. In L. Poon, W. Chodzko-Zajko, & P.D. Tomporowski (Eds.), *Active living, cognitive functioning, and aging,* Vol. 1 (pp. 15-32). Champaign, IL: Human Kinetics.

Underwood, B.J. (1975). Individual differences as a crucible in theory construction. *American Psychologist, 30,* 128-134.

Ursin, H. (1986). Energetics and the self regulation of activation. In G.R.J. Hockey, A.W.K. Gaillard, & M.G.H. Coles (Eds.), *Energetics and human information processing* (pp. 53-70). Boston: Martinus Nijhoff.

Van Doornen, L.J.P., & De Geus, E.J.C. (1993). Stress, physical activity and coronary disease. *Work and Stress, 7,* 121-139.

Van Gerven, P.W.M., Paas, F.G.W.C., Van Merrienboer, J.J.G., & Schmidt, H.G. (2000). Cognitive load theory and the acquisition of complex cognitive skills in the elderly: Towards an integrative framework. *Educational Gerontology, 26,* 503-521.

Welford, A.T. (1965). Performance, biological mechanisms, and age: A theoretical sketch. In A.T. Welford & J.E. Birren (Eds.), *Behavior, aging and the nervous system.* Springfield, IL: Charles C Thomas.

Wessely, A., Hotopt, M., & Sharpe, M. (1998). *Chronic fatigue and its syndromes.* Oxford, UK: Oxford University Press.

West, R.L. (1996). An application of prefrontal cortex function theory to cognitive aging. *Psychological Bulletin, 120,* 272-292.

Woodruff-Pak, D.S., Coffin, J.M., & Sasse, D.K. (1991). Learning, memory, and aging: Neural changes and drug actions. In K.W. Schaie (Ed.), *Annual review of gerontology and geriatrics* (Vol. 11, pp. 23-44). New York: Springer.

Woodruff-Pak, D.S., & Papka, M. (1999). Theories of neuropsychology and aging. In V.L. Bengtson & K.W. Schaie (Eds.), *Handbook of theories of aging* (pp. 113-132). New York: Springer.

Chapter 8

Bartus, R.T. (1990). Drugs to treat age-related neurodegenerative problems. The final frontier of medical science? *Journal of the American Geriatrics Society, 38,* 680-695.

Bartus, R.T., Dean, R.L., Beer, B., & Lippa A.S. (1982). The cholinergic hypothesis of geriatric memory dysfunction. *Science, 217,* 408-417.

Bickford, P. (1993). Motor learning deficits in aged rats are correlated with loss of cerebellar noradrenergic function. *Brain Research, 620,* 133-138.

Bickford, P.C., Chadman, K., Williams, B., Shukitt-Hale, B., Holmes, D., Taglialatela, G., et al. (1999). Effect of normobaric hyperoxia on two indexes of synaptic function in Fischer 344 rats. *Free Radical Biology and Medicine, 26,* 817-824.

Bickford, P., Heron, C., Young, D.A., Gerhardt, G.A., & De La Garza, R. (1992). Impaired acquisition of novel locomotor tasks in aged and norepinephrine-depleted F344 rats. *Neurobiology and Aging, 13,* 475-481.

Brandeis, R., Brandys, Y., & Yehuda, S. (1989). The use of the Morris water maze in the study of memory and learning. *International Journal of Neuroscience, 48,* 29-69.

Cantuti-Castelvetri, I., Shukitt-Hale, B., & Joseph, J.A. (2000). Neurobehavioral aspects of antioxidants in aging. *International Journal of Developmental Neuroscience, 18,* 367-381.

Cantuti-Castelvetri, I., Shukitt-Hale, B., & Joseph, J.A. (2003). Dopamine neurotoxicity: Age-dependent behavioral and histological effects. *Neurobiology and Aging, 24,* 697-706.

Cao, G., Sofic, E., & Prior, R.L. (1996). Antioxidant capacity of tea and common vegetables. *Journal of Agriculture and Food Chemistry, 44,* 3426-3431.

Carney, J.M., Smith, C.D., Carney, A.M., & Butterfield, D.A. (1994), Aging- and oxygen-induced modifications in brain biochemistry and behavior. *Annals of the New York Academy of Sciences, 738,* 44-53.

Chang, H.N., Wang, S.R., Chiang, S.C., Teng, W.J., Chen, M.L., Tsai, J.J., et al. (1996). The relationship of aging to endotoxin shock and to production of TNFa. *Journal of Gerontology, 51,* M220-M222.

References

Chang, R.C., Chen, W., Hudson, P., Wilson, B., Han, D.S., & Hong, J.S. (2001). Neurons reduce glial responses to lipopolysaccharide (LPS) and prevent injury of microglial cells from over-activation by LPS. *Journal of Neurochemistry, 76,* 1042-1049.

Cheng, Y., Wixom, P., James-Kracke, M.R., & Sun, A.Y. (1994). Effects of extracellular ATP on Fe^{2+}-induced cytotoxicity in PC-12 cells. *Journal of Neurochemistry, 66,* 895-902.

Denisova, N.A., Erat, S.A., Kelly, J.F., & Roth, G.S. (1998). Differential effect of aging on cholesterol modulation of carbachol stimulated low-Km GTPase in striatal synaptosomes. *Experimental Gerontology, 33,* 249-265.

Devan, B.D., Goad, E.H., & Petri, H.L. (1996). Dissociation of hippocampal and striatal contributions to spatial navigation in the water maze. *Neurobiology of Learning and Memory, 66,* 305-323.

Egashira, T., Takayama, F., & Yamanaka, Y. (1996). Effects of bifemelane on muscarinic receptors and choline acetyltransferase in the brains of aged rats following chronic cerebral hypoperfusion induced by permanent occlusion of bilateral carotid arteries. *Japanese Journal of Pharmacology, 72,* 57-65.

Floyd, R.A. (1999). Antioxidants, oxidative stress, and degenerative neurological disorders. *Proceedings of the Society for Experimental and Biological Medicine, 222,* 236-245.

Frick, K.M., Baxter, M.G., Markowska, A.L., Olton, D.S., & Price, D.L. (1995). Age-related spatial reference and working memory deficits assessed in the water maze. *Neurobiology of Aging, 16,* 149-160.

Gilissen, E.P., Jacobs, R.E., & Allman, J.M. (1999). Magnetic resonance microscopy of iron in the basal forebrain cholinergic structures of the aged mouse lemur. *Journal of Neurological Sciences, 168,* 21-27.

Gould, T.J., & Bickford, P. (1997). Age-related deficits in the cerebellar beta-adrenergic signal transduction cascade in Fischer 344 rats. *Journal of Pharmacology and Experimental Therapeutics, 281,* 965-971.

Hauss-Wegrzyniak, B., Dobrzanski, P., Stoehr, J.D., & Wenk G.L. (1998). Chronic neuroinflammation in rats reproduces components of the neurobiology of Alzheimer's disease. *Brain Research, 780,* 294-303.

Hauss-Wegrzyniak, B., Vannucchi, M.G., & Wenk G.L. (2000). Behavioral and ultrastructural changes induced by chronic neuroinflammation in young rats. *Brain Research, 859,* 157-166.

Hauss-Wegrzyniak, B., Vraniak, P., & Wenk, G.L. (1999). The effects of a novel NSAID on chronic neuroinflammation are age dependent. *Neurobiology of Aging, 20,* 305-313.

Hauss-Wegrzyniak, B., Willard, L.B., Del Soldato, P., Pepeu, G., & Wenk, G.L. (1999). Peripheral administration of novel anti-inflammatories can attenuate the effects of chronic inflammation within the CNS. *Brain Research, 815,* 36-43.

Ingram, D.K., Jucker, M., & Spangler, E. (1994). Behavioral manifestations of aging. In U. Mohr, D.L. Cungworth, & C.C. Capen (Eds.), *Pathobiology of the aging rat* (Vol. 2, pp. 149-170). Washington, DC: ILSI Press.

References

Joseph, J.A. (1992). The putative role of free radicals in the loss of neuronal functioning in senescence. *Integrative Physiological and Behavioral Science, 27*, 216-227.

Joseph, J.A., Bartus, R.T., Clody, D.E., Morgan, D., Finch, C., Beer, B., et al. (1983). Psychomotor performance in the senescent rodent: Reduction of deficits via striatal dopamine receptor up-regulation. *Neurobiology of Aging, 4*, 313-319.

Joseph, J.A., Berger, R.E., Engel, B.T., & Roth, G.S. (1978). Age-related changes in the nigrostriatum: A behavioral and biochemical analysis. *Journal of Gerontology, 33*, 643-649.

Joseph, J.A., Denisova, N., Fisher, D., Bickford, P., Prior, R., & Cao, G. (1998). Age-related neuro-degeneration and oxidative stress: Putative nutritional intervention. *Neurologic Clinics, 16*, 747-755.

Joseph, J.A., Denisova, N.A., Fisher, D., Shukitt-Hale, B., Bickford, P., Prior, R., et al. (1998). Membrane and receptor modifications of oxidative stress vulnerability in aging: Nutritional considerations. *Annals of the New York Academy of Sciences, 854*, 268-276.

Joseph, J.A., Erat, S., & Rabin, B.M. (1998). CNS effects of heavy particle irradiation in space: Behavioral implications. *Advances in Space Research, 22*, 209-216.

Joseph, J.A., Hunt, W.A., Rabin, B.M., & Dalton, T.K. (1992). Possible "accelerated striatal aging" induced by ^{56}Fe heavy-particle irradiation: Implications for manned space flights. *Radiation Research, 130*, 88-93.

Joseph, J.A., Kowatch, M.A., Maki, T., & Roth, G.S. (1990). Selective cross activation/inhibition of second messenger systems and the reduction of age-related deficits in the muscarinic control of dopamine release from perfused rat striata. *Brain Research, 537*, 40-48.

Joseph, J.A., Shukitt-Hale, B., Denisova, N.A., Bielinski, D., Martin, A., McEwen, J.J., et al. (1999). Reversals of age-related declines in neuronal signal transduction, cognitive and motor behavioral deficits with blueberry, spinach or strawberry dietary supplementation. *Journal of Neuroscience, 19*, 8114-8121.

Joseph, J.A., Shukitt-Hale, B., Denisova, N.A., Martin, A., Perry, G., & Smith, M.A. (2001). Copernicus revisited: Amyloid beta in Alzheimer's disease. *Neurobiology of Aging, 22*, 131-146.

Joseph, J.A., Shukitt-Hale, B., Denisova, N.A., Prior, R.L., Cao, G., Martin, A., et al. (1998). Long-term dietary strawberry, spinach or vitamin E supplementation retards the onset of age-related neuronal signal-transduction and cognitive behavioral deficits. *Journal of Neuroscience, 18*, 8047-8055.

Joseph, J.A., Shukitt-Hale, B., McEwen, J., & Rabin, B.M. (2000). CNS-induced deficits of heavy particle irradiation in space: The aging connection. *Advances in Space Research, 25*, 2057-2064.

Kluger, A., Gianutsos, J.G., Golomb, J., Ferris, S.H., George, A.E., Frannssen, E., et al. (1997). Patterns of motor impairment in normal aging, mild cognitive decline, and early Alzheimer's disease. *Journal of Gerontology, 52*, 28-39.

Kornhuber, J., Schoppmeyer, K., Bendig, C., & Riederer, P. (1996). Characterization of [3H] pentazocine binding sites in post-mortem human frontal cortex. *Journal of Neural Transmission, 103*, 45-53.

References

Kushner, I. (2001). C-reactive protein elevation can be caused by conditions other than inflammation and may reflect biologic aging. *Cleveland Clinic Journal of Medicine, 68*, 535-537.

Landfield, P.W., & Eldridge, J.C. (1994). The glucocorticoid hypothesis of age-related hippocampal neurodegeneration: Role of dysregulated intraneuronal Ca^{2+}. *Annals of the New York Academy of Sciences, 746*, 308-321.

Levine, M.S., & Cepeda, C. (1998). Dopamine modulation of responses mediated by excitatory amino acids in the neostriatum. *Advances in Pharmacology, 42*, 724-729.

Lo, Y.Y., Conquer, J.A., Grinstein, S., & Cruz, T.F. (1998). Interleukin-1 beta induction of c-fos and collagenase expression in articular chondrocytes: Involvement of reactive oxygen species. *Journal of Cellular Biochemistry, 69*, 19-29.

Luine, V.N., Richards, S.T., Wu, V.Y., & Beck, K.D. (1998). Estradiol enhances learning and memory in a spatial memory task and effects levels of monoaminergic neurotransmitters. *Hormones and Behavior, 34*, 149-162.

Manev, H., & Uz, T. (1999). Primary cultures of rat cerebellar granule cells as a model to study neuronal 5-lipoxygenase and FLAP gene expression. *Annals of the New York Academy of Sciences, 890*, 183-190.

McDonald, R.J., & White, N.M. (1994). Parallel information processing in the water maze: Evidence for independent memory systems involving dorsal striatum and hippocampus. *Behavioral and Neural Biology, 61*, 260-270.

McGeer, P.L., & McGeer, E.G. (1995). The inflammatory response system of the brain: Implications for therapy of Alzheimer and other neurodegenerative diseases. *Brain Research Reviews, 21*, 195-218.

Muir, J.L. (1997). Acetylcholine, aging, and Alzheimer's disease. *Pharmacology, Biochemistry, and Behavior, 56*, 687-696.

Olanow, C.W. (1992). An introduction to the free radical hypothesis in Parkinson's disease. *Annals of Neurology, 32*, S2-S9.

Oliveira, M.G.M., Bueno, O.F.A., Pomarico, A.C., & Gugliano, E.B. (1997). Strategies used by hippocampal- and caudate-putamen-lesioned rats in a learning task. *Neurobiology of Learning and Memory, 68*, 32-41.

Piette, J., Piret, B., Bonizzi, G., Schoonbroodt, S., Merville, M.P., Legrand-Poels, S., et al. (1997). Multiple redox regulation in NF-kappaB transcription factor activation. *Biological Chemistry, 378*, 1237-1245.

Prior, R.L., Cao, G., Martin, A., Sofic, E., McEwen, J., O'Brien, C., et al. (1998). Antioxidant capacity as influenced by total phenolic and anthocyanin content, maturity and variety of Vaccinium species. *Journal of Agricultural and Food Chemistry, 46*, 2586-2593.

Rabin, B.M., Joseph, J.A., & Erat, S. (1998). Effects of exposure to different types of radiation on behaviors mediated by peripheral or central systems. *Advances in Space Research, 22*, 217-225.

Rabin, B.M., Joseph, J.A., Shukitt-Hale, B., & McEwen, J. (2000). Effects of exposure to heavy particles on a behavior mediated by the dopaminergic system. *Advances in Space Research, 25*, 2065-2074.

References

Rosenman, S.J., Shrikant, P., Dubb, L., Benveniste, E.N., & Ransohoff, R.M. (1995). Cytokine induced expression of vascular cell adhesion molecule-1 (VCAM-1) by astrocytes and astrocytoma cell lines. *Journal of Immunology, 154,* 1888-1899.

Rozovsky, I., Finch, C.E., & Morgan, T.E. (1998). Age-related activation of microglia and astrocytes: In vitro studies show. *Neurobiology and Aging, 19,* 97-103.

Sadoul, R. (1998). Bcl-2 family members in the development and degenerative pathologies of the nervous system. *Cell Death and Differentiation, 5,* 805-815.

Savory, J., Rao, J.K., Huang, Y., Letada, P.R., & Herman, M.M. (1999). Age-related hippocampal changes in Bcl-2:Bax ratio, oxidative stress, redox-active iron and apoptosis associated with aluminum-induced neurodegeneration: Increased susceptibility with aging. *Neurotoxicology, 20,* 805-817.

Schipper, H.M. (1996). Astrocytes, brain aging, and neurodegeneration. *Neurobiology and Aging, 17,* 467-480.

Shukitt-Hale, B. (1999). The effects of aging and oxidative stress on psychomotor and cognitive behavior. *Age, 22,* 9-17.

Shukitt-Hale, B., Casadesus, G., McEwen, J.J., Rabin, B.M., & Joseph, J.A. (2000). Spatial learning and memory deficits induced by exposure to iron-56-particle radiation. *Radiation Research, 154,* 28-33.

Shukitt-Hale, B., Denisova, N.A., Strain, J.G., & Joseph, J.A. (1997). Psychomotor effects of dopamine infusion under decreased glutathione conditions. *Free Radical Biology and Medicine, 23,* 412-418.

Shukitt-Hale, B., Erat, S.A., & Joseph, J.A. (1998). Spatial learning and memory deficits induced by dopamine administration with decreased glutathione. *Free Radical Biology and Medicine, 24,* 1149-1158.

Shukitt-Hale, B., McEwen, J.J., Szprengiel, A., and Joseph, J.A. (2004). *Effect of age on the radial arm water maze—A test of spatial learning and memory.*

Shukitt-Hale, B., Mouzakis, G., & Joseph, J.A. (1998). Psychomotor and spatial memory performance in aging male Fischer 344 rats. *Experimental Gerontology, 33,* 615-624.

Spaulding, C.C., Walford, R.L., & Effros, R.B. (1997). Calorie restriction inhibits the age-related dysregulation of the cytokines TNF-alpha and IL-6 in C3B10RF1 mice. *Mechanisms of Ageing and Development, 93,* 87-94.

Steffen, B., Breier, G., Butcher, E., Schulz, M., & Engelhardt, B. (1996). VCAM-1, and MAdCAM-1 are expressed on choroid plexus epithelium but not endothelium and mediate binding of lymphocytes in vitro. *American Journal of Pathology, 148,* 1819-1838.

Stella, N., Estelles, A., Siciliano, J., Tence, M., Desagher, S., Piomelli, D., et al. (1997). Interleukin-1 enhances the ATP-evoked release of arachidonic acid from mouse astrocytes. *Journal of Neuroscience, 17,* 2939-2946.

Volpato, S., Guralnik, J.M., Ferrucci, L., Balfour, J., Chaves, P., Fried, L.P., et al. (2001). Cardiovascular disease, interleukin-6, and risk of mortality in older women: The women's health and aging study. *Circulation, 103,* 947-953.

Wang, H., Cao, G., & Prior, R. (1996). Total antioxidant capacity of fruits. *Journal of Agricultural and Food Chemistry, 44,* 701-705.

West, R.L. (1996). An application of pre-frontal cortex function theory to cognitive aging. *Psychological Bulletin, 120,* 272-292.

Woodroofe, M. (1995). Cytokine production in the central nervous system. *Neurology, 45,* S6-S10.

Yamada, K., Komori, Y., Tanaka, T., Senzaki, K., Nikai, T., Sugihara, H., et al. (1999). Brain dysfunction associated with an induction of nitric oxide synthase following an intracerebral injection of lipopolysaccharide in rats. *Neuroscience, 88,* 281-294.

Youdim, K.A., & Joseph, J.A. (2001). A possible emerging role of phytochemicals in improving age-related neurological dysfunctions: A multiplicity of effects. *Free Radical Biology and Medicine, 30,* 583-594.

Youdim, K.A., Martin, A., & Joseph, J.A. (2000). Essential fatty acids and the brain: Possible health implications. *International Journal of Developmental Neuroscience, 18,* 383-399.

Youdim, K.A., Shukitt-Hale, B., Martin, A., Wang, H., Denisova, N., & Joseph, J.A. (2000). Short-term dietary supplementation of blueberry polyphenolics: Beneficial effects on aging brain performance and peripheral tissue function. *Nutritional Neuroscience, 3,* 383-397.

Yu, B.P. (1994). Cellular defenses against damage from reactive oxygen species. *Physiological Reviews, 76,* 139-162.

Zyzak, D.R., Otto, T., Eichenbaum, H., & Gallagher, M. (1995). Cognitive decline associated with normal aging in rats: A neuropsychological approach. *Learning and Memory, 2,* 1-16.

Chapter 9

Adam, K., & Oswald, I. (1983). Protein synthesis, bodily renewal, and the sleep-wake cycle. *Clinical Science, 65,* 561-567.

Bassetti, C., & Aldrich, M.S. (1999). Sleep apnea in acute cerebrovascular disease: Final report on 128 patients. *Sleep, 22,* 217-223.

Bosselli, M., Parrino, L., Smerieri, A., & Terzano, M.G. (1998). Effects of age on EEG arousals in normal sleep. *Sleep, 21,* 351-357.

Brosse, A., Sheets, E.S., Lett, H.S., & Blumenthal, J.A. (2002). Exercise and the treatment of clinical depression in adults: Recent findings and future directions. *Sports Medicine, 32*(12), 741-760.

Brugere, D., Barrit, J., Butat, C., Cosset, M., & Volkoff, S. (1997). Shiftwork, age, and health: An epidemiologic investigation. *International Journal of Occupational and Environmental Health, 3*(Suppl. 2), 15-19.

Campbell, S.S., Kripke, D.F., Gillin, J.C., & Hrubovcak, J.C. (1988). Exposure to light in healthy elderly subjects and Alzheimer's patients. *Physiology and Behavior, 42*(2), 141-144.

Colcombe, S., & Kramer, A.F. (2003). Fitness effects on the cognitive function of older adults: A meta-analytic study. *Psychological Science, 14*(2), 125-130.

References

Chesson, A.L., Littner, M., Davila, D., Anderson, W.M., Grigg-Damberger, M., Hartse, K., et al. (1999). Practice parameters for the use of light therapy in the treatment of sleep disorders. *Sleep, 22*(5), 641-660.

Cooley, S., Deitch, I., Harper, M., Hinrichsen, G., Lopez, M., & Molinari, V. (1998). What practitioners should know about working with older adults. *Professional Psychology, Research, and Practice, 29*(5), 413-427.

Dement, W.C., & Mitler, M.M. (1993). It's time to wake up to the importance of sleep disorders. *Journal of the American Medical Association, 269*(12), 1548-1550.

Dement, W., Seidel, W.G., Cohen, S.A., Bliwise, N.G., & Carskadon, M.A. (1986). Sleep and wakefulness in aircrew before and after transoceanic flights. *Aviation, Space, and Environmental Medicine, 57*(Suppl. 12), B14-B28.

Dinges, D.F., Pack, F., Williams, K., Gillen, K.A., Powell, J.W., Ott, G.E., et al. (1997). Cumulative sleepiness, mood disturbance, and psychomotor vigilance performance decrements during a week of sleep restricted to 4-5 hours per night. *Sleep, 20*(4), 267-277.

Djik, D.J., Duffy, J.F., & Czeisler, C.A. (2000). Contribution of circadian physiology and sleep homeostasis to age-related changes in human sleep. *Chronobiology International, 17*, 285-311.

Dorsey, C.M., Lukas, S.E., Teicher, M.H., Harper, D., Winkelman, J.W., Cunningham, S.L., et al. (1996). Effects of passive body heating on the sleep of older female insomniacs. *Journal of Geriatric Psychiatry and Neurology, 9*(2), 83-90.

Dorsey, C.M., Teicher, M.H., Cohen-Zion, M., Stefanovic, L., Satlin, A., Tartarini, W., et al. (1999). Core body temperature and sleep of older female insomniacs before and after passive body heating. *Sleep, 22*(7), 891-898.

Douglas, N.J. (2000). Chronic obstructive pulmonary disease. In M.H. Kryger, T. Roth, & W.C. Dement (Eds.), *Principles and practice of sleep medicine* (3rd ed., pp. 965-975). Philadelphia: Saunders.

Driver, H., & Taylor, S. (2000). Exercise and sleep. *Sleep Medicine Reviews, 4*, 387-402.

Edinger, J.D., Stout, A.L., & Hoelscher, T.J. (1988). Cluster analysis of insomniacs' MMPI profiles: Relation of subtypes to sleep history and treatment outcome. *Psychosomatic Medicine, 50*, 77-87.

Foley, D.J., Monjan, A.A., Brown, S.L., & Simonsick, E.M. (1995). Sleep complaints among elderly persons: An epidemiologic study of three communities. *Sleep, 18*, 425-432.

The Gallup Organization. (1991). *Sleep in America*. Los Angeles: National Sleep Foundation.

Glotzbach, S.F., & Heller, H.D. (1994). Temperature regulation. In M.H. Kryger, T. Roth, & W.C. Dement (Eds.), Principles and practice of sleep medicine (pp. 260-275). Philadelphia: Saunders.

Guilleminault, C., Clerk, A., Black, J., Labanowski, M., Pelayo, R., & Claman, D. (1995). Nondrug treatment trials in psychophysiologic insomnia. *Archives of Internal Medicine, 155*(8), 838-844.

References

Guilleminault, C., Quera-Salva, M.A., & Goldberg, M.P. (1993). Pseudo-hypersomnia and pre-sleep behavior with bilateral paramedian thalamic lesions. *Brain, 116,* 1549-1563.

Hohagen, F., Kappler, C., Schramm, E., Rink, K., Weyerer, S., Riemann, D., et al. (1994). Prevalence of insomnia in elderly general practice attenders and the current treatment modalities. *Acta Psychiatrica Scandinavica, 90,* 102-108.

Horne, J.A., & Staff, L.H.E. (1983). Exercise and sleep: Body heating effects. *Sleep, 6,* 36-46.

Javaheri, S. (1999). A mechanism of central sleep apnea in patients with heart failure. *New England Journal of Medicine, 341,* 949-954.

Johnson, L.C., & Spinweber, C.L. (1983). Good and poor sleepers differ in Navy performance. *Military Medicine, 148,* 727-731.

Katz, D.A., & McHorney, C.A. (1988). Clinical correlates of insomnia in patients with chronic illness. *Archives of Internal Medicine, 158,* 1101-1107.

King, A.C., Baumann, K., O'Sullivan, P., Wilcox, S., & Castro, C. (2002). Effects of moderate-intensity exercise on physiological, behavioral, and emotional responses to family caregiving: A randomized controlled trial. *Journals of Gerontology. Series A, Biological Sciences and Medical Sciences, 57*(1), 1079-5006.

King, A.C., Oman, R.F., Brassington, G.S., Bliwise, D.L., & Haskell, W.L. (1997). Moderate-intensity exercise and self-rated quality of sleep in older adults: A randomized controlled trial. *Journal of the American Medical Association, 277,* 32-37.

Kubitz, K., Landers, D., Petruzzello, S., & Han, M. (1996). The effects of acute and chronic exercise on sleep: A meta-analytic review. *Sports Medicine, 21,* 4.

Longobardo, G., Gothe, B., Goldman, M., & Cherniak, N. (1982). Sleep apnea considered as a control system instability. *Respiratory Physiology, 50,* 311-333.

Lichstein, K.L., Means, M.K., Noe, S.L., & Aguillard, R.N. (1997). Fatigue and sleep disorders. *Behaviour Research and Therapy, 35,* 733-740.

Mahowald, M.L., & Mahowald, M.K. (2000). Nighttime sleep and daytime functioning sleepiness and fatigue in well-defined chronic rheumatic diseases. *Sleep Medicine, 1,* 179-193.

McGinty, D., & Szymusiak, R. (1990). Keeping cool: A hypothesis about the mechanisms and functions of slow wave sleep. *Trends in Neuroscience, 13,* 480-487.

Mellinger, G.D., Balter, M.B., & Uhlenhuth, E.H. (1985). Insomnia and its treatment. *Archives of General Psychiatry, 42,* 225-232B.

Moldofsky, H. (1989). Sleep influences on regional and diffuse pain syndromes associated with osteoarthritis. *Seminars in Arthritis and Rheumatism, 18*(4, Suppl. 2): 18-21.

Monk, T.H., Leng, V.C., Folkard, S., & Weitzman, E.D. (1983). Circadian rhythms in subjective alertness and core body temperature. *Chronobiology, 10,* 49-55.

Monk, T.H., & Moline, M.L. (1989). The timing of bedtime and waketime decisions in free-running subjects. *Psychophysiology, 26,* 304-310.

References

Ohayon, M.M. (2002). Epidemiology of insomnia: What we know and what we still need to learn. *Sleep Medicine Reviews, 6*(2), 97-111.

Petruzzello, S.J., Landers, D.M., Hatfield, B.D., Kubitz, K.A., & Salazar, W. (1991). A meta-analysis on the anxiety reducing effects of acute and chronic exercise: Outcomes and mechanisms. *Sports Medicine, 11*(3), 143-182.

Phillips, B., & Ancoli-Israel, S. (2001). Sleep disorders in the elderly. *Sleep Medicine, 2*, 99-114.

Pollak, C.P., Perlick, D., Linsner, J.P., Wenston, J., & Hsieh, F. (1990). Sleep problems in the community elderly as predictors of death and nursing home placement. *Journal of Community Health, 15*(2), 123-135.

Porkka-Heiskanen, T., Strecker, R.E., Thakkar, M., Bjorkum, A.A., Greene, R.W., & McCarley, R.W. (1997). Adenosine: A mediator of the sleep-inducing effects of prolonged wakefulness. *Science, 276*, 1265-1268.

Prinz, P.N., Peskind, E.R., Vitaliano, P.P., Raskind, M.A., Eisdorfer, C., Zemcuznikov, N., et al. (1982). Changes in the sleep and waking EEGs of nondemented and demented elderly subjects. *Journal of the American Geriatrics Society, 30*, 86-93.

Riedel, B.W., & Lichstein, K.L. (1998). Objective sleep measures and subjective sleep satisfaction: How do older adults with insomnia define a good night's sleep? *Psychology and Aging, 13*, 159-163.

Sandek, K., Andersson, T., Bratel, T., Hellstrom, G., & Lagerstrand, L. (1999). Sleep quality, carbon dioxide responsiveness and hypoxaemic patterns in nocturnal hypoxaemia due to chronic obstructive pulmonary disease (COPD) without daytime hypoxaemia. *Respiratory Medicine, 93*, 79-87.

Schenck, C.H., Bundlie, S.R., Ettinger, M.G., & Mahowald, M. (1986). Chronic behavioral disorders of human REM sleep: A new category of parasomnia. *Sleep, 9*, 293-308.

Schwartz, S., Anderson, W.M., Cole, S.R., Cornoni-Huntley, J., Hays, J.C., & Blazer, D. (1999). Insomnia and heart disease: A review of epidemiologic studies. *Journal of Psychosomatic Research, 47*, 313-333.

Sherrill, D.L., Kotchou, K., & Quan, S.F. (1998). Association of physical activity and human sleep disorders. *Archives of Internal Medicine, 158*, 1894-1898.

Simon, G.E., & VonKorff, M. (1997). Prevalence, burden, and treatment of insomnia in primary care. *American Journal of Psychiatry, 154*, 1417-1423.

Singh, N., Clements, K., & Fiatarone, M. (1997). A randomized controlled trial of the effect of exercise on sleep. *Sleep, 20*(2), 95-101.

Stepanski, E., Lamphere, J., Badia, P., Zorick, F., & Roth, T. (1984). Sleep fragmentation and daytime sleepiness. *Sleep, 7*, 18-26.

Stepanski, E., Rybarczyk, B., Lopez, M., & Stevens, S. (2003). Assessment and treatment of sleep disorders in older adults: A review for rehabilitation psychologists. *Rehabilitation Psychology, 48*(1), 23-36.

Van Reeth, O., Sturis, J., Byrne, M.M., Blackman, J.D., L'Hermite-Baleriaux, M., Leproult, R., et al. (1994). Nocturnal exercise phase delays circadian rhythms of melatonin and thyrotropic secretion in normal men. *American Journal of Physiology, 266*, E964-E974.

Van Someren, E.J. (2000). More than a marker: Interaction between the circadian regulation temperature and sleep, age-related changes, and treatment possibilities. *Chronobiology International, 17*, 113-354.

Vitiello, M.V., Moe, K.E., & Prinz, P.N. (2002). Sleep complaints cosegregate with illness in older adults: Clinical research informed by and informing epidemiological studies of sleep. *Journal of Psychosomatic Research, 53*(1), 555-559.

Vitiello, M.V., Prinz, P.N., & Schwartz, R.S. (1994). Slow wave sleep but not overall sleep quality of healthy older men and women is improved by increased aerobic fitness. *Sleep Research, 23*, 149.

Vuori, I., Urponen, H., Hasan, J., & Partinen, M. (1988). Epidemiology of exercise effects on sleep. *Acta Physiologica Scandinavica, 133*(Suppl. 574), 3-7.

Webb, W.B. (1981). Sleep stage responses of older and younger subjects after sleep deprivation. *Electroencephalography and Clinical Neurophysiology, 52*, 368-371.

Weitzman, E.D., Moline, M.L., Czeisler, C.A., & Zimmerman, J.C. (1982). Chronobiology of aging: Temperature, sleep-wake rhythms and entrainment. *Neurobiology and Aging, 3*, 299-309.

Youngstedt, S.D. (2000). The exercise-sleep mystery. *International Journal of Sport Psychology, 10*, 241-255.

Youngstedt, S.D. (2003). Ceiling and floor effects in sleep research. *Sleep Medicine Reviews, 7*(4), 351-365.

Youngstedt, S.D., Kripke, D., & Elliott, J. (1999). Is sleep disturbed by vigorous late-night exercise? *Medicine and Science in Sports and Exercise, 31*(6), 864-869.

Youngstedt, S., Kripke, D., & Elliott, J. (2001). Circadian phase-delaying effects of bright light alone and combined with exercise in humans. *American Journal of Physiology: Regulatory, Integrative, and Comparative Physiology, 282*(1), R259-R266.

Youngstedt, S.D., Kripke, J.A., Elliott, J.A., & Klauber, M.R. (2001). Circadian abnormalities in older adults. *Journal of Pineal Research, 31*(3), 264-269.

Youngstedt, S., O'Connor, P., & Dishman, R. (1997). The effects of acute exercise on sleep: A quantitative synthesis. *Sleep, 20*(3), 203-214.

Chapter 10

Adem, A., Jossan, S., d'Argy, R., Gillberg, P.G., Nordberg, A., Winblad, B., et al. (1989). Insulin-like growth factor 1 (IGF-I) receptors in the human brain: Quantitative autoradiographic localization. *Brain Research, 503*, 299-303.

Aleman, A., Verhaar, H., de Haan, E., De Vries, W.R., Samson, M.M., Drent, M.L., et al. (1999). Insulin-like growth factor-I and cognitive function in healthy older men. *Journal of Clinical Endocrinology and Metabolism, 84*(2), 471-475.

Ambrosini, M.V., & Giuditta, A. (2001). Learning and sleep: The sequential hypothesis. *Sleep Medicine Reviews, 5*(6), 477-490.

Aström, C., & Lindholm, J. (1990). Growth hormone-deficient young adults have decreased deep sleep. *Neuroendocrinology, 51*(1), 82-84.

References

Aström, C., & Trojaborg, W. (1992). Effect of growth hormone on human sleep EEG energy. *Clinical Endocrinology, 36*(3), 241-245.

Baum, H., Katznelson, L., Sherman, J., Biller, B.M., Hayden, D.L., Schoenfeld, D.A., et al. (1998). Effects of physiological growth hormone (GH) therapy on cognition and quality of life in patients with adult-onset GH deficiency. *Journal of Clinical Endocrinology and Metabolism, 83*(9), 3184-3189.

Bjorntorp, P. (2002). Alterations in the ageing corticotropic stress-response axis. *Novartis Foundation Symposium, 242,* 46-65.

Blumenthal, J.A., Emery, C.F., Madden, D.J., George, L.K., Coleman, R.E., Riddle, M.W., et al. (1989). Cardiovascular and behavioral effects of aerobic exercise training in healthy older men and women. *Journal of Gerontology, 44*(5), M147-M157.

Blumenthal, J.A., & Madden, D.J. (1988). Effects of aerobic exercise training, age, and physical fitness on memory-search performance. *Psychology and Aging, 3*(3), 280-285.

Blunden, S., Lushington, K., & Kennedy, D. (2001). Cognitive and behavioural performance in children with sleep-related obstructive breathing disorders. *Sleep Medicine Reviews, 5*(6), 447-461.

Bonnet, M.H., & Arand, D.L. (1997). Hyperarousal and insomnia. *Sleep Medicine Reviews, 1*(2), 97-108.

Bonnet, M.H., & Arand, D.L. (1998). Heart rate variability in insomniacs and matched normal sleepers. *Psychosomatic Medicine, 60,* 610-615.

Clarkson-Smith, L., & Hartley, A.A. (1989). Relationships between physical exercise and cognitive abilities in older adults. *Psychology and Aging, 4*(2), 183-189.

Charlton, G.A., & Crawford, M.H. (1997). Physiologic consequences of training. *Cardiology Clinics, 15*(3), 345-354.

Colcombe, S., & Kramer, A.F. (2003). Fitness effects on the cognitive function of older adults: A meta-analytic study. *Psychological Sciences, 14*(2), 125-130.

Connor, B., Beilharz, E., Williams, C., Synek, B., Gluckman, P.D., Faull, R.L., et al. (1997). Insulin-like growth factor-I (IGF-I) immunoreactivity in the Alzheimer's disease temporal cortex and hippocampus. *Molecular Brain Research, 49,* 283-290.

Connor, B., & Dragunow, M. (1998). The role of neuronal growth factors in neurodegenerative disorders of the human brain. *Brain Research Reviews, 27,* 1-39.

de Diego Acosta, A.M., Garcia, J.C., Fernandez-Pastor, V.J., Peran, S., Ruiz, M., & Guirado, F. (2001). Influence of fitness on the integrated neuroendocrine response to aerobic exercise until exhaustion. *Journal of Physiology and Biochemistry, 57*(4), 313-320.

Deijen, J., de Boer, H., Blok, G., & van der Veen, E. (1996). Cognitive impairments and mood disturbances in growth hormone deficient men. *Psychoneuroendocrinology, 21,* 313-322.

References

Deijen, J., de Boer, H., & van der Veen, E. (1998). Cognitive changes during growth hormone replacement in adult men. *Psychoneuroendocrinology, 23*, 45-55.

Drewnowski, A., & Evans, W.J. (2001). Nutrition, physical activity, and quality of life in older adults: Summary. *Journals of Gerontology. Series A, Biological Sciences and Medical Sciences, Spec No 2*(2):89-94.

Driver, H., & Taylor, S. (2000). Exercise and sleep. *Sleep Medicine Reviews, 4*(4), 387-402.

Drucker-Colin, R.R., Spanis, C.W., Hunyadi, J., Sassin, J.F., & McGaugh, J.L. (1975). Growth hormone effects on sleep and wakefulness in the rat. *Neuroendocrinology, 18*(1), 1-8.

Edinger, J.D., Fins, A.I., Glenn, M., Sullivan, R.J., Bastian, L.A., Marsh, G.R., et al. (2000). Insomnia and the eye of the beholder: Are there clinical markers of objective sleep disturbances among adults with and without insomnia complaints? *Journal of Consulting and Clinical Psychology, 68*(4), 586-593.

Elzinga, B.M., & Bremner, J.D. (2002). Are the neural substrates of memory the final common pathway in posttraumatic stress disorder (PTSD)? *Journal of Affective Disorders, 70*(1), 1-17.

Fabre, C., Chamari, K., Mucci, P., Masse-Biron, J., & Prefaut, C. (2002). Improvement of cognitive function by mental and/or individualized aerobic training in healthy elderly subjects. *International Journal of Sports Medicine, 23*(6), 415-421.

Fulda, S., & Shulz, H. (2001). Cognitive dysfunction in sleep disorders. *Sleep Medicine Reviews, 5*(6), 423-445.

Garry, P., Roussel, B., Cohen, R., Biot-Laport, S., Charfi, A.E., Jouvet, M., et al. (1985). Diurnal administration of human growth hormone-releasing factor does not modify sleep and sleep-related growth hormone secretion in normal young men. *Acta Endocrinologica, 110*(2), 158-163.

Goldsmith, R.L., Bloomfield, D.M., & Rosenwinkel, E.T. (2000). Exercise and autonomic function. *Coronary Artery Diseases, 11*(2), 129-135.

Guldner, J., Schier, T., Friess, E., Colla, M., Holsboer, F., & Stieger, A. (1997). Reduced efficacy of growth hormone-releasing hormone in modulating sleep endocrine activity in the elderly. *Neurobiology and Aging, 18*(5), 491-495.

Hakkinen, K., Pakarinen, A., Kraemer, W.J., Hakkinen, A., Valkeinen, H., & Alen, M. (2001). Selective muscle hypertrophy, changes in EMG and force, and serum hormones during strength training in older women. *Journal of Applied Physiology, 91*(2), 569-580.

Hibberd, C., Yau, J.L., & Seckl, J.R. (2000). Glucocorticoids and the ageing hippocampus. *Journal of Anatomy, 197*(Pt 4), 553-562.

Hill, R.D., Storant, M., & Malley, M. (1993). The impact of long-term exercise training on psychological function in older adults. *Journal of Gerontology, 48*(1), P12-P17.

Hoschl, C., & Hajek, T. (2001). Hippocampal damage mediated by corticosteroids—A neuropsychiatric research challenge. *European Archives of Psychiatry and Clinical Neuroscience, 251*(Suppl 2), II81-II88.

Johansson, J., Larson, G., Andersson, M., Elmgren, A., Hynsjo, L., Lindahl, A., et al. (1995). Treatment of growth hormone-deficient adults with recombinant human growth hormone increases in concentration of growth hormone in the cerebrospinal fluid and affects neurotransmitters. *Neuroendocrinology, 61*, 57-66.

Jones, K., & Harrison, Y. (2001). Frontal lobe function, sleep loss and fragmented sleep. *Sleep Medicine Reviews, 5*(6), 463-475.

Karani, R., McLaughlin, M.A., & Cassel, C.K. (2001). Exercise in the healthy older adult. *American Journal of Geriatric Cardiology, 10*(5), 269-273.

Kerkhofs, M., Van Cauter, E. Van Onderbergen, A., Caufriez, A., Thorner, M.O., & Copinschi, G. (1993). Sleep-promoting effects of growth hormone-releasing hormone in normal men. *American Journal of Physiology, 264*, E594-E598.

Kerr, B., Scott, M., & Vitiello, M.V. (1993). Can aerobic exercise influence cognitive and motor function for older individuals? *Proceedings of thes Psychonomic Society, 34*, 3.

King, A.C., Oman, R.F., Brassington, G.S., Bliwise, D.L., & Haskell, W.L. (1997). Moderate-intensity exercise and self-rated quality of sleep in older adults. *Journal of the American Medical Association, 277*(1), 32-37.

Kramer, A.F., Hahn, S., Cohen, N.J., Banich, M.T., McAuley, E., Harrison, C.R., et al. (1999). Ageing, fitness and neurocognitive function. *Nature, 400*(6743), 418-419.

Krueger, J.M., Obal, F., & Fang, J. (1999). Humoral regulation of physiological sleep: Cytokines and GHRH. *Journal of Sleep Research, 8*(Suppl 1), 53-59.

Kubitz, K.A., Landers, D.M., Petruzzello, S.J., & Han, M. (1996). The effects of acute and chronic exercise on sleep: A meta-analytic review. *Sports Medicine, 21*, 277-291.

Kupfer, D.J., Jarrett, D.B., & Ehlers, C.L. (1991). The effect of GRF on the EEG sleep of normal males. *Sleep, 14*(1), 87-88.

Lai, Z., Roos, P., Zhai, O., Olsson, Y., Fholenhag, K., Larsson, C., et al. (1993). Age-related reduction of human growth hormone-binding sites in the human brain. *Brain Research, 621*, 260-266.

Laurin, D., Verreault, R., Lindsay, J., MacPherson, K., & Rockwood, K. (2001). Physical activity and risk of cognitive impairment and dementia in elderly persons. *Archives of Neurology, 58*(3), 498-504.

Lee, A.L., Ogle, W.O., & Sapolsky, R.M. (2002). Stress and depression: Possible links to neuron death in the hippocampus. *Bipolar Disorders, 4*(2), 117-128.

Lichtenwalner, R., Forbes, M., Bennett, S., Lynch, C.D., Sonntag, W.E., & Riddle, D.R. (2001). Intercerebroventricular infusion of insulin-like growth factor-I ameliorates the age-related decline in hippocampal neurogenesis. *Neuroscience, 107*(4), 603-613.

Lupien, S.J., Nair, N.P., Briere, S., Maheu, F., Tu, M.T., Lemay, M., et al. (1999). Increased cortisol levels and impaired cognition in human aging: Implication for depression and dementia in later life. *Reviews in the Neurosciences, 10*(2), 117-139.

Lynch, C., Lyons, D., Khan, A., Bennett, S.A., & Sonntag, W.E. (2001). Insulin-like growth factor-1 selectively increases glucose utilization in brains of aged animals. *Endocrinology, 142*(1), 506-509.

Madden, D.J., Blumenthal, J.A., Allen, P.A., & Emery, C.F. (1989). Improving aerobic capacity in healthy older adults does not necessarily lead to improved cognitive performance. *Psychology and Aging, 4*(3), 307-320.

Marshall, L., Boes, N., Strasburger, C., Born, J., & Fehm, H.L. (1997). Differential influences in sleep of growth hormone-releasing hormone at different concentrations. *Experimental and Clinical Endocrinology and Diabetes*, (Suppl 1), 113.

Marshall, L., Molle, M., Boschen, G., Stieger, A., Fehm, H.L., & Born, J. (1996). Greater efficacy of episodic than continuous growth hormone-releasing hormone (GHRH) administration in promoting slow-wave sleep (SWS). *Journal of Endocrinology and Metabolism, 81*(3), 1009-1013.

Morin, C.M. (2000). The nature of insomnia and the need to refine out diagnostic criteria. *Psychosomatic Medicine, 62*, 483-485.

Murck, H., Frieboes, R.M., Schier, T., & Steiger, A. (1997). Longtime administration of growth hormone-releasing hormone (GHRH) does not restore the reduced efficiency of GHRH on sleep endocrine activity in 2 old-aged subjects—A preliminary study. *Pharmacopsychology, 30*(4), 122-124.

Nyberg, F. (1997). Aging effects on growth hormone receptor binding in the brain. *Experimental Gerontology, 32*, 521-528.

Nyberg, F., & Burman, P. (1996). Growth hormone and its receptors in the central nervous system: Location and functional significance. *Hormone Research, 45*, 18-22.

Obal, F., Alfoldi, P., Cady, A.B., Johannsen, L., Sary, G., & Kreuger, J.M. (1988). Growth hormone-releasing factor enhances sleep in rats and rabbits. *American Journal of Physiology, 255*(2 Pt 2), R310-R316.

Obal, F., Floyd, R., Kapas, L., Bodosi, B., & Krueger, J.M. (1996). Effects of systemic GHRH on sleep in intact and hypophysectomized rats. *American Journal of Physiology, 270*(2 Pt 1), E230-E237.

Obal, F., & Krueger, J.M. (2001). The somatotropic axis and sleep. *Revue Neurologique, 157*(11 Pt 2), S12-S15.

Obal, F., Payne, L., Kapas, L., Opp, M., & Krueger, J.M. (1991). Inhibition of growth hormone-releasing factor suppresses both sleep and growth hormone secretion in the rat. *Brain Research, 557*, 149-153.

O'Sullivan, S.E., & Bell, C. (2000). The effects of exercise and training on human cardiovascular reflex control. *Journal of the Autonomic Nervous System, 81*(1-3), 16-24.

Papadakis, M., Grady, D., Black, D., Tierney, M.J., Gooding, G.A., Schambelen, M., et al. (1996). Growth hormone replacement in healthy older men improves body composition but not functional ability. *Annals of Internal Medicine, 124*, 708-716.

References

Papadakis, M., Grady, D., Tierney, M., Black, D., Wells, L., & Grunfeld, C. (1995). Insulin-like growth factor 1 and functional status in healthy older men. *Journal of the American Geriatrics Society, 43*(12), 1350-1355.

Perlis, M.L., Smith, M.T., Andrews, P.J., Orff, H., & Giles, D.E. (2001). Beta/gamma EEG activity in patients with primary and secondary insomnia and good sleeper controls. *Sleep, 24*(1), 110-117.

Poehlman, E.T., & Copeland, K.C. (1990). Influence of physical activity on insulin-like growth factor-I in healthy younger and older men. *Journal of Clinical Endocrinology and Metabolism, 71*(6), 1468-1473.

Prinz, P.N., Weitzman, E.D., Cunningham, G.R., Karacan, I. (1983). Plasma growth hormone during sleep in young and aged men. *Journal of Gerontology, 38*(5):519-524.

Richards, M., Hardy, R., & Wadsworth, M.E. (2003). Does active leisure protect cognition? Evidence from a national birth cohort. *Social Science and Medicine, 56*(4), 785-792.

Richardson, G.S., Poe, G.R., Seymour, A., & Roth, T. (2001). Objective and subjective sleep disruption following dietary salt restriction in normal subjects. *Sleep, 24*(Suppl.), A114-A115.

Rikli, R.E., & Edwards, D.J. (1991). Effects of a three-year exercise program on motor function and cognitive processing speed in older women. *Research Quarterly for Exercise and Sport, 62*(1), 61-67.

Rollero, A., Murialdo, G., Fonzi, S., Garrone, S., Gianelli, M.V., Gazzerro, E., et al. (1998). Relationship between cognitive function, growth hormone and insulin-like growth factor I plasma levels in aged subjects. *Neuropsychobiology, 23*, 45-55.

Rosa, R.R., & Bonnet, M.H. (2000). Reported chronic insomnia is independent of poor sleep as measured by electroencephalography. *Psychosomatic Medicine, 62*, 474-482.

Sapolsky, R.M. (1989). Hypercortisolism among socially subordinate wild baboons originates at the CNS level. *Archives of General Psychiatry, 46*(11), 1047-1051.

Sapolsky, R.M. (2002). Chickens, eggs and hippocampal atrophy. *Nature Neuroscience, 5*(11), 1111-1113.

Sartorio, A., Conti, A., Molinari, E., Riva, G., Morabito, F., & Faglia, G. (1996). Growth, growth hormone and cognitive functions. *Hormone Research, 45*, 23-29.

Seals, D.R., Taylor, J.A., Ng, A.V., & Esler, M.D. (1994). Exercise and aging: Autonomic control of the circulation. *Medicine and Science in Sports and Exercise, 26*(5), 568-576.

Shier, T., Guldner, J., Colla, M., Holsboer, F., & Steiger, A. (1997). Changes in sleep-endocrine activity after growth hormone-releasing hormone depend on time of administration. *Journal of Neuroendocrinology, 9*, 201-205.

Singh, N., Clements, K., & Fiatarone, M. (1997). Sleep, sleep deprivation, and daytime activities. *Sleep, 20*(2), 95-101.

Smith, C. (2001). Sleep states and memory processes in humans: Procedural versus declarative memory systems. *Sleep Medicine Reviews, 5*(6), 491-506.

References

Soares, C.d.N., Musolino, N.R., Cunha Neto, M., Caires, M.A., Rosenthal, M.C., Camarqo, C.P., et al. (1999). Impact of recombinant human growth hormone (RH-GH) treatment on psychiatric, neuropsychological and clinical profiles of GH deficient adults. A placebo-controlled trial. *Arquivos de Neuro-Psiquiatria, 57*(2A), 182-189.

Sonntag, W., Brunso-Bechtold, J., & Riddle, D. (2001). Age-related decreases in growth hormone and insulin-like growth factor (IGF)-1: Implications for brain aging. *Journal of Anti-Aging Medicine, 4*(4), 311-330.

Sonntag, W., Lynch, C., Cooney, P., & Hutchins, P. (1997). Decreases in cerebral microvasculature with age are associated with the decline of growth hormone and insulin like growth factor 1. *Endocrinology, 138*(8), 3515-3520.

Sonntag, W., Lynch, C., Thornton, P., Khan, A., Bennett, S., & Ingram, R. (2000). The effects of growth hormone and IGF-I deficiency on cerebrovascular and brain aging. *Journal of Anatomy, 197*(Pt 4), 575-585.

Steiger, A. (2003). Sleep and endocrine regulation. *Frontiers in Bioscience, 1*(8), S358-S376.

Steiger, A., Guldner, J., Hemmeter, U., Rothe, B., Wiedemann, K., & Holsboer, F. (1992). Effects of growth hormone-releasing hormone and somatostatin on sleep EEG and nocturnal hormone secretion in male controls. *Neuroendocrinology, 56*(4), 566-573.

Strickgold, R. (2001). Toward a cognitive neuroscience of sleep. *Sleep Medicine Reviews, 5*(6), 417-421.

Thornton, P., Ingram, R., & Sonntag, W. (2000). Chronic [D-Ala2]-growth hormone-releasing hormone administration attenuates age-related deficits in spatial memory. *Journals of Gerontology. Series A, Biological Sciences and Medical Sciences, 55*(2), B106-B112.

Thornton, P., Ng, A., & Sonntag, W. (1999). Insulin-like growth factor-1 modulates learning and memory in young and old rats. *Society for Neuroscience Abstracts, 25*, 1064.

Tworoger, S.S., Yasui, Y., Vitiello, M.V., Schwartz, R.S., Ulrish, C.M., Aiello, E.J., et al. (2003). Effects of a year-long moderate intensity exercise or stretching intervention on sleep quality in post-menopausal women. *Sleep, 26*(7), 830-836.

Uno, H., Tarara, R., Else, J.G., Suleman, M.A., & Sapolsky, R.M. (1989). Hippocampal damage associated with prolonged and fatal stress in primates. *Journal of Neuroscience, 9*(5), 1705-1711.

Van Dam, P., Aleman, A., de Vries, W., Deijen, J.B., van der Veen, E.A., de Haan, E.H., et al. (2000). Growth hormone, insulin-like growth factor I and cognitive function in adults. *Growth Hormone and IGF Research, 10*(Suppl. B), S69-S73.

van der Reijden-Lakeman, I.E., de Sonneville, L.M., Swaab-Barneveld, H.J., Slijper, F.M., Verhulst, F.C. (1997). Evaluation of attention before and after 2 years of growth hormone treatment in intrauterine growth retarded children. *Journal of Clinical and Experimental Neuropsychology, 19*(1), 101-118.

Vgontzas, A.N., Bixler, E.O., Lin, H., Prolo, P., Mastorakos, G., Vela-Bueno, A., et al. (2001). Chronic insomnia is associated with nyctohemeral activation of the hypothalamic-pituitary-adrenal axis: Clinical implications. *Journal of Clinical Endocrinology and Metabolism*, 86(8), 3787-3794.

Vgontzas, A.N., Bixler, E.O., Wittman, A.M., Zachman, K., Lin, H.M., Vela-Bueno, A., et al. (2001). Middle-aged men show higher sensitivity of sleep to the arousing effects of corticotropin-releasing hormone than young men: Clinical implications. *Journal of Clinical Endocrinology and Metabolism*, *86*(4), 1489-1495.

Vgontzas, A.N., Tsigos, C., Bixler, E.O., Stratakis, C.A., Zachman, K., Kales, A., et al. (1998). Chronic insomnia and activity of the stress system: A preliminary study. *Journal of Psychosomatic Research*, *45*(1 Spec No), 21-31.

Vitiello, M.V., Mazzoni, G., Moe, K.E., Drolet, G., Barsness, S., Merriam, G.R., et al. (2002). Growth hormone releasing hormone improves the cognitive function of healthy older men and women. *Journal of Clinical Psychiatry*, *63*(11), 1084.

Vitiello, M., Merriam, G., Moe, K., Droplet, G., Barsness, S., & Schwartz, R.S. (1999). IGF-I correlates with cognitive function in healthy older men and estrogenized women. *The Gerontologist*, *39*(1), 6.

Vitiello, M., Mazzoni, G., Moe, K., Droplet, G., Barsness, S., & Schwartz, R.S. (2000). GHRH treatment may improve cognitive function in the healthy elderly. *The Gerontologist*, *40*(1), 39.

Vitiello, M.V., Moe, K.E., Larsen, L.H., Merriam, G.R., & Schwartz, R.S. (2003). Long-term growth hormone releasing hormone administration does not improve the sleep quality of healthy older men and women. *Sleep*, *26*(Abstract Suppl.), A154.

Vitiello, M.V., Moe, K.E., Merriam, G.R., Mazzoni, G., Buchner, D.H., & Schwartz, R.S. (2006). Growth hormone releasing hormone improves the cognition of healthy older adults. *Neurobiology of Aging*, *27*(2), 318-323.

Vitiello, M.V., Prinz, P.N., & Halter, J.B. (1983). Sodium-restricted diet increases nighttime plasma norepinephrine and impairs sleep patterns in man. *Journal of Clinical Endocrinology and Metabolism*, 56(3), 553-556.

Vitiello, M.V., Prinz, P.N., & Schwartz, R.S. (1994a). Slow wave sleep but not overall sleep quality of healthy older men and women is improved by increased aerobic fitness. *Sleep Research*, *23*, 149.

Vitiello, M.V., Prinz, P.N., & Schwartz, R.S. (1994b). The subjective sleep quality of healthy older men and women is enhanced by participation in two fitness training programs: A nonspecific effect. *Sleep Research*, *23*, 148.

Vitiello, M.V., Ralph, D.D., Veith, R.C., & Prinz, P.N. (1990). Suppression of nighttime sympathetic activity does not affect the sleep quality of healthy young men. In J. Horne (Ed.), *Sleep '90* (pp. 34-36). Bochum: Pontenagel Press.

Vitiello, M.V., Schwartz, R.S., Buchner, D.M., Moe, K.E., Mazzoni, G., & Merriam, G.R. (2001). Treating age-related changes in somatotrophic hormones, sleep and cognition. *Dialogues in Clinical Neuroscience*, *3*(3), 229-236.

Vitiello, M.V., Veith, R.C., Ralph, D.D., Frommlet, M.S., & Prinz, P.N. (1989). Low sodium diet elevates plasma norepinephrine and impairs sleep patterns in man: A replication. In J. Horne (Ed.), *Sleep '88* (pp. 206-207). New York: Gustav Fischer Verlag.

Vitiello, M.V., Veith, R.C., Ralph, D.D., & Prinz, P.N. (1992). Nighttime plasma norepinephrine and sleep fragmentation. In S. Smirne, M. Franceschi, L. Ferini-Strambi, & M. Zucconi (Eds.), *Sleep, hormones and the immunological system* (pp. 155-170). Milan: Masson.

Vitiello, M.V., Wilkinson, C.W., Merriam, G.R., Moe, K.E., Prinz, P.N., Ralph, D.D., et al. (1997). Successful 6-month endurance training does not alter insulin-like growth factor-I in healthy older men and women. *Journals of Gerontology. Series A, Biological Sciences and Medical Sciences, 52*(3), M149-M154.

Vuori, I., Urponen, H., Hasan, J., & Partinen, M. (1988). Epidemiology of exercise effects on sleep. *Acta Physiologica Scandinavica Supplementum, 574*, 3-7.

Wang, R.Y., Tsai, S.C., Chen, J.J., & Wang, P.S. (2001). The simulation effects of mountain climbing training on selected endocrine responses. *Chinese Journal of Physiology, 44*(1), 13-8.

Woo, S., Morris, S., Castro, C.M., Thomson, J., Morton, J., Wu, J., et al. (2003). Associations between physical fitness and sleep in older adults. *Sleep, 26*(Abstract Suppl.), A162.

Chapter 11

Alves de Moraes, S., Szklo, M., Knopman, D., & Sato, R. (2002). The relationship between temporal changes in blood pressure and changes in cognitive function: Atherosclerosis Risk in Communities (ARIC) study. *Preventive Medicine, 35*(3), 258-263.

American Heart Association. (2003). *Heart disease and stroke statistics—2003 update*. Dallas: American Heart Association.

Applegate, R.J., & Little, W.C. (1994). Alteration of autonomic influence on left ventricular contractility by epicardial superfusion with hexamethonium and procaine. *Cardiovascular Research, 28*(7), 1042-1048.

Barnes, D.E., Yaffe, K., Satariano, W.A., & Tager, I.B. (2003). A longitudinal study of cardiorespiratory fitness and cognitive function in healthy older adults. *Journal of the American Geriatrics Society, 51*(4), 459-465.

Bassuk, S.S., Wypij, D., & Berkman, L.F. (2000). Cognitive impairment and mortality in the community-dwelling elderly. *American Journal of Epidemiology, 151*(7), 676-688.

Colcombe, S.J., Erickson, K.I., Raz, N., Webb, A.G., Cohen, N.J., McAuley, E., et al. (2003). Aerobic fitness reduces brain tissue loss in aging humans. *Journal of Gerontology, 58*(2), 176-180.

Collins, R., Peto, R., MacMahon, S., Hebert, P., Fiebach, N.H., Eberlein, K.A., et al. (1990). Blood pressure, stroke, and coronary heart disease: Part 2, short-term reductions in blood pressure: Overview of randomized drug trials in their epidemiological context. *Lancet, 335*, 827-838.

DeSouza, C.A., Shapiro, L.F., Clevenger, C.M., Dinenno, F.A., Monahan, K.D., Tanaka, H., et al. (2000). Regular aerobic exercise prevents and restores age-related declines in endothelium-dependent vasodilation in healthy men. *Circulation, 102*, 1351-1357.

Elias, M.F., Wolf, P.A., D'Agostino, R.B., Cobb, J., & White, L.R. (1993). Untreated blood pressure level is inversely related to cognitive functioning: The Framingham Study. *American Journal of Epidemiology, 138*(6), 353-364.

Erickson, C.A., & Barnes, C.A. (2003). The neurobiology of memory changes in normal aging. *Experimental Gerontology, 38*(1-2), 61-69.

Fagard, R., & Amery, A. (1995). Physical exercise in hypertension. In J.H. Laragh & B.M. Brenner (Eds.), *Hypertension: Pathophysiology, diagnosis, and management* (2nd ed., pp. 2669-2681). New York: Raven Press.

Farmer, M.E., White, L.R., Abbott, R.D., Kittner, S.J., Kaplan, E., Wolz, M.M., et al. (1987). Blood pressure and cognitive performance. The Framingham Study. *American Journal of Epidemiology, 126*(6), 1103-1114.

Forette, F., Seux, M.L., Staessen, J.A., Thijs, L., Babarskiene, M.R., Babeanu, S., et al. (2002). The prevention of dementia with antihypertensive treatment: New evidence from the Systolic Hypertension in Europe (Syst-Eur) study. *Archives of Internal Medicine, 162*(18), 2046-2052.

Forette, F., Seux, M.L., Staessen, J.A., Thijs, L., Birkenhager, W.H., Babarskiene, M.R., et al. (1998). Prevention of dementia in randomised double-blind placebo-controlled Systolic Hypertension in Europe (Syst-Eur) trial. *Lancet, 352*(9137), 1347-1351.

Guo, Z., Fratiglioni, L., Winblad, B., & Viitanen, M. (1997). Blood pressure and performance on the Mini-Mental State Examination in the very old. Cross-sectional and longitudinal data from the Kungsholmen Project. *American Journal of Epidemiology, 145*(12), 1106-1113.

Hagberg, J.M., Montain, S.J., Martin, W.H., & Ehsani, A.A. (1989). Effect of exercise training in 60- to 69-year-old persons with essential hypertension. *American Journal of Cardiology, 64*, 348-353.

Ishikawa, K., Ohta, T., Zhang, J., Hashimoto, S., & Tanaka, H. (1999). Influence of age and gender on exercise training-induced blood pressure reduction in systemic hypertension. *American Journal of Cardiology, 84*(2), 192-196.

Jennings, J.R. (2003). Autoregulation of blood pressure and thought: Preliminary results of an application of brain imaging to psychosomatic medicine. *Psychosomatic Medicine, 65*(3), 384-395.

Johansson, B.B. (1994). Pathogenesis of vascular dementia: The possible role of hypertension. *Dementia, 5*(3-4), 174-176.

Joint National Committee on Prevention, Evaluation, and Treatment of High Blood Pressure. (1997). The sixth report of the Joint National Committee on Prevention, Detection, Evaluation, and Treatment of High Blood Pressure. *Archives of Internal Medicine, 157*(24), 2413-2446.

Kannel, W.B. (1999). Historic perspectives on the relative contributions of diastolic and systolic blood pressure elevation to cardiovascular risk profile. *American Heart Journal, 138*(3 Pt 2), 205-210.

References

Kannel, W.B., D'Agostino, R.B., & Silbershatz, H. (1997). Blood pressure and cardiovascular morbidity and mortality rates in the elderly. *American Heart Journal, 134*, 758-763.

Kenny, R.A., Kalaria, R., & Ballard, C. (2002). Neurocardiovascular instability in cognitive impairment and dementia. *Annals of the New York Academy of Sciences, 977*, 183-195.

Keunen, R.W.M., Vliegen, J.H.R., Stam, C.J., & Tavy, D.L.J. (1996). Nonlinear transcranial Doppler analysis demonstrates age-related changes of cerebral hemodynamics. *Ultrasound in Medicine and Biology, 22*(4), 383-390.

Kilander, L., Nyman, H., Boberg, M., Hansson, L., & Lithell, H. (1998). Hypertension is related to cognitive impairment: A 20-year follow-up of 999 men. *Hypertension, 31*(3), 780-786.

Launer, L.J., Masaki, K., Petrovitch, H., Foley, D., & Havlik, R.J. (1995). The association between midlife blood pressure levels and late-life cognitive function. The Honolulu-Asia Aging Study. *Journal of the American Medical Association, 274*(23), 1846-1851.

Laurin, D., Verreault, R., Lindsay, J., MacPherson, K., & Rockwood, K. (2001). Physical activity and risk of cognitive impairment and dementia in elderly persons. *Archives of Neurology, 58*(3), 498-504.

Lavi, S., Egbarya, R., Lavi, R., & Jacob, G. (2003). Role of nitric oxide in the regulation of cerebral blood flow in humans: Chemoregulation versus mechanoregulation. *Circulation, 107*(14), 1901-1905.

Lipsitz, L.A. (1989). Orthostatic hypotension in the elderly. *New England Journal of Medicine, 321*(14), 952-957.

MacMahon, S., & Rodgers, A. (1993). The effects of blood pressure reduction in older patients: An overview of five randomized controlled trials in elderly hypertensives. *Clinical and Experimental Hypertension, 15*(6), 967-978.

Monahan, K.D., Dinenno, F.A., Seals, D.R., Clevenger, C.M., Desouza, C.A., & Tanaka, H. (2001). Age-associated changes in cardiovagal baroreflex sensitivity are related to central arterial compliance. *American Journal of Physiology, Heart and Circulatory Physiology, 281*(1), H284-H289.

Monahan, K.D., Dinenno, F.A., Tanaka, H., Clevenger, C.M., DeSouza, C.A., & Seals, D.R. (2000). Regular aerobic exercise modulates age-associated declines in cardiovagal baroreflex sensitivity in healthy men. *Journal of Physiology, 529*(1), 263-271.

Monahan, K.D., Tanaka, H., Dinenno, F.A., & Seals, D.R. (2001). Central arterial compliance is associated with age- and habitual exercise-related differences in cardiovagal baroreflex sensitivity. *Circulation, 104*, 1627-1632.

Nichols, W.W., & O'Rourke, M.F. (1998). *McDonald's blood flow in arteries: Theoretical, experimental and clinical principles* (4th ed.). London: Arnold.

O'Rourke, M. (1990). Arterial stiffness, systolic blood pressure, and logical treatment of arterial hypertension. *Hypertension, 15*, 339-347.

Paffenbarger, R.S., Jr., Wing, A.L., Hyde, R.T., & Jung, D.L. (1983). Physical activity and incidence of hypertension in college alumni. *American Journal of Epidemiology, 117*(3), 245-257.

Panerai, R.B., Carey, B.J., & Potter, J.F. (2003). Short-term variability of cerebral blood flow velocity responses to arterial blood pressure transients. *Ultrasound in Medicine and Biology, 29*(1), 31-38.

Patterson, J.C., II (2001). Cerebellar perfusion abnormalities correlated with change in cognitive and affective state in a 78-year-old man. *American Journal of Geriatric Psychiatry, 9*(3), 309-314.

Pavan, L., Casiglia, E., Braga, L.M., Winnicki, M., Puato, M., Pauletto, P., et al. (1999). Effects of a traditional lifestyle on the cardiovascular risk profile: The Amondava population of the Brazilian Amazon. Comparison with matched African, Italian and Polish populations. *Journal of Hypertension, 17*(6), 749-756.

Phillips, S.J., & Whisnant, J.P. (1992). Hypertension and the brain. The National High Blood Pressure Education Program. *Archives of Internal Medicine, 152*(5), 938-945.

Pierce, T.W., Madden, D.J., Siegel, W.C., & Blumenthal, J.A. (1993). Effects of aerobic exercise on cognitive and psychosocial functioning in patients with mild hypertension. *Health Psychology, 12*(4), 286-291.

PROGRESS Collaborative Group. (2001). Randomised trial of a perindopril-based blood-pressure-lowering regimen among 6,105 individuals with previous stroke or transient ischaemic attack. *Lancet, 358*(9287), 1033-1041.

PROGRESS Collaborative Group. (2003). Effects of blood pressure lowering with perindopril and indapamide therapy on dementia and cognitive decline in patients with cerebrovascular disease. *Archives of Internal Medicine, 163*, 1069-1075.

Qiu, C., Winblad, B., Viitanen, M., & Fratiglioni, L. (2003). Pulse pressure and risk of Alzheimer disease in persons aged 75 years and older: A community-based, longitudinal study. *Stroke, 34*(3), 594-599.

Rao, R. (2002). The role of carotid stenosis in vascular cognitive impairment. *Journal of the Neurological Sciences, 203-204*, 103-107.

Rogers, R.L., Meyer, J.S., & Mortel, K.F. (1990). After reaching retirement age physical activity sustains cerebral perfusion and cognition. *Journal of the American Geriatrics Society, 38*(2), 123-128.

Safar, M.E., & London, G.M. (2000). Therapeutic studies and arterial stiffness in hypertension: Recommendations of the European Society of Hypertension. The Clinical Committee of Arterial Structure and Function. *Journal of Hypertension, 18*(11), 1527-1535.

Seals, D.R., & Reiling, M.J. (1991). Effect of regular exercise on 24-hour arterial pressure in older hypertensive humans. *Hypertension, 18*, 583-592.

Seals, D.R., Silverman, H.G., Reiling, M.J., & Davy, K.P. (1997). Effect of regular aerobic exercise on elevated blood pressure in postmenopausal women. *American Journal of Cardiology, 80*(1), 49-55.

Seals, D.R., Stevenson, E.T., Jones, P.P., DeSouza, C.A., & Tanaka, H. (1999). Lack of age-associated elevations in 24-h systolic and pulse pressures in women who exercise regularly. *American Journal of Physiology, 277*, H947-H955.

Seals, D.R., Tanaka, H., Clevenger, C.M., Monahan, K.D., Reiling, M.J., Hiatt, W.R., et al. (2001). Blood pressure reductions with exercise and sodium restriction in postmenopausal women with elevated systolic pressure: Role of arterial stiffness. *Journal of the American College of Cardiology, 38*(2), 506-513.

Seux, M.L., & Forette, G. (1999). Effects of hypertension and its treatment on mental function. *Current Hypertension Reports, 1*, 232-237.

Seux, M.L., Thijs, L., Forette, F., Staessen, J.A., Birkenhager, W.H., Bulpitt, C.J., et al. (1998). Correlates of cognitive status of old patients with isolated systolic hypertension: The Syst-Eur Vascular Dementia Project. *Journal of Hypertension, 16*(7), 963-969.

Shapiro, A.P., Miller, R.E., King, H.E., Ginchereau, E.H., & Fitzgibbon, K. (1982). Behavioral consequences of mild hypertension. *Hypertension, 4*, 355-360.

Sharrett, A.R., Sorlie, P.D., Chambless, L.E., Folsom, A.R., Hutchinson, R.G., Heiss, G., et al. (1999). Relative importance of various risk factors for asymptomatic carotid atherosclerosis versus coronary heart disease incidence: The Atherosclerosis Risk in Communities Study. *American Journal of Epidemiology, 149*(9), 843-852.

Spirduso, W.W., & Clifford, P. (1978). Replication of age and physical activity effects on reaction and movement time. *Journal of Gerontology, 33*(1), 26-30.

Starr, J.M. (1999). Blood pressure and cognitive decline in the elderly. *Current Opinion in Nephrology and Hypertension, 8*(3), 347-351.

Tanaka, H., Bassett, D.R., Howley, E.T., Thompson, D.L., Ashraf, M., & Rawson, F.L. (1997). Swimming training lowers the resting blood pressure in individuals with hypertension. *Journal of Hypertension, 15*(6), 651-657.

Tanaka, H., DeSouza, C.A., & Seals, D.R. (1998). Absence of age-related increase in central arterial stiffness in physically active women. *Arteriosclerosis, Thrombosis, and Vascular Biology, 18*(1), 127-132.

Tanaka, H., DeSouza, C.A., & Seals, D.R. (1999). Exercise and hypertension in older adults. In H. Tanaka & M. Shindo (Eds.), *Exercise for preventing common diseases* (pp. 45-50). Tokyo: Springer-Verlag.

Tanaka, H., Dinenno, F.A., Hunt, B.E., Jones, P.P., DeSouza, C.A., & Seals, D.R. (1998). Hemodynamic sequelae of age-related increases in arterial stiffness in healthy humans. *American Journal of Cardiology, 82*, 1152-1155.

Tanaka, H., Dinenno, F.A., Monahan, K.D., Clevenger, C.M., DeSouza, C.A., & Seals, D.R. (2000). Aging, habitual exercise, and dynamic arterial compliance. *Circulation, 102*, 1270-1275.

Tanaka, H., Reiling, M.J., & Seals, D.R. (1998). Regular walking increases peak limb vasodilatory capacity of older hypertensive humans: Implications for arterial structure. *Journal of Hypertension, 16*, 423-428.

Taylor, J.O., Cornoni-Huntley, J., Curb, J.D., Manton, K.G., Ostfeld, A.M., Scherr, P., et al. (1991). Blood pressure and mortality risk in the elderly. *American Journal of Epidemiology*, *134*(5), 489-501.

Chapter 12

Allen, S.C., Jain, M., Ragab, S., & Malik, N. (2003). Acquisition and retention of inhaler techniques require intact executive function in elderly subjects. *Age and Ageing*, *32*, 299-302.

Awad, I.A., Spetzler, R.F., Hodak, J.A., Awad, C.A., & Carey, R. (1986). Incidental subcortical lesions identified on magnetic resonance imaging in the elderly: I. Correlation with age and cerebrovascular risk factors. *Stroke*, *17*, 1084-1089.

Barnes, D.E., Yaffe, K., Satariano, W.A., & Tager, I.B. (2003). A longitudinal study of cardiorespiratory fitness and cognitive function in healthy older adults. *Journal of the American Geriatrics Society*, *51*, 459-465.

Baxter, L.R., Schwartz, J.M., Phelps, M.E., Mazziotta, J.C., Guze, B.H., Selin, C.E., et al. (1989). Reduction of prefrontal cortex glucose metabolism common to three types of depression. *Archives of General Psychiatry*, *49*, 243-250.

Beck, A.T., Steer, R.A., & Brown, G.K. (1996). *Manual for Beck Depression Inventory–II*. San Antonio, TX: Psychological Corporation.

Binder, E.F., Storandt, M., & Birge, S.J. (1999). The relation between psychometric test performance and physical performance in older adults. *Journals of Gerontology. Series A, Biological Sciences and Medical Sciences*, *54*, M428-M432.

Blackman, J.D., Towle, V.L., Sturis, J., Lewis, G.F., Spire, J.P., & Polonsky, K.S. (1992). Hypoglycemic thresholds for cognitive dysfunction in IDDM. *Diabetes*, *41*, 392-399.

Blumenthal, J.A., Emery, C.F., Madden, D.J., George, L.K., Coleman, R.E., Riddle, M.W., et al. (1989). Cardiovascular and behavioural effects of aerobic exercise training in healthy older men and women. *Journals of Gerontology. Series A, Biological Sciences and Medical Sciences*, *44*, M147-M157.

Bootsma-van der Wiel, A., Gussekloo, J., De Craen, A.J., Van Exel, E., Bloem, B.R., & Westendorp, R.G. (2002). Common chronic diseases and general impairments as determinants of walking disability in the oldest-old population. *Journal of the American Geriatrics Society*, *50*, 1405-1410.

Brink, T.L. (1987). Why depression scales should not include all diagnostic criteria [Letter]. *Journal of the American Geriatrics Society*, *35*, 368.

Colcombe, S.J., Erickson, K.I., Raz, N., Webb, A.G., Cohen, N.J., McAuley, E., et al. (2003). Aerobic fitness reduces brain tissue loss in aging humans. *Journals of Gerontology. Series A, Biological Sciences and Medical Sciences*, *58*, 176-180.

Desmond, D.W., Tatemichi, T.K., Paik, M., & Stern, Y. (1993). Risk factors for cerebrovascular disease as correlates of cognitive function in a stroke free cohort. *Archives of Neurology*, *50*, 162-166.

References

Fan, E., Royall, D.R., Chiodo, L.K., Polk, M.J., & Mouton, C. (2003). Insight into financial capacity in non-institutionalized retirees [Abstract]. *Journal of the American Geriatrics Society, 50*, S80.

Fazekas, F., Niederhorn, K., Schmidt, R., Offenbach, H., Horner, S., Bertha, G., et al. (1988). White matter signal abnormalities in normal individuals: Correlation with carotid ultrasonography, cerebral blood flow measurements and cerebrovascular risk factors. *Stroke, 19*, 1285-1288.

Fillenbaum, G.G. (1985). Screening the elderly: A brief instrumental activities of daily living measure. *Journal of the American Geriatrics Society, 33*, 698-706.

Fillit, H.M., Butler, R.N., O'Connell, A.W., Albert, M.S., Birren, J.E., Cotman, C.W., et al. (2002). Achieving and maintaining cognitive vitality with aging. *Mayo Clinic Proceedings, 77*, 681-696.

Folstein, M.F., Folstein, S.E., & McHugh, P.R. (1975). Mini-Mental State: A practical method for grading the cognitive state of patients for the clinician. *Journal of Psychiatric Research, 12*, 198.

Fried, L.P., Ettinger, W.H., Lind, B., Newman, A.B., & Gardin, J. (1994). Physical disability in older adults: A physiological approach. *Journal of Clinical Epidemiology, 47*, 747-760.

Gavard, J.A., Lustman, P.J., & Clouse, R.E. (1993). Prevalence of depression in adults with diabetes: An epidemiological evaluation. *Diabetes Care, 16*, 1167-1178.

Grigsby, J., Kaye, K., Shetterly, S.M., Baxter, J., Morgenstern, N.E., & Hamman, R.F. (2002). Prevalence of disorders of executive cognitive functioning among the elderly: Findings from the San Luis Valley Health and Aging Study. *Neuroepidemiology, 21*, 213-220.

Hollenberg, M., Ngo, L.H., Turner, D., & Tager, I.B. (1998). Treadmill exercise testing in an epidemiological study of elderly subjects. *Journals of Gerontology. Series A, Biological Sciences and Medical Sciences, 53A*, B259-B267.

Ishii, N., Nishihara, Y., & Imamura, T. (1986). Why do frontal lobe symptoms predominate in vascular dementia with lacunes? *Neurology, 36*, 340-345.

Keymeulen, B., Jacobs, A., deMetz, K., de Sadeleer, C., Bossuyt, A., & Somers, G. (1995). Regional cerebral hypoperfusion in long-term type-1 (insulin dependent) diabetic patients: Relation to hypoglycaemic events. *Nuclear Medicine Communications, 16*, 10-16.

Kramer, A.F., Hahn, S., Cohen, N.J., Banich, M.T., McAuley, E., Harrison, C.R., et al. (1999). Aging, fitness and neurocognitive function. *Nature, 400*, 418-419.

La Rue, A., Romero, L.J., Ortiz, I.E., Liang, H.C., & Lindeman, R.D. (1999). Neuropsychological performance of Hispanic and non-Hispanic older adults: An epidemiologic survey. *Clinical Neuropsychology, 13*, 474-486.

Lauterbach, E.C., Jackson, J.G., Price, S.T., Wilson, A.N., Kirsh, A.D., & Dever, G.E. (1997). Clinical, motor, and biological correlates of depressive disorders after focal sub-cortical lesions. *Journal of Neuropsychiatry and Clinical Neurosciences, 9*, 259-266.

Leedom, L., Meehan, W.P., Procci, W., & Zeidler, A. (1991). Symptoms of depression in patients with type II diabetes mellitus. *Psychosomatics, 32,* 280-286.

Lustman, P.J., Griffith, L.S., Clouse, R.E., & Cryer, P.E. (1986). Psychiatric illness in diabetes mellitus: Relationship to symptoms and glucose control. *Journal of Nervous and Mental Disorders, 174,* 736-742.

Martin, K.A., Rejeski, W.J., Miller, M.E., James, M.K., Ettinger, W.H., Jr., & Messier, S.P. (1999). Validation of the PASE in older adults with knee pain and physical disability. *Medicine and Science in Sports and Exercise, 31,* 627-633.

Meneilly, G.S., Cheung, E., Tessier, D., Yakura, C., & Tuokko, H. (1993). The effects of improved glycemic control on cognitive functions in the elderly patient with diabetes. *Journals of Gerontology. Series A, Biological Sciences and Medical Sciences, 48,* M117-M121.

New England Research Institute. (1991). *PASE: Physical activity scale for the elderly: Administration and scoring instruction manual.* Watertown, MA: New England Research Institute.

Ott, A., Stolk, R.P., van Harskamp, F., Pols, H., Hofman, A., & Breteler, M. (1999). Diabetes mellitus and the risk of dementia: The Rotterdam Study. *Neurology, 53,* 1937-1942.

Palmer, R., Royall, D.R., Chiodo, L.K., & Polk, M.J. (2000). Growth curve models of longitudinal change in ECF: Relationship to functional status [Abstract]. *Gerontology, 47*(Suppl. 1), 50.

Perlmuter, L.C., Tun, P., Sizer, N., McGlinchey, R.E., & Nathan, D.M. (1987). Age and diabetes related changes in verbal fluency. *Experimental Aging Research, 13,* 9-14.

Radloff, L.S. (1977). The Center for Epidemiological Study–Depression Scale: A self-report depression scale for use in the general adult population. *Applied Psychological Assessments, 3,* 385-401.

Reaven, G.M., Thompson, L.W., Nahum, D., & Haskins, E. (1990). Relationship between hyperglycemia and cognitive function in older NIDDM patients. *Diabetes Care, 13,* 16-21.

Robinson, R.G., Kubos, K.L., Starr, L.B., Rao, K., & Price, T.R. (1984). Mood disorders in stroke patients: Importance of location of the lesion. *Brain, 107,* 81-93.

Royall, D.R. (1997). Some "depressive" symptoms may not imply depression [Letter]. *Journal of the American Geriatrics Society, 45,* 891-892.

Royall, D.R. (1999). Executive cognitive impairment: A novel perspective on dementia. *Neuroepidemiology, 19,* 293-299.

Royall, D.R. (2002). Bedside assessment of vascular dementia. In S. Gautier & T. Erkinjuntti (Eds.), *Vascular cognitive impairment* (pp. 307-322). London, UK: Martin Dunitz.

Royall, D.R., Chiodo, L.K., & Polk, M.J. (2000). Correlates of disability among elderly retirees with "sub-clinical" cognitive impairment. *Journals of Gerontology: Medical Sciences, 55A,* M541-M546.

Royall, D.R., Chiodo, L.K., & Polk, M.J. (2001). Executive impairment: Cross-sectional prevalence and relationship to level of care [Abstract]. *Gerontology*, 47(Suppl.), 50.

Royall, D.R., Cordes, J., & Polk, M.J. (1998). CLOX: An Executive Clock-Drawing Task. *Journal of Neurology, Neurosurgery, and Psychiatry, 64*, 588-594.

Royall, D.R., Espino, D.V., Polk, M., Palmer, R., & Markides, K.S. (2004). Prevalence and patterns of executive impairment in the Hispanic EPES Study. *International Journal of Geriatric Psychiatry, 19*, 926-934.

Royall, D.R., Espino, D.V., Polk, M., Verdeha, R., Vale, S., Gonzales, H., et al. (2003). Validation of a Spanish translation of the CLOX for use in Hispanic samples: The Hispanic EPESE Study. *International Journal of Geriatric Psychiatry, 18*, 135-141.

Royall, D.R., Lauterbach, E.C., Cummings, J.L., Reeve, A., Rummans, T.A., Kaufer, D.I., et al. (2002). Executive control function: A review of its promise and challenges to clinical research. *Journal of Neuropsychiatry and Clinical Neurosciences, 14*, 377-405.

Royall, D.R., Mulroy, A., Chiodo, L.K., & Polk, M.J. (1999). Clock drawing is sensitive to executive control: A comparison of six methods. *Journals of Gerontology. Series B, Psychological Sciences and Social Sciences, 54B*, P328-P333.

Royall, D.R., Palmer, R., Chiodo, L.K., & Polk, M.J. (2000). Declining executive control in normal aging predicts change in functional status: The Freedom House Study. *Journal of the American Geriatrics Society, 52*, 346-352.

Royall, D.R., Palmer, R., Chiodo, L.K., & Polk, M.J. (2005). Executive control mediates memory's association with change in instrumental activities of daily living: The Freedom House Study. *Journal of the American Geriatrics Society, 53*, 11-17.

Royall, D.R., Palmer, R., Chiodo, L.K., & Polk, M.J. (in press). Wisconsin card sort performance fails to predict change in functional status in old age: The Freedom House Study. *Journal of Clinical and Experimental Neuropsychology*.

Royall, D.R., & Polk, M.J. (1998). Dementias that present with and without posterior cortical features: An important clinical distinction. *Journal of the American Geriatrics Society, 46*, 98-105.

Schmidt, R. (1992). Comparison of magnetic resonance imaging in Alzheimer's disease, vascular dementia and normal aging. *European Neurology, 32*, 164-169.

Sheikh, J.I., & Yesavage, J.A. (1996). Geriatric Depression Scale (GDS): Recent evidence and development of a shorter version. *Clinical Gerontology, 5*, 165-173.

Schuit, A.J., Schouten, E.G., Westerterp, K.R., & Saris, W.H.M. (1997). Validity of the physical activity scale for the elderly (PASE): According to energy expenditure assessed by the doubly labeled water method. *Journal of Clinical Epidemiology, 50*, 541-546.

Shay, K.A., & Roth, D.L. (1992). Association between aerobic fitness and visuospatial performance in healthy older adults. *Psychology of Aging, 7*, 15-24.

Starkstein, S.E., Robinson, R.G., & Price, T.R. (1988). Comparison of patients with and without poststroke major depression matched for size and location of lesion. *Archives of General Psychiatry, 45,* 247-252.

Steer, R.A., Ball, R., Ranieri, W.F., & Beck, A.T. (1999). Dimensions of the Beck Depression Inventory–II in clinically depressed outpatients. *Journal of Clinical Psychology, 55,* 117-128.

Steingart, A., Hachinski, V.C., Lau, C., Fox, A.J., Diaz, F., Cape, R., et al. (1987). Cognitive and neurologic findings in subjects with diffuse white matter lucencies on computed tomographic scan (leukoariosis). *Archives of Neurology, 44,* 32-35.

Tombaugh, T.N., & McIntyre, N.J. (1992). The mini-mental state examination: A comprehensive review. *Journal of the American Geriatrics Society, 40,* 922-935.

Tribl, G., Howorka, K., Heger, G., Anderer, P., Thoma, H., & Zeithofer, J. (1996). EEG topology during insulin-induced hypoglycemia in patients with insulin-dependent diabetes mellitus. *European Neurology, 36,* 303-309.

Tun, P.A., Perlmuter, L.C., Russo, P., & Nathan, D.M. (1987). Memory self-assessment and performance in aged diabetics and non-diabetics. *Experimental Aging Research, 13,* 151-157.

Van Boxtel, M.P., Buntinx, F., Houx, P.J., Metsemakers, J.F., Knottnerus, A., & Jolles, J. (1998). The relationship between morbidity and cognitive performance in a normal aging population. *Journals of Gerontology. Series A, Biological Sciences and Medical Sciences, 53,* M147-M154.

Wang, L., van Belle, G., Kukull, W.B., & Larson, E.B. (2002). Predictors of functional change: A longitudinal study of nondemented people aged 65 and older. *Journal of the American Geriatrics Society, 50,* 1525-1534.

Washburn, R.A., & Ficker, J.L. (1999). Physical activity scale for the elderly (PASE): The relationship with activity measured by a portable accelerometer. *Journal of Sports Medicine and Physical Fitness, 39,* 336-340.

Washburn, R.A., McAuley, E., Katula, J., Mihalko, S.L., & Boileau, R.A. (1999). The physical activity scale for the elderly (PASE): Evidence for validity. *Journal of Clinical Epidemiology, 52,* 643-651.

Wilson, R.S., Bennett, D.A., Bienias, J.L., Aggarwal, N.T., Mendes De Leon, C.F., Morris, M.C., et al. (2002). Cognitive activity and incident AD in a population-based sample of older persons. *Neurology, 59,* 1910-1914.

Chapter 13

Agle, D.P., & Baum, G.L. (1977). Psychological aspects of chronic obstructive pulmonary disease. *Medical Clinics of North America, 61,* 749-758.

ACCP/AACVPR. (1997). Pulmonary rehabilitation: Evidence based guidelines. *Chest, 112,* 1363-1396.

Albert, M.S., Jones, K., Savage, C.R., Berkman, L., Seeman, T., Blazer, D., et al. (1995). Predictors of cognitive change in older persons: MacArthur studies of successful aging. *Psychology and Aging, 10,* 578-589.

References

American Lung Association. (2004). *Trends in chronic bronchitis and emphysema: Morbidity and mortality. Epidemiology and statistical unit.* New York: American Lung Association.

Berry, D.T.R., & Block, A.J. (1988). Sleep-disordered breathing in patients with COPD. In A.J. McSweeny & I. Grant (Eds.), *Chronic obstructive pulmonary disease: A behavioral perspective* (pp. 1-18). New York: Marcel Dekker.

Blair, S.N., Horton, E., Leon, A.S., Lee, I.-M., Drinkwater, B.L., Dishman, R., et al. (1996). Physical activity, nutrition, and chronic disease. *Medicine and Science in Sports and Exercise, 28,* 335-349.

Blumenthal, J.A., Emery, C.F., Madden, D.J., George, L.K., Coleman, R.E., Riddle, M.W., et al. (1989). Cardiovascular and behavioral effects of aerobic exercise training in healthy older men and women. *Journal of Gerontology: Medical Sciences, 44,* M147-M157.

Chapman, K.M., & Winter, L. (1996). COPD: Using nutrition to prevent respiratory function decline. *Geriatrics, 51,* 37-42.

Colcombe, S.J., Erickson, K.I., Raz, N., Webb, A.G., Cohen, N.J., McAuley, E., et al. (2003). Aerobic fitness reduces brain tissue loss in aging humans. *Journal of Gerontology: Medical Sciences, 58,* 176-180.

Cugell, D.W. (1988). COPD: A brief introduction for behavioral scientists. In A.J. McSweeny & I. Grant (Eds.), *Chronic obstructive pulmonary disease: A behavioral perspective* (pp. 1-18). New York: Marcel Dekker.

Decary, A., Rouleau, I., & Montplaisir, J. (2000). Cognitive deficits associated with sleep apnea syndrome: A proposed neuropsychological test battery. *Sleep, 23,* 369-381.

Dustman, R.E., Emmerson, R.Y., Ruhling, R.O., Shearer, D.E., Steinhaus, L.A., Johnson, S.C., et al. (1990). Age and fitness effects on EEG, ERPs, visual sensitivity, and cognition. *Neurobiology of Aging, 11,* 193-200.

Dustman, R., Ruhling, R., Russell, E., Shearer, D., Bonekat, W., Shigeoka, J., et al. (1984). Aerobic exercise training and improved neuropsychological function of older individuals. *Neurobiology of Aging, 5,* 35-42.

Emery, C.F., & Gatz, M. (1990). Psychological and cognitive effects of an exercise program for community-residing older adults. *Gerontologist, 30,* 184-188.

Emery, C.F., Honn, J.L., Diaz, P.T., Lebowitz, K.R., & Frid, D.J. (2001). Acute effects of exercise on cognitive function among patients with chronic obstructive pulmonary disease. *American Journal of Respiratory and Critical Care Medicine, 164,* 1624-1627.

Emery, C.F., Huppert, F.A., & Schein, R.L. (1997). Do smoking and pulmonary function predict cognitive function? Findings from a British sample. *Psychology and Health, 12,* 265-275.

Emery, C.F., Leatherman, N.E., Burker, E.J., & MacIntyre, N.R. (1991). Psychological outcomes of a pulmonary rehabilitation program. *Chest, 100,* 613-617.

Emery, C.F., Pedersen, N.L., Svartengren, M., & McClearn, G.E. (1998). Longitudinal and genetic effects in the relationship of pulmonary function and cognitive function. *Journal of Gerontology: Psychological Sciences, 53B,* P311-P317.

Emery, C.F., Schein, R.L., Hauck, E.R., & MacIntyre, N.R. (1998). Psychological and cognitive outcomes of a randomized trial of exercise among patients with chronic obstructive pulmonary disease. *Health Psychology, 17*, 232-240.

Emery, C.F., Shermer, R.L., Hauck, E.R., Hsiao, E.T., & MacIntyre, N.R. (2003). Cognitive and psychological outcomes of exercise in a one-year follow up study of patients with chronic obstructive pulmonary disease. *Health Psychology, 22*, 598-604.

Etnier, J.L., & Berry, M. (2001). Fluid intelligence in an older COPD sample after short- or long-term exercise. *Medicine and Science in Sports and Exercise, 33*, 1620-1628.

Etnier, J.L., Johnston, R., Dagenbach, D., Pollard, R.J., Rejeski, W.J., & Berry, M. (1999). The relationships among pulmonary function, aerobic fitness, and cognitive functioning in older COPD patients. *Chest, 116*, 953-960.

Goldstein, R.S., Gort, E.H., Stubbing, D., Avendano, M.A., & Guyatt, G.H. (1994). Randomised controlled trial of respiratory rehabilitation. *Lancet, 344*, 1394-1397.

Grant, I., Heaton, R.K., McSweeny, A.J., Adams, K.M., & Timms, R.M. (1982). Neuropsychologic findings in hypoxemic chronic obstructive pulmonary disease. *Archives of Internal Medicine, 142*, 1470.

Grant, I., Prigatano, G.P., Heaton, R.K., McSweeny, A.J., Wright, E.C., & Adams, K.M. (1987). Progressive neuropsychologic impairment and hypoxemia. *Archives of General Psychiatry, 44*, 999-1006.

Heaton, R.K., Grant, I., McSweeny, A.J., Adams, K.M., & Petty, T.L. (1983). Psychologic effects of continuous and nocturnal oxygen therapy in hypoxemic chronic obstructive pulmonary disease. *Archives of Internal Medicine, 143*, 1941-1945.

Incalzi, R.A., Gemma, A., Marra, C., Capparella, O., Fuso, L., & Carbonin, P. (1997). Verbal memory impairment in COPD: Its mechanisms and clinical relevance. *Chest, 112*, 1506-1513.

Kaplan, R., Ries, A., Prewitt, L., & Eakin, E. (1994). Self-efficacy expectations predict survival for patients with chronic obstructive pulmonary disease. *Health Psychology, 13*, 366-368.

Khatri, P., Blumenthal, J.A., Babyak, M.A., Craighead, W.E., Herman, S., Baldewicz, T., et al. (2001). Effects of exercise training on cognitive functioning among depressed older men and women. *Journal of Aging and Physical Activity, 9*, 43-57.

Kozora, E., Filley, C.M., Julian, L.J., & Cullum, C.M. (1999). Cognitive functioning in patients with chronic obstructive pulmonary disease and mild hypoxemia compared with patients with mild Alzheimer disease and normal controls. *Neuropsychiatry, Neuropsychology, and Behavioral Neurology, 12*, 178-183.

Kozora, E., Tran, Z.V., & Make, B. (2002). Neurobehavioral improvement after brief rehabilitation in patients with chronic obstructive pulmonary disease. *Journal of Cardiopulmonary Rehabilitation, 22*, 426-430.

Kramer, A.F., Hahn, S., Cohen, N.J., Banich, M.T., McAuley, E., Harrison, C.R., et al. (1999). Aging, fitness and neurocognitive function. *Nature, 400*, 418-419.

Krop, H., Block, A.J., & Cohen, E. (1973). Neuropsychologic effects of continuous oxygen therapy in chronic obstructive pulmonary disease. *Chest, 64*, 317.

Lake, F.R., Henderson, K., Briffa, T., Openshaw, J., & Musk, A.W. (1990). Upper-limb and lower-limb exercise training in patients with chronic airflow obstruction. *Chest, 97*, 1077-1082.

McSweeny, A.J., Grant, I., Heaton, R.K., Adams, K.M., & Timms, R.M. (1982). Life quality of patients with chronic obstructive pulmonary disease. *Archives of Internal Medicine, 142*, 473-478.

Prigatano, G.P., Parsons, O., Wright, E., Levin, D.C., & Hawryluk, G. (1983). Neuropsychological test performance in mildly hypoxemic patients with chronic obstructive pulmonary disease. *Journal of Consulting and Clinical Psychology, 51*, 108-116.

Ries, A.L., Kaplan, R.M., Limberg, T.M., & Prewitt, L.M. (1995). Effects of pulmonary rehabilitation on physiologic and psychosocial outcomes in patients with chronic obstructive pulmonary disease. *Annals of Internal Medicine, 122*, 823-832.

Sassi-Dambron, D.E., Eakin, E.G., Ries, A.L., & Kaplan, R.M. (1995). Treatment of dyspnea in COPD: A controlled clinical trial of dyspnea management strategies. *Chest, 107*, 724.

Chapter 14

Colcombe, S., & Kramer, A.F. (2003). Fitness effects on the cognitive function of older adults: A meta-analytic study. *Psychological Science, 2*, 125-130.

INDEX

Note: The italicized *f* and *t* following page numbers refer to figures and tables, respectively.

ABOUT THE EDITORS

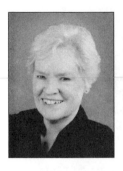

Waneen W. Spirduso, EdD, is the Oscar and Anne Mauzy Regents Professor in the department of kinesiology and health education at The University of Texas (UT) at Austin. She was chair of the UT department of kinesiology and health education for 14 years and served as interim dean of the College of Education for 2 1/2 years. Since 1975 her academic interests, research, and presentations have focused on issues central to gerontology and kinesiology, and her research programs have been sponsored by four of the National Institutes of Health and several local foundations.

A widely published author, Dr. Spirduso is also a popular speaker at conferences across the United States. She is the recipient of many honors and awards, including recognition as the Texas Association for Health, Physical Education, Recreation and Dance Scholar in 1986 and the American Alliance for Health, Physical Education, Recreation and Dance Scholar (AAHPERD) in 1987. She served two terms as president of the North American Society for the Psychology of Sport and Physical Activity (NASPSPA) and one term as president of the American Academy of Kinesiology and Physical Education (AAKPE).

Dr. Spirduso is a fellow of the Gerontological Society of America and a member of AAHPERD, ACSM, and AAKPE.

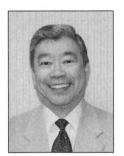

Leonard W. Poon, PhD, is a professor of public health and psychology, chair of the faculty of gerontology, and director of the Gerontology Center at the University of Georgia at Athens. He received his PhD in experimental psychology in 1972 from the University of Denver and has studied aging and cognition for over 30 years with specific emphasis on environmental and lifestyle influences that enhance cognitive functioning in older adults.

A fellow of the American Psychological Association, American Psychological Society, Association of Gerontology in Higher Education, and the Gerontology Society of America, Poon was a Fulbright senior research scholar in Sweden and a senior visiting research scientist to Japan. In 2000, Poon received an honorary doctorate of philosophy from Lund University in Sweden. Among his research awards are the NIA Special Research Award, VA Medical Research Service Achievement Award, North American Leader in Psychogeriatrics, and Southern Gerontological Society Academic Gerontologist Award.

Poon's primary research areas are normal and pathological changes of memory processes in aging, clinical assessment of memory (including assessment of early stages of dementia of the Alzheimer's type), and survival characteristics and adaptation of centenarians. He is currently directing a nine-university, NIA-funded program studying the genetic basis of longevity, relationships between the brain and behavior in Alzheimer's disease, and daily functioning capacities of the oldest-old.

Poon currently resides in Athens, Georgia. In his free time he enjoys cycling, photography, and traveling.

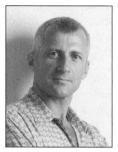

Wojtek Chodzko-Zajko, PhD, serves as both department head and professor of kinesiology and community health at the University of Illinois at Urbana-Champaign. He served on the World Health Organization Scientific Advisory Committee, which issued guidelines for physical activity in older adults. Chodzko-Zajko chairs the Active Aging Partnership, a national coalition in the area of healthy aging linking the American College of Sports Medicine, the National Institute of Aging, the Centers for Disease Control and Prevention, the American Geriatrics Society, the National Council on the Aging, the American Association of Retired Persons, and the Robert Wood Johnson Foundation.

Since 2002, Chodzko-Zajko has served as principal investigator of the National Blueprint Project, a coalition of more than 50 national organizations with a joint commitment to promoting independent, active aging in the 50+ population. He was founding editor of the *Journal of Aging and Physical Activity* and president of the International Society for Aging and Physical Activity.

He is frequently invited to speak about healthful aging at national and international meetings. Chodzko-Zajko has appeared often on television and radio, including the NBC "Today Show," National Public Radio, and CNN.

ABOUT THE CONTRIBUTORS

Jennifer Etnier, PhD, is an assistant professor of exercise science at Arizona State University, where she received the Rousseau Award for Research in Gerontology. She specializes in the effects of exercise and exercise training on cognition and psychomotor learning in older adults. Her work has been published in journals such as *Research Quarterly for Exercise and Sport, Chest, Journal of Sport and Exercise Psychology, Medicine and Science in Sports and Exercise,* and *Journal of Aging and Physical Activity.* She is a frequent speaker to national associations such as the American College of Sports Medicine (ACSM) and currently serves on the ACSM Strategic Health Initiative on Aging and Exercise and on the Gerontology Executive Committee for Arizona State University. Her most recent grant, from the Arizona Biomedical Center, supports a collaborative research project with Mayo Clinic Scottsdale and is designed to examine the effects of physical fitness and ApoE-4 genotype on cognitive functioning in postmenopausal women.

John B. Bartholomew, PhD, is an associate professor in the Department of Kinesiology and Health Education at the University of Texas at Austin. He received his BA in psychology from Harvard University and a PhD in exercise science from Arizona State University. He was selected as a research fellow for the Research Direction and Strategies in Physical Activity and Public Health course that is offered by the Centers for Disease Control and Prevention. Dr. Bartholomew's primary area of research is the use of exercise to regulate psychological states, including depression, stress, and affect. His most recent work is focused on the use of acute bouts of exercise to relieve the negative moods that are associated with clinical depression. He has multiple grants from the Texas Department of Health and has published in *Journal of Sport and Exercise Psychology, Research Quarterly for Exercise and Sport, Journal of Behavioral Medicine, Journal of Applied Sport Psychology, Journal of Sport Science,* and *International Journal of Sport Psychology.* Joseph T. Ciccolo, PhD, who completed his master's degree in health psychology under Dr. Bartholomew's supervision, assisted in the writing of this chapter.

Nicole C. Berchtold, PhD, is a postdoctoral researcher with Dr. Carl Cotman, director of the Institute for Brain Aging and Dementia at the University of California, Irvine. Previously, she completed 2 years of neurobiology research at the Institute of Physiology in Lausanne, Switzerland. Since 1995, her research interests have been on how behavioral and environmental factors such as exercise, diet, and stress influence brain health and function, particularly on understanding exercise-related molecular changes that occur in the hippocampus, a brain region of central importance to learning and memory function. One of her notable accomplishments has been the characterization of exercise-dependent regulation of neurotrophins in the hippocampus, especially brain-derived neurotrophic factor (BDNF). BDNF, a neurotrophic factor up-regulated by exercise, has emerged as a pivotal factor underlying learning and memory formation as well as vulnerability to depression. Her work is published in *Neurobiology of Aging, Journal of Neuroscience Research,* and *Brain Research and Molecular Research.*

Edward McAuley, PhD, is currently a professor in the Departments of Kinesiology, Psychology, and the Beckman Institute for Advanced Science and Technology at the University of Illinois at Urbana-Champaign. His research interests are in the psychology antecedents and consequences of physical activity, particularly in older adults. This work, driven primarily by social cognitive theory, is an extensive examination of the role played by self-efficacy in physical activity and physcial and psychological function. He has published over 130 referred publications and serves on the editorial boards of the *Journal of Behavioral Medicine, Journal of Aging and Physical Activity,* and *Health Psychology.* He is the recipient of Early Career Distinguished Scholar Award from the North American Society for the Psychology of Physcial Activity, the King James McCrystal Distinguished Scholar Award, the University of Illinois University Scholar Award, as well as College and University Awards for Excellence in Undergraduate Teaching.

Phillip D. Tomporowski received his PhD in experimental psychology at the University of Mississippi. His primary research interests focus on the relationship between exercise and cognitive functioning. While he was at the University of Alabama, the Alabama Department of Mental Health provided support for a multiyear project that assessed the effects of aerobic exercise training on adult intelligence and behavior. He has held positions in the Department of Psychology at the University of Florida and in the Department of Kinesiology at the University of Connecticut. Presently, he is an associate professor in the Department of Exercise Science and a member of the Faculty of Gerontology at the University of Georgia. His ongoing research focuses on the effects of acute bouts of physical activity on older adults' cognitive functioning. He has been published in *Psychological Bulletin, Acta Psychologica, Journal of Aging and Physical Activity,* and *Educational Gerontology.*

Timothy A. Salthouse, PhD, is Brown–Forman Professor of Psychology in the Department of Psychology at the University of Virginia. He previously was professor of psychology at the University of Missouri–Columbia and Regents Professor of Psychology at the Georgia Institute of Technology. He is a fellow of the American Association for the Advancement of Science (AAAS), the American Psychological Association (APA), the American Psychological Society (APS), and the Gerontological Society of America and a member of the Psychonomic Society. He received the APA Division 20 Distinguished Contribution Award in 1995 and was named an APS William James Fellow in 1998. He was editor of the journal *Psychology and Aging* from 1991 through 1996 and has published eight books and more than 150 chapters and journal articles. Dr. Salthouse has previously served on the NRC Panel on Human Factors Research Needs for an Aging Population and on the NRC Panel on Future Directions for Cognitive Research on Aging, and he is currently serving on the NRC Panel on Health and Safety Needs of Older Workers. His research has been supported by the National Institute on Aging since 1978 and has included a Research Career Development Award and a MERIT Award.

James Joseph received his PhD in behavioral neuroscience from the University of South Carolina in 1976. He was a postdoctoral fellow at the Gerontology Research Center/NIH from 1976 to 1982 and a senior scientist at Lederle Research Laboratories from 1982 to 1985 when he joined the Armed Forces Radiobiology Institute. In 1988 he returned to the GRC as a senior scientist and in 1993 joined the USDA Human Nutrition Research Center on Aging at Tufts University as chief of the neuroscience laboratory. He is the author or coauthor of more than 165 publications and has shared in the Sandoz Award in Gerontology. He has received a JAFEH fellowship from the National Institute for Longevity Science, the Stephanie Overstreet Award in Alzheimer Research from the Alzheimer Foundation, the Alex Wetherbee Award from the North American Blueberry Council, and the Glenn Foundation Award for Aging Research.

Martita Lopez received her PhD in clinical psychology from Syracuse University. She has held positions at Virginia Tech and at Rush–Presbyterian–St. Luke's Medical Center in Chicago, where she directed the clinical geropsychology program and the psychology internship program. While there, she served as the coprincipal investigator of an NCNR grant that studied the relationship between aerobic exercise and physical and cognitive functioning in older adults. More recently, Dr. Lopez and colleagues have been studying insomnia and aging. She was the coinvestigator on a grant from the National Institute on Aging to explore the efficacy of behavioral techniques for insomnia with older adults who are medically ill, a group until now excluded from most sleep research. Dr. Lopez is now clinical associate professor and director of the Clinical Psychology Training Clinic of the Department of Psychology at the University of Texas at Austin. She is a fellow of the Society of Behavioral Medicine.

Michael V. Vitiello, PhD, is professor and senior scientist, Sleep Research Group, Department of Psychiatry and Behavioral Sciences, University of Washington, Seattle. He holds an Independent Scientist (K02) Research Career Award from the National Institute of Mental Health, is a fellow of the Gerontological Society of America, is a member of the board of directors and circadian rhythms section head of the Sleep Research Society, and is editor in chief (for the Americas) of *Sleep Medicine Reviews*. Federally funded for more than 20 years, he studies the causes, consequences, and treatments of sleep disturbance in the elderly and is the author of nearly 300 scientific papers, chapters, abstracts, and editorials. He has been or is an investigator on five prospective fitness intervention studies in the elderly examining a variety of outcome measures. Among Dr. Vitiello's completed research projects are two prospective randomized intervention studies that assessed the impact of either aerobic fitness training or growth hormone–releasing hormone on both the sleep quality and cognitive function of noncomplaining older men and women.

Hiro Tanaka received his PhD in exercise physiology from the University of Tennessee and completed postdoctoral training in cardiovascular physiology at the University of Colorado. An assistant professor in the Department of Kinesiology and Health Education at the University of Texas at Austin, he has directed his research toward the influence of aging and lifestyle modifications on cardiovascular disease risk and functions in humans. In particular, he studies the efficacy of regular physical activity for primary and secondary prevention of age-related changes in arterial function and structure. His research has been supported by the National Institutes of Health and the American Heart Association. He is a recipient of various awards, including a New Investigator Award from the American College of Sports Medicine and a Research Career Enhancement Award from the American Physiological Society.

Donald R. Royall, MD, completed residency training in both internal medicine and psychiatry at Johns Hopkins Hospital. He is certified by the American Board of Internal Medicine and the American Board of Psychiatry and Neurology, with added qualifications in geriatric psychiatry. He is currently chief of the Geriatric Psychiatry Division at the University of Texas Health Sciences Center in San Antonio. He is a professor in the departments of psychiatry, internal medicine, and pharmacology. Dr. Royall is internationally known for his research on executive control functions and their associations with aging, dementia, disability, and medical conditions such as diabetes. He has developed bedside measures of executive function, including the Executive Interview (EXIT25) and CLOX: An Executive Clock-Drawing Task. Dr. Royall was recently listed in the 2002-2003 Consumers' Research Council of America Guide to America's Top Psychiatrists. He has published many book chapters and research papers in journals such as *Journal of the American Geriatrics Society, American Journal of Psychiatry, International Journal of Geriatric Psychiatry, Neuroepidemiology, Experimental Aging Research,* and *Journal of Gerontology.* He is an associate editor of *Journal of the American Geriatrics Society.*

Charles F. Emery, PhD, is associate professor of psychology and internal medicine at Ohio State University (OSU) and director of the Cardiopulmonary Behavioral Medicine Program at OSU's Center for Wellness and Prevention. His research program, supported by the NIH and by fellowships from the Fulbright Foundation and the American–Scandinavian Foundation, addresses psychological and physiological outcomes of exercise interventions among healthy older adults and among adults with chronic illness and has documented cognitive improvements associated with exercise among patients with chronic obstructive pulmonary disease. Ongoing work in his laboratory is now evaluating cognitive and neuropsychological outcomes among patients participating in the National Emphysema Treatment Trial. Dr. Emery is on the editorial boards of *Health Psychology* and *Journal of Cardiopulmonary Rehabilitation.* He is a fellow of the American Psychological Association, the American Association of Cardiovascular and Pulmonary Rehabilitation, and the Society of Behavioral Medicine.